PROFESSIONS, WORK
AND CAREERS

PROFESSIONS, WORK
AND CAREERS

BY
ANSELM L. STRAUSS

ta

Transaction Books
New Brunswick, New Jersey

Printed in the United States of America
Library of Congress Catalog Card Number: 73-168948
ISBN: 0-87855-128-X

To Herbert Blumer, Everett C. Hughes and
Alfred R. Lindesmith, friends and colleagues
without whom . . .

CONTENTS

PREFACE *

The research papers and chapters that comprise this book originally appeared in several journals and books. Why, now, bring them all together? One answer is that almost every author would like to see some of his work collected in one spot "for handy reference," and to remind readers that they may just possibly have missed the ones he likes best. They may also have overlooked some continuities in his work, having read it cross-sectionally rather than longitudinally. All those reasons have prompted this re-publication, plus the equally relevant rationale that if put between two covers these writings might reach a wider audience than hitherto. I have in mind especially graduate and undergraduate students who are interested in the sociology of work or in the sociology of medicine. It is my hope also that sociologists who are concerned with the development of theory may find this collection pertinent to their own interests. All the writings are based on research (mainly through fieldwork or qualitative interviewing), and virtually all are focused not only on substantive concerns but on the development of theory.

The book itself can be read in at least three ways. Probably it will be most frequently read *topically*. Its major topics are profession, career, work and organization — and various associated matters such as ideology, socialization, occupational identity, social mobility, professional relationships, negotiated order; also more specific referents such as hospitals, wards, nurses, physicians, chemists, executives, students of art, nursing, doctoring, and terminal care. Since all those topics can be researched and discussed from many different perspectives, it is incumbent on me to indicate my own past and current perspectives. This will be done more fully below, but not before I hazard a guess that most American sociologists would label my approach as "social psychological" and as derived from "the Chicago

* I am grateful to various of my co-authors for their permission to reprint work done with them: Howard Becker, Rue Bucher, Danuta Ehrlich, Barney Glaser, Norman Martin, Lee Rainwater, Melvin Sabshin, Leonard Schatzman.

1

School." Perhaps some also would say that I write like a symbolic interactionist. That labeling would be only partly correct — an assertion that brings me to the second and third ways of reading this book.

Besides topically, it can be read as mirroring the development of one sociologist's *intellectual biography* — itself a commentary on the foregoing labels — as well as read *thematically* ("interaction," "identity," "structural process"). The biographical details are easily outlined, and anyone interested enough to read the reprinted articles chronologically can trace something of the development for himself. While an undergraduate I had discovered Dewey and Thomas, had been much influenced in graduate school by Herbert Blumer and later also by Alfred Lindesmith. As a graduate student, I thought of myself as in the tradition of these men. In 1952, I returned to the University of Chicago after eight years of teaching courses in social psychology, anthropology and sociology. At Chicago there still was great ferment around the work of Everett Hughes and his students in occupational sociology (Becker and Goffman were there, and others who had left were finishing their theses elsewhere). I found myself drawn to these men and their research topics, and my first attempt at this research style (which remained unpublished but is included here) was a brief paper on the recruitment of art students to the Chicago Art Institute. The paper is very much in the Hughes tradition.

Meanwhile I was attempting to work out in *Mirrors and Masks* some amalgam of Meadian social psychology and the more recently developed structural sociology: with a focus on identity, and on the relationship of person to social organization. During this period, Howard Becker and I collaborated on "Careers, Personality, and Adult Socialization," attempting to theorize about careers a bit further than had been done previously. A year or two later, after about two months of fieldwork at the University of Kansas Medical Center, I wrote a long background paper for Becker-Geer-Hughes, who were later to co-author *Boys in White*. The unpublished paper placed considerable emphasis on structured interaction, on patterned tactics and on a process basic to many organizations: the rotation of personnel. This paper still strikes me as quite different in emphasis than *Boys In White*, and reflects my effort at that time "to put social psychology and social organization together." (Earlier, Norman Martin and I had collaborated on an analysis of his field data, bearing on the horizontal and vertical mobility of executives in a large business corporation; the emphases again were on organization in relation to career processes, and on consequences for identity as well as for organization.)

2

In 1958, I left the University of Chicago and did a study which resulted in *Psychiatric Ideologies and Institutions*. On the research team were two students of mine, Rue Bucher and Leonard Schatzman — rather symbolically, the first was trained mainly in the sociology of work and the second in Meadian social psychology. (Bucher was also a student of Hughes.) Our goal was to explore the impact of three psychiatric ideologies on the relationships of personnel and patients within two mental hospitals. Other than the idea that those ideologies might exist (the idea was Melvin Sabshin's, a psychiatrist who also was on the research team), we entered the field like most fieldworkers without specific hypotheses; but with a consciously applied framework derived from the sociology of work and from sociological social psychology. The final result was a complex comparative analysis with emphasis on such matters as careers, work relationships, ideologies, professional biographies, work sites viewed as arenas, and social order as negotiated. Social structure was viewed as "in process." The years of our research covered 1958 through 1962, and they are treated as a point in time, a cross-section of a set of complex and evolving social-intellectual movements within psychiatry and its allied health specializations. Before the research was finished, Rue Bucher and I had written "Professions in Process," underlining the segmentalization of professions, and noting some of the range of relationships that existed among evolving segments. Bucher, meanwhile, had finished a thesis about pathologists, using this processual framework.

While *Psychiatric Ideologies and Institutions* was being written (1960-62), I had embarked on a study of terminal care in hospitals. Barney Glaser (also a nurse, Jeanne Quint) soon joined me. Glaser and I published two books, including the portion of *Time for Dying* which is reprinted here. That book reflects our concern with temporal aspects of work and of organizations, as well as with developing the inseparability of structure and process ("structural process"). This research project also helped us to develop the notions of theoretical sampling, theoretical coding, and the type of comparative analysis based on them; all discussed in *The Discovery of Grounded Theory*. The type of theory developed in the books on terminal care was "substantive," but in a recently published volume *(The Contexts of Social Mobility)*, I have used a formal theory of Status Passage evolved by Glaser and me (see *Status Passage*) to develop a partial substantive theory of social mobility: one chapter of that book is reproduced here because it has direct implications for mobility within organizations, occupations and professions. A pertinent part of this intellectual development also is that Glaser recently had analyzed much of the literature on careers, including that produced by the Chicago sociologists, and had developed a formal theory of organiza-

3

tional careers by analyzing comparatively the available substantive theories of careers *(Organizational Careers)*.

And last, I should mention that an earlier interest in using historical material for sociological purposes had led, around 1963-65, to looking at firsthand data bearing on the evolution of American Nursing. The resulting "Ideology and Structure of American Nursing" reflects not only that interest but my preoccupation with professions-in-process, ideology, careers, and with the various kinds of relationships which exist between given professionals and other groups of people.

The third mode of reading this book is now very easy to reintroduce: it can be read *thematically*. Some of the major themes, of course, are structure, interaction, processual analysis, and "time" as the sociologist might profitably view it. These themes, I anticipate, will emerge by themselves via reading of this book, if they have not already been sufficiently adumbrated by the foregoing narrative. Perhaps in this preface I need only to capture, however briefly, those themes in one net, by an extended quotation from *Awareness of Dying* (pp. 13-15):

> Our own approach to the problem of interaction is much affected by a set of convictions about the maintenance of social order. Concerning social order, Norton Long, a political scientist, recently wrote that there is a sociology of John Locke and a sociology of Thomas Hobbes: the one emphasizes a realm of stable, unquestioned values underlying the social order, and the other, the highly problematic character of social order. George Mead earlier rephrased the Hobbesian view by noting that social changes occur constantly; he argued that the human task is 'to bring those changes about in an orderly fashion,' to direct change so that it is not chaotic, or in Hobbes' language, anarchistic. Our vision, which combines both views of this overdrawn dichotomy, is that the bases of social order must be reconstituted continually, must be 'worked at,' both according to established values and with the purpose of establishing values to preserve order. The maintenance of social order, whether in society, organizations, groups or interaction, we believe, turns about handling relatively unforeseen consequences in this twofold manner.
>
> Our assumptions about social order have naturally led us to explore the developmental possibilities of interaction though our assumptions need not be accepted to legitimate this aim as of immense sociological importance. In his re-

4

cent *Behavior in Public Places,* Erving Goffman analyzed interaction in terms of the social regulations that subtly govern it and make it the genuine embodiment of social order; in contrast, we are cognizant of rules but are principally interested in analyzing interaction in terms of its open-ended and problematic character. Rather than focusing on interactional *stability,* we shall be preoccupied . . . with *changes* that may occur during the course of interaction. However, relatively stable or purely repetitive interaction also demands analysis beyond detailing the governing regulations: that is, one must combine both the rule and the 'working at' basis of social order. Thus, we are interested not only in the social regulations and other structural conditions entering into the interaction, but also in the tendency for interaction to move out of regulated bounds and into new interactional modes.

To this, I would add only one more theme — or perhaps better said, add one not-so-hidden agenda embodied by these reprinted papers whether they are read individually or collectively. I owe to Herbert Blumer, whose argument first convinced me, the belief that a primary task of the next generation of sociologists was to close the embarrassing gap between theory and data. Now, as in the 1940s, our literature is replete both with simple "low-level" description and with speculative theory. The first certainly has some value; the second, I believe, has no enduring value whatever. Rather than argue the point here, I merely emphasize that all work reported in this volume is directed in one way or other at "grounded theory" (an adjective one would blush to use except that other kinds of "theory" do exist); that means that all of the writing was based on research and yet aimed at developing theory. To coin a possibly inept aphoristic imperative — but the best I can do at this moment — "keep your head in the clouds but *please* keep your feet on the ground." Or alternatively, a Chinese proverb of great predictive power: "He whose head is in the clouds but whose feet are not on the ground is likely to float, all disembodied head; and wander, all undirected feet."

PART I

IDEOLOGIES AND PROFESSIONS

PROFESSIONS IN PROCESS[1]

(With Rue Bucher)

The "process" or "emergent" approach to the study of professions developed in the following pages bears considerable resemblance to a common-sense point of view. It utilizes common language to order the kinds of events that professionals informally discuss among themselves — frequently with great animation. It is even used by sociologists in their less professional moments when they are personally challenged by their own colleagues or by persons from other fields. What is different here is that we shall take the first steps toward developing an explicit scheme of analysis out of these common-place materials. In addition, it will become apparent that this approach differs from the prevailing "functionalism" because it focuses more pointedly upon conflicting interests and upon change.

Functionalism sees a profession largely as a relatively homogeneous community whose members share identity, values, definitions of

[1]The intellectual origins of this scheme of analysis are both our own research and various writings of our predecessors and colleagues. Its specific ideas occurred to us when Miss Bucher, several years ago, had occasion to analyze a number of specialty journals and interview a sample of pathologists. Since then we have both been engaged in a study which brings us much information about psychiatrists and psychiatric nurses in Chicago, and we have had available also Everett C. Hughes's interviews with the medical staff at the University of Kansas medical school. The writings to which we are most indebted are those of Everett Hughes on work and professions (cf. *Men and Their Work* [Glencoe, Ill.: Free Press 1958]) and the symbolic-interaction position in social psychology (cf. George Herbert Mead's *Mind, Self, and Society* [Chicago: University of Chicago Press. 1934]). Because the materials on occupations, work, and professions are well known and readily available, we have not cited all references to pertinent literature; the files of various specialty journals in all the professions are useful to anyone interested in further illustrations.

Reprinted by permission from
THE AMERICAN JOURNAL OF SOCIOLOGY
Vol. LXVI, January 1961, pp. 325-34
Copyright 1961 by the University of Chicago

role, and interests.[2] There is room in this conception for some variation, some differentiation, some out-of-line members, even some conflict; but, by and large, there is a steadfast core which defines the profession, deviations from which are but temporary dislocations. Socialization of recruits consists of induction into the common core. There are norms, codes, which govern the behavior of the professional to insiders and outsiders. In short, the sociology of professions has largely been focused upon the mechanics of cohesiveness and upon detailing the social structure (and/or social organization) of given professions. Those tasks a structural-functional sociology is prepared to do, and do relatively well.

But this kind of focus and theory tends to lead one to overlook many significant aspects of professions and professional life. Particularly does it bias the observer against appreciating the conflict — or at least difference—of interests within the profession; this leads him to overlook certain of the more subtle features of the profession's "organization" as well as to fail to appreciate how consequential for changes in the profession and its practitioners differential interests may be.

In actuality, the assumption of relative homogeneity within the profession is not entirely useful: there are many identities, many values, and many interests. These amount not merely to differentiation or simple variation. They tend to become patterned and shared; coalitions develop and flourish — and in opposition to some others. We shall call these groupings which emerge within a profession "segments." (Specialties might be thought of as major segments, except that a close look at a specialty betrays its claim to unity, revealing that specialties, too, usually contain segments, and, if they ever did have common definitions along all lines of professional identity, it was probably at a very special, and early, period in their development.) We shall develop the idea of professions as loose amalgamations of segments pursuing different objectives in different manners and more or less delicately held together under a common name at a particular period in history.

Our aim in this paper, then, is to present some initial steps in formulating a "process" model for studying professions. The model can be considered either as a supplement of, or an alternative to, the prevailing functional model. Some readers undoubtedly will prefer to consider the process model as supplementary. If so, then there will be a need for a further step, that is, for a transcending model. But we ourselves are concerned here only with sketching the outlines of a process approach, suggesting a few potentially useful concepts,

[2]Cf. William J. Goode, "Community within a Community: The Professions," *American Sociological Review*, XX (1957), 194-200.

and pointing to certain research problems that flow from our framework and concepts.

"ORGANIZED MEDICINE"

Medicine is usually considered the prototype of the professions, the one upon which current sociological conceptions of professions tend to be based; hence, our illustrative points in this paper will be taken from medicine, but they could just as pertinently have come from some other profession. Of the medical profession as a whole a great deal could be, and has been, said: its institutions (hospitals, schools, clinics); its personnel (physicians and paramedical personnel); its organizations (the American Medical Association, the state and county societies); its recruitment policies; its standards and codes; its political activities; its relations with the public; not to mention the profession's informal mechanisms of sociability and control. All this minimal "structure" certainly exists.

But we should also recognize the great divergency of enterprise and endeavor that mark the profession; the cleavages that exist along with the division of labor; and the intellectual and specialist movements that occur within the broad rubric called "organized medicine." It might seem as if the physicians certainly share common ends, if ever any profession did. When backed to the wall, any physician would probably agree that his long-run objective is better care of the patient. But this is a misrepresentation of the actual values and organization of activity as undertaken by various segments of the profession. Not all the ends shared by all physicians are distinctive to the medical profession or intimately related to what many physicians do as their work. What is distinctive of medicine belongs to certain segments of it — groupings not necessarily even specialties — and may not actually be shared with other physicians. We turn now to a consideration of some of those values which these segments do *not* share and about which they may actually be in conflict.

The sense of mission.—It is characteristic of the growth of specialties that early in their development they carve out for themselves and proclaim unique missions. They issue a statement of the contributions that the specialty, and it alone, can make in a total scheme of values and, frequently, with it an argument to show why it is peculiarly fitted for this task. The statement of mission tends to take a rhetorical form, probably because it arises in the context of a battle for recognition and institutional status. Thus, when surgical specialties, such as urology and proctology, were struggling to attain identities independent of general surgery, they developed the argument that the particular anatomical areas in which they were interested required special attention and that only physicians with their particular background were competent to give it. Anesthesiologists developed a

11

similar argument. This kind of claim separates a given area out of the general stream of medicine, gives it special emphasis and a new dignity, and, more important for our purposes, separates the specialty group from other physicians. Insofar as they claim an area for themselves, they aim to exclude others from it. It is theirs alone.

While specialties organize around unique missions, as time goes on segmental missions may develop within the fold. In radiology, for example, there are groups of physicians whose work is organized almost completely around diagnosis. But there is a recently burgeoning group of radiologists whose mission is to develop applications of radiation for therapeutic purposes. The difference of mission is so fundamental that it has given rise to demands for quite different residency training programs and to some talk of splitting off from the parent specialty. In pathology — one of the oldest medical specialties, whose traditional mission has been to serve as the basic science of medicine with relatively little emphasis upon clinical applications — lately a whole new breed of pathologists has come to the fore, dedicated to developing pathology as a specialized service to clinical practitioners and threatening those who cling to the traditional mission.

The split between research mission and clinical practice runs clear through medicine and all its specialties. Pediatrics has been one of the most rapidly growing fields of practice, but it has also attracted a number of young people, particularly at some centers in the Northeast, specifically for research. They are people who have no conceptions of themselves as family pediatricians at all; they are in this field because of what they can do in the way of research. In the two oldest specialties, surgery and internal medicine, one finds throughout the literature considerable evidence of this kind of split. One finds an old surgeon complaining that the young men are too much interested in research, and in internal medicine there are exhortations that they should be doctors, not scientists. This latter lament is particularly interesting in view of the traditional mission of the internist to exemplify the finest in the "art of medicine": it is a real betrayal when one of them shows too much interest in controlled research.

Work Activities.—There is great diversity in the tasks performed in the name of the profession. Different definitions may be found between segments of the profession concerning what kinds of work the professional should be doing, how work should be organized, and which tasks have precedence. If, for example, the model physician is taken as one who sees patients and carries out the diagnosis and treatment of illness, then an amazing variety of physicians do not fit this model. This diversity is not wholly congruent with the or-

12

ganization of practice by medical specialties, although there are certain specialties — like pathology, radiology, anesthesiology, and public health — whose practitioners for the most part do not approach the model. Within a core specialty like internal medicine there are many different kinds of practice, ranging from that of a "family doctor" to highly specialized consultation, a service to other doctors. These differences in the weights assigned to elements of practice do not begin to take into account the further diversity introduced when professionals assign different weights to such activities as research, teaching, and public service.

This point can be made more clearly by considering some of the different organizations of work activities that can be found within single specialties. The people who organize their work life as follows all call themselves "pathologists:" (a) time nearly equally divided between research and teaching, with little or no contact with patient care; (b) time divided (ideally) equally between research, teaching, and diagnostic services to other doctors; (c) administration of a hospital service, diagnostic services and consultants with other physicians and educational activities. (The objects of educational activities are not only medical students and residents but other practitioners of the hospital. These pathologists may also actually examine patients face-to-face and consult on a course of treatment.)

Again, consider the radiologist. There is considerable range in the scope and kind of practice subsumed under radiology. The "country radiologist" tends to function as an all-around diagnostic consultant, evaluating and interpreting findings concerning a broad spectrum of medical conditions. In the large medical center the diagnostic radiologist either does limited consultation concerning findings or else specializes in one area such as neurological radiology or pediatric radiology. Then there is the radiologist whose work is not primarily diagnostic at all but involves the application of radiation for therapeutic purposes. This man may have his own patients in course of treatment, much like an internist or urologist.

These illustrations suggest that members of a profession not only weigh auxiliary activities differently but have different conceptions of what constitutes the core — *the most characteristic professional act* — of their professional lives. For some radiologists it is attacking tumors with radiation; for others it is interpreting X-ray pictures. For many pathologists it is looking down the barrel of a microscope; for others it is experimental research. A dramatic example of the difference in characteristic professional acts is to be found in psychiatry, which for many of its practitioners means psychotherapy, an intricate set of interactions with a single patient. This is what a psychiatrist does. Yet many practitioners of psychiatry have as little face-to-face interaction with a patient as possible and concentrate upon physical therapies. Still others may spend a good deal of their time administering or directing the activities of other people who actually carry out various therapies.

Not all segments of profession can be said to have this kind of core — a most characteristic activity; many are not so highly identified with a single work activity. But, to the extent that segments develop divergent core activities, they also tend to develop characteristic associated and auxiliary activities, which may introduce further diversity in commitment to major areas, like practice, research, or public health.

Methodology and techniques.—One of the most profound divisions among members of a profession is in their methodology and technique. This, again, is not just a division between specialties within a profession. Specialties frequently arise around the exploitation of a new method or technique, like radiology in medicine, but as time goes by they may segmentalize further along methodological perspectives. Methodological differences can cut across specialty — and even professional — lines with specialists sharing techniques with members of other specialties which they do not share with their fellows.

Insofar as these methodological differences reflect bitter disagreements over the reality that the profession is concerned with, the divisions are deep indeed, and communication between the factions is at a minimum. In psychiatry the conflict over the biological versus the psychological basis of mental illness continues to produce men who speak almost totally different languages. In recent years the situation has been further complicated by the rise of social science's perspectives on mental illness. Focusing upon different aspects of reality, psychiatrists of these various persuasions do different kinds of research and carry out various kinds of therapy. They read a variety of journals, too; and and the journals a man reads, in any branch of medicine, tend to reflect his methodological as well as his substantive interests.

Social scientists must not suppose that, since psychiatry is closer in subject matter to the social sciences, it is the only branch of medicine marred by bitter methodological disputes (we do not mean to imply that such disputes ought to be avoided). Pathologists are currently grappling with methodological issues which raged in some of the biological sciences, particularly anatomy, some years ago. The central issue has to do with the value of morphology, a more traditional approach which uses microscopic techniques to describe the structure of tissues, as against experimental approaches based upon more dynamic biochemical techniques. While the proponents of the

14

two methodologies appear to understand each other somewhat better than do the psychiatrists, they still do not wholly appreciate each other: the morphologists are disposed to be highly defensive, and the experimentalists a little embarrassed by the continued presence of those purely morphologically inclined. Then, in the primarily clinical specialties, those combining medical and surgical techniques offer their own peculiar possibilities for dispute. Men can differ as to how highly they value and emphasize the medical or surgical approach to treatment; for example, an older urologist complained in a journal article that the younger men in the field are "knife-happy." An analogous refrain can be heard among clinicians who frown upon too great a dependence upon laboratory techniques for diagnosis and accuse many of their colleagues of being unable to carry out a complex physical examination in the grand clinical manner.

Clients.—Characteristically, members of professions become involved in sets of relationships that are distinctive to their own segment. Wholly new classes of people may be involved in their work drama whom other segments do not have to take into account. We shall confine ourselves for the moment to considering relationships with clients.

We suspect that sociologists may too easily accept statements glorifying "the doctor-patient relationship" made by segments of the medical profession who have an interest in maintaining a particular relationship to patients. In actuality, the relationships between physicians and patients are highly varied. It does appear that an image of a doctor-patient relationship pervades the entire medical profession, but it is an image which, if it fits any group of physicians in its totality, comes closest to being the model for the general practitioner or his more modern counterpart, the family-practice internist. It seems to set an ideal for other physicians, who may incorporate whatever aspects of it are closest to their own working conditions into an image of the doctor-patient relationship peculiar to their own segment.

Specialties, or segments of specialties, develop images of relationships with patients which distinguish them from other medical groupings. Their own sense of mission and their specialized jobs throw them into new relationships with patients which they eventually formulate and refer to in idealized ways. Moreover, they do not simply define the relationship, but may highly elaborate a relation which this particular kind of doctor, and this kind alone, can have with patients. The pediatricians, for example, have created an image of family practitioner to whom not only the child but the parents and the whole family group surrounding the sick child are patients. According to a spokesman of the pediatricians, the peculiar involve-

15

ment of parents in the illness of the child creates the conditions under which the pediatrician can evolve his relationship to the family unit. Something similar exists in psychiatry, where it is not the mentally ill patient who may be regarded as the sole or even main client but the family. It is probably in psychiatry, too, that the most highly elaborated doctor-patient relationships exist, since the psychotherapeutic practitioner uses his relationships to patients as a conscious and complex therapeutic tool. The most significant point here is that the young psychiatrist, learning the art of psychotherapy, has to unlearn approaches to the patient that he acquired in medical school.

In addition, there are the physicians who only in a special sense can be said to have patients at all. We are likely to think of pathologists, anesthesiologists, and radiologists as doctors without patients: they may have little or no contact with patients, but they do have a relationship to them. The pathologist practicing in a hospital has a well-developed set of obligations to the patient whom he may never confront, and interest groups among the pathologists are concerned with making the lay public aware of the functions of the pathologist behind the scenes. Practitioners in all three of these specialties appear to be concerned with defining their own relationship to patients.

Colleagueship.—Colleagueship may be one of the most sensitive indicators of segmentation within a profession. Whom a man considers to be his colleagues is ultimately linked with his own place within his profession. There is considerable ambiguity among sociologists over the meaning of the term "colleague." Occasionally the word is used to refer to co-workers, and other times simply to indicate formal membership in an occupation — possession of the social signs. Thus, all members of the occupation are colleagues. But sociological theory is also likely to stress colleagueship as a brotherhood. Gross, for example, writes about the colleague group characterized by *esprit de corps* and a sense of "being in the same boat." This deeper colleague relationship, he says, is fostered by such things as control of entry to the occupation, development of a unique mission, shared attitudes toward clients and society, and the formation of informal and formal association.[3]

This conception of colleagueship stresses occupational unity. Once entry to the occupation is controlled, it is assumed that all members of the occupation can be colleagues; they can rally around common symbols. However, the difficulty is that the very aspects of occupational life which Gross writes about as unifying the profession also break it into segments. What ties a man more closely to one member

[3]Edward Gross, *Work and Society* (New York: Thomas Y. Crowell Co., 1958), pp. 223-35.

of his profession may alienate him from another: when his group develops a unique mission, he may no longer share a mission with others in the same profession.

Insofar as colleagueship refers to a relationship characterized by a high degree of shared interests and common symbols, it is probably rare that all members of a profession are even potentially colleagues. It is more feasible, instead, to work with a notion of circles of colleagueship. In the past, sociologists have recognized such circles of colleagueship, but from the viewpoint of the selective influence of such social circumstances as class and ethnicity. The professional identity shared by colleagues, though, contains far more than the kinds of people they desire as fellows. More fundamentally, they hold in common notions concerning the ends served by their work and attitudes and problems centering on it. The existence of what we have called segments thus limits and directs colleagueship.

Identification with segments not only directs relationships within a profession but has a great deal to do with relations with neighboring and allied occupations. We might use the term "alliances" to distinguish this phenomenon from colleagueship within a profession. Alliances frequently dramatize the fact that one branch of a profession may have more in common with elements of a neighboring occupation than with their own fellow professionals. For example, experimentally minded pathologists consult and collaborate with biochemists and other basic scientists, while pathologists oriented toward practice make common cause with clinicians of various specialties.

Interests and associations.—to what extent, and under what conditions, can we speak of professionals as having interests in common? (Here we mean "interests" in the sense of fate, not merely that they are "interested in" different matters.) Sociologists have been overlooking a very rich area for research because they have been too readily assuming unity of interest among professionals. That interests do diverge within a profession is clear enough when the observer looks for it; not only may interests run along different lines, but they may be, and frequently are, in direct conflict.

Pathologists present a particularly striking illustration of conflict of fateful interest between segments of a specialty. The practitioner pathologists are intent upon promulgating an image of the pathologist that undermines the identity of the research-oriented pathologist. The more the practitioners succeed in promoting the notion of the pathologist as a person who performs invaluable services to the clinician, and succeeds in enlarging the area of service, the more do the pathologists who want to do research have to ward off demands from their institutions for more and more service. Fee-splitting in surgery is

17

an example of another kind of conflict of interest: many surgeons can make a living only by engaging in fee-splitting relationships. The more successful surgeons who dominate the professional associations see the practice as tarnishing the reputation of the specialty as a whole and attempt to discredit it in codes of ethics, but they cannot, and even dare not, attempt to stamp it out.

Probably the areas in which professionals come most frequently into conflicts of interest are in gaining a proper foothold in institutions, in recruitment, and in relations with the outside. Here there are recurrent problems which segments and emerging specialties have with their fellow professionals. In order to survive and develop, a segment must be represented in the training centers. The medical-school curriculum today is crowded as the medical specialties compete for the student's time and attention, seeking to recruit or, at least, to socialize the budding professional into the correct attitudes toward themselves. Some specialties regard themselves as having so little lien on the student's time that they use that time primarily, in some medical schools, to impress upon him that only specialists can safely do certain procedures — in short, how important and necessary is the particular specialty of the instructor.

Then, too, segments require different understandings, even different contractual relations, with clients and institutions. Many a professional association has arisen out of just such conflicts as this. In the 1920's there was a great deal of ferment between the rising specialty of pediatrics and the American Medical Association over governmental ventures into child health legislation, the pediatricians favoring the Shepherd-Towner Act. The pediatricians, recognizing a need for an organization which would represent their own interests independent of the American Medical Association, eventually formed the American Academy of Pediatrics. The big professional associations in the specialty of pathology are all dominated by, and exist for, practitioners in pathology. Therefore, when leading research-oriented pathologists recently became concerned with increasing research potential in the field, and incidentally with capturing some of the funds which the National Institutes of Health were dispensing to pathology, they formed committees especially for this purpose to function as temporary associations. Recently, a Society of Medical Psychiatry has been formed, undoubtedly in response to the growing power of psychoanalytic psychiatry and to the lessening importance, in many academic settings, of somatic psychiatrists.

Looking at professional associations from this perspective, it seems that associations must be regarded in terms of just whose fateful interests within the profession are served. Associations are not everybody's association but represent one segment or a particular alliance

18

of segments. Sociologists may ask of medicine, for example: Who has an interest in thinking of medicine as a whole, and which segments take on the role of spokesmen to the public?

Spurious unity and public relations.—There remain to be considered the relations of professions to the lay public and the seeming unity presented by such arrangements as codes of ethics, licensure, and the major professional associations. These products of professional activity are not necessarily evidence of internal homogeneity and consensus but rather of the power of certain groups: established associations become battlegrounds as different emerging segments compete for control. Considered from this viewpoint, such things as codes of ethics and procedures of certification become the historical deposits of certain powerful segments.

Groups that control the associations can wield various sanctions so as to bring about compliance of the general membership with codes which they have succeeded in enacting. The association concerned with the practice of pathology, for example, has recently stipulated specific contractual relations which the pathologist should enter into with his hospital and is moving toward denying critical services of the association to non-complying members — despite the fact that a goodly proportion of practicing pathologists neither have such contractual relations nor even consider them desirable. But more or less organized opposition to the code-writing of intrenched groups can lead to revision of codes from time to time. Changes occur as the composition of critical committees is altered. Thus, since the clinically oriented pathologists have gained power, they have succeeded in making certification examinations more and more exacting along applied lines, making it steadily more difficult for young pathologists trained for research to achieve certification. Certification procedures thus shift with the relative power of segments, putting a premium on some kinds of training and discriminating against others.

Those who control the professional associations also control the organs of public relations. They take on the role of spokesmen to the public, interpreting the position of the profession, as they see it. They also negotiate with relevant special publics. The outsider coming into contact with the profession tends to encounter the results of the inner group's efforts; he does not necessarily become aware of the inner circle or the power struggles behind the unified front. Thus, in considering the activities of professional associations the observer must continually ask such questions as: Who handles the public and what do they represent? Whose codes of ethics are these? What does the certification stand for? We should also ask, wherever a profession seems to the general public to be relatively unified, why it seems so — for this, too, is a pertinent problem.

19

SEGMENTS AS SOCIAL MOVEMENTS

Our mode of presentation might lead the reader to think of segments as simple differentiation along many rubrics. On the contrary, the notion of segments refers to organized identities. A position taken on one of the issues of professional identity discussed above entails taking corresponding positions along other dimensions of identity. Segments also involve shared identities, manifested through circles of colleagueship. This allows one to speak of types of pathologist or types of pediatrician — groups of people who organize their professional activity in ways which distinguish them from other members of their profession.

Segments are not fixed, perpetually defined parts of the body professional. They tend to be more or less continually undergoing change. They take form and develop, they are modified, and they disappear. Movement is forced upon them by changes in their conceptual and technical apparatus, in the institutional conditions of work, and in their relationship to other segments and occupations. Each generation engages in spelling out, again, what it is about and where it is going. In this process, boundaries become diffuse as generations overlap, and different loci of professional activity articulate somewhat different definitions of the work situation. Out of this fluidity new groupings may emerge.

If this picture of diversity and movement is a realistic description of what goes on within professions, how can it be analyzed? As a beginning, the movement of segments can fruitfully be analyzed as analogous to social movements. Heretofore, the analysis of social movements has been confined to religious, political, and reform movements, to such problems as the conditions of their origin, recruitment, leadership, the development of organizational apparatus, ideologies, and tactics. The same questions can be asked of movements occurring within professions. Professional identity may be thought of as analogous to the ideology of a political movement; in this sense, segments have ideology. We have seen that they have missions. They also tend to develop a brotherhood of colleagues, leadership, organizational forms and vehicles, and tactics for implementing their position.

At any one time the segments within a profession are likely to be in different phases of development and engaging in tactics appropriate to their position. In pathology, for example, the clinically oriented segment, which one of its antagonists termed "evangelistic" and which is still expanding, has already created strong organizations, captured many academic departments, promulgated codes of ethics, and is closing in on the battle to secure desirable status for pathologists in hospitals. The more scientifically oriented segment, on the other hand, finds itself in a somewhat defensive position, forced to reaffirm some aspects of its identity and modify others and to engage in tactics to hold its institutional supports. Possibly the acme for some expanding segments is the recognized status of specialty or subspecialty. Certainly, this is the way specialties seem to develop. But the conditions under which segments will become formal specialties is in itself a fascinating research problem. (So also is the whole question of relative development, degree of change, influence, and power — matters expressively alluded to when professionals speak of "hot" areas and dead ones.)

We have said that professions consist of a loose amalgamation of segments which are in movement. Further, professions involve a number of social movements in various kinds of relationship to each other. Although the method of analysis developed for studying political and reform movements provides a viewpoint on phenomena of professional life neglected in contemporary research, some differences must be noted between professional movements and the traditional subject matter of analysis. First of all, professional movements occur within institutional arrangements, and a large part of the activity of segments is a power struggle for the possession of them or of some kind of place within them. Second, the fates of segments are closely intertwined: they are possibly more interdependent and responsive to one another than are other kinds of movements. It is probably impossible to study one segment in movement adequately without taking into account what is happening to others. Third, the leaders are men who have recognized status in the field, operate from positions of relative institutional power, and command the sources of institutionalized recruitment. Finally, it must be pointed out that not all segments display the character of a social movement. Some lack organized activities, while others are still so inchoate that they appear more as a kind of backwash of the profession than as true segments.

In any case, the existence of segments, and the emergence of new segments, takes on new significance when viewed from the perspective of social movements within a profession. Pockets of resistance and embattled minorities may turn out to be the heirs of former generations, digging in along new battle lines. They may spearhead new movements which sweep back into power. What looks like backwash, or just plain deviancy, may be the beginnings of a new segment which will acquire an institutional place and considerable prestige and power. A case in point is that of the progenitors of the clinical pathologists, who today are a threat to the institutional position of research-oriented pathologists but who were considered the failures, or poor cousins, of the specialty thirty years ago.

We have indicated what new kinds of research might originate from the conception of professions that we have presented. However, this perspective has implications for several quite traditional areas of research.

1. *Work situation and institution as arenas.*—The work situation and the institution itself are not simply places where people of various occupations and professions come together and enact standard occupational roles, either complimentary or conflicting. These locales constitute the arenas wherein such roles are forged and developed. Work situation and institution must be regarded in the light of the particular professional segments represented there: where the segments are moving and what effect these arenas have on their further development. Since professions are in movement, work situations and institutions inevitably throw people into new relationships.

2. *Careers.*—The kinds of stages and the locales through which a man's career moves must be considered in terms of the segment to which he "belongs." Further, the investigator must be prepared to see changes not only in stages of career but in the ladder itself. The system that the career is moving through can change along the way and take on entirely new directions. The fate of individual careers is closely tied up with the fate of segments, and careers that were possible for one generation rarely are repeatable for the next generation.

3. *Socialization.*—An investigator should not focus solely upon how conceptions and techniques are imparted in the study of socialization; he should be equally interested in the clash of opinions among the socializers, where students are among the prizes. Segments are in competition for the allegiance of students: entire schools as well as single departments can be the arena of, and weapons in, this conflict. During their professional training, students pick their way through a maze of conflicting models and make momentous commitments thereby.

4. *Recruitment.*—The basic program of recruitment probably tends to be laid down by powerful segments of the profession. Yet different segments require different kinds of raw material to work upon, and their survival depends upon an influx of candidates who are potential successors. Thus, recruitment can be another critical battleground upon which segments choose candidates in their own image or attempt to gain sufficient control over recruitment procedures to do so. Defection by the recruited and recruiters, by the sponsored and the sponsors, is also well worth studying, being one way that new careers take form.

5. *Public Images.*—We have seen that images beamed to the public tend to be controlled by particular segments of the profession.

22

However, sometimes segments reject these public images as inappropriate — either to themselves, specifically, or to the profession at large. If only the former, then they may require that the public acquire specialized images for themselves. In any case, segments from time to time must engage in tactics to project their own images to the public. The situation is more complicated when the whole profession is considered as a public for particular specialties or for segments of specialties. Segments may be at pains to counteract the images which other people in the profession have of them, and attempt to create alternative images.

6. *Relations with other professions.*—Different segments of the profession come into contact with different occupations and professions. They might have quite special problems with other occupations which they do not share with other members of their profession. In considering the handling of relations with other professions, it is thus necessary to ask such questions as: Who in the profession is concerned with this problem and what difference does it make to them? Who does the negotiating and in what ways?

7. *Leadership.*—Most leadership is associated less with the entire profession than with restricted portions of it. Certainly, it is linked with intellectual movements, and with the fates and fortunes of certain segments. Leadership, strategies, and the fates of segments deserve full focus in our studies of professionalization.

STRUCTURE AND IDEOLOGY OF THE
NURSING PROFESSION

Every occupation has its own particular history that, in some respect at least, is unique. If scrutinized, closely enough, each occupation also possesses a unique contemporary pattern of structural and ideological features; for instance, its particular modes of, and ideas about, recruitment and education, its predominant types and places of work, its prevailing internal divisions of labor. Ordinarily when discussing occupations, historians pay strict attention to historical narrative but leave structural aspects implicitly or entirely secondary to the painstaking hunt for chronological accuracy; while sociologists, their gaze mainly upon the contemporary scene, confront the occupaiton on its own contemporary grounds, and use occupational history only as a backdrop to the current drama. Additional insight can be gained by fusing both approaches. This chapter is an interpretation of how certain prominent structural and ideologies features of American nursing have evolved from certain historical conditions pertaining to the occupation and to the country at large.

I shall discuss first the structural profile of the occupation: its complex of structural features which seem both to characterize the occupation and to hang together in a complicated pattern. I shall trace how various parts of the pattern and their associated ideological elements seem to have emerged historically, because of structural conditions once characteristic of the country and of the occupation.

Before turning to these tasks, it may be necessary to emphasize that I have not attempted to write a history of nursing but to give an interpretation of nursing's past history and current status. It is based on what historians of nursing say about the profession as well as on some issues and events not noted in traditional accounts or highlighted in contemporary commentary. I use the term "interpretation" advisedly, thus inviting argument, and anticipating that many readers will disagree — perhaps almost totally — with this particular reading of the profession. I would only hope that the resulting argument generates light rather than merely heat, with the effect of deepening our knowledge of this fascinating, and important, profession.

STRUCTURAL FEATURES OF THE OCCUPATION

Whether we read through the various journals devoted to the activities of nurses or observe those activities at the various sites where nurses work, we will immediately be stuck by certain features of nursing. Nursing is almost wholly a woman's province. Nurses are found at the bedside ministering to the sick, but also behind the desks and office doors shuffling papers and administering the institution's affairs. Nurses are found everywhere in the United States — although the greatest ratio are in cities — and they are of all ages. Although a considerable number of nurses work for a fee, as private duty nurses, the majority work for a salary in various kinds of institutions (notably hospitals, physicians' offices, public health agencies, schools, and as teachers in universities, colleges, and hospital schools). Nurses seem to work in subordination to physicians. These cursory observations can be the starting point for a discussion of this occupation's structural profile which, in total detail, is unlike any other occupation.

In more precise terms, let us examine each of the foregoing characteristics, then add others that are less obvious to the casual eye. To begin with, nursing is one of the greatest *women's occupations* of the nation, paralleled by teaching, social welfare, and the more amorphous white-collar "jobs."

In 1960, there were approximately 500,000 practicing licensed graduate nurses (this figure does not include the almost 250,000 nonpracticing R.N.'s or the sizable number of practical nurses and nursing aides); whereas there were approximately 225,000 physicians and 90,000 chemists.

A third feature of nursing, as noted earlier, is that it is now predominantly, and increasingly, a *salaried* occupation, although a substantial proportion still work as private duty nurses for fees.

A fourth feature is the *relatively open recruitment* of nurses. Some occupations maintain tight control over their recruitment (such as the medical profession in America) but others cannot maintain such control. Almost any woman can enter some kind of nursing school and if graduated can nurse legitimately for money. During wartime, there is great pressure upon the occupation to open its gates and admit floods of new candidates, a pressure accompanied by perennial cries of "lowered standards" versus "national requirements."

A fifth feature is the great *geographical mobility* of nurses: traditionally and currently a licensed nurse could migrate from one city to another, one region to another, and easily find employment.[1] The point is not merely the relatively open market for nursing skills, but the spatial transferability of these skills.

A sixth feature of the occupation pertains to the establishments where nurses work. Traditionally and currently the *majority* of *nurses work predominately* at three locales: hospitals, public health agencies, and to some extent still in private homes. To these nurses must be added a sizable number of "nurse educators" who teach in various educational establishments. (Others work in industry, public schools, and physicians' offices.)

A seventh feature of nursing pertains to the work of nurses. They *teach*. They *administer*. Traditionally, and despite increasing administrative duties, they also do the *bedside-nursing* that is thought generally to be nursing's main rationale for existence. As will later be seen, these three job functions have been characteristically blurred, but now are becoming increasingly distinct. An eighth feature is that nurses tend to *look upward to physicians* for orders and *downward to assistants* (practical nurses or aides) for response to their own orders. Said another way, this occupation is scarcely autonomous, but *embedded within a hierarchy of authority*.

A ninth feature is that *specialization* within nursing *tends both to follow the hierarchical lines of hospitals or agencies and the clinical specializations of medicine itself*. To this we must add another specialization: teaching. However, these nursing specialties tend not to be tightly constraining, since the lines among them are relatively permeable (though probably growing less so). Many nurses seem somewhat hestitant to overemphasize specialization and prefer to overemphasize the all-purpose or generally "well-trained" nurse. Even the specialization due to use of nurses for administration is hardly recognized as a specialty, worth separate education: nurses rise in the ranks and frequently demote themselves because of distaste for administration, distaste for the particular post, or because they migrate to another locale and accept whatever position is available

[1]Cf., "Committee on the Grading of Nursing Schools," *Nurses, Patients and Pocketbooks* (New York: Committee on the Grading of Nursing Schools, 1928), pp. 100-101; also, Ruth Pape, "Touristy: A Type of Occupational Mobility," *Social Problems* (1964) pp. 336-344.

there. However, the current strain between "education" and "nursing service," based on increased career specialization, is notable.

A _tenth_ feature of nursing is its curious _melange of educational institutions and nursing degrees._ Traditionally nurses were educated in one type of establishment, the so-called "hospital school," which will be discussed shortly. Currently these schools range greatly in quality (although in the past decade an accrediting system has sharply cut off those below a certain level and probably raised the educational level of the mass of schools). Over the years, nursing has affiliated with colleges and universities, and under such a variety of circumstances that the range of "degree programs" offered can be staggering to the naive university scholar, familiar only with a simple tricotomy of B.S., M.S., and Ph.D, when he first learns about nursing programs.

In summary then, American nursing is a woman's occupation that is massive in scope. Salaries are increasing, recruitment is relatively open, and there is a high degree of geographical mobility. Work occurs mainly in three or four types of establishments, where there is strong tendency to control by the medical profession and where three job functions (teaching, administering, and bedside nursing) are characteristically blurred. However, they are becoming more distinct, but bedside nursing is still believed to be the chief rationale for "nursing." There is a tendency for specialization to follow hierarchical lines up the administrative ladder or to follow medical specialization itself; there are a host of educational programs which seem to represent both the occupation's attempt to get "professional" legitimation through higher education and a genuine desire to improve the services which the occupation offers to its clients.

Unquestionably more features could be added to this list, but these few should provide enough problems for discussion. These structural features of the occupation should not be taken for granted; they must be explained. Why these particular features? And why all of these, in what probably can be termed a pattern?

SOME ASPECTS OF NATIONAL DEVELOPMENT

To answer these questions requires, as already mentioned, an historical approach. Let us begin with a framework, noting particular and well-known aspects of American national development. These few aspects are not selected by random; they will function prominently, although implicitly, in the structurally oriented narrative itself. A convenient initial fact worth noting is that the story of American nursing as a self-conscious claimant to professional title began roughly in the 1880's.

Since that date, one striking characteristic of national development has been the massive shift from a predominantly agricultural economy to industrialization. This shift has been accompanied by significant changes in the organization of work, work site, and the services provided by people who work. Expressed in polar terms: Americans moved from the farm and small town into sizable cities and metropoli; they moved from small farms and small businesses to large factories, corporations, and agri-business systems. Mass production of consumer goods eventually predominated, and the services afforded only by the rich before the twentieth century became the common property of a substantial proportion of Americans. Associated with all this has been a tremendous expansion of population resulting from immigration and internal growth, for our kind of industrial development has both rested upon and made possible an increased population. This development also required a rising level of education. Industrialized nations need educated manpower to run industries, to manage corporations, governmental agencies, and hospitals, and to educate new generations of manpower. "The advancing industrial economy must have a fully developed system of general education, and at the same time its educational institutions must become more functionally oriented to the training of skilled technicians, engineers, scientists, and administrators."[2]

Higher education, therefore, has become a prominent feature of American life. Our universities are something quite different from Cardinal Newman's idea of the university. They have become crucial training grounds for emergent professions and occupational specializations undreamed of by earlier educators. Finally, and here the consumer theme touched upon earlier is repeated, the whole surge of the economy over the past several decades has brought hospitalization, medication, and medical services to the verge of being every citizen's right, whether obtained through private purchase, insurance plans, or federal support. All these national developments are well known. They are listed only because they are, as a cluster, vital to any understanding of either the structure or the functioning of American nursing as an occupation.

THE NURSING REFORM MOVEMENT

The origins of organized nursing in America are inseparable from the tide of reform which swept middle-class America during the 1870's, 1880's, and 1890's. During these decades America seemed destined to become an urban nation, and with urbanism came reform. By 1880, there were eight cities with populations over 250,000, and

2Clark Kerr, et al., *Industrialism and Industrial Man* (Cambridge, Mass.: Harvard University Press, 1960), p. 159.

the Middle West was building up fast behind the Eastern Seaboard. These crowded cities were composed of rural migrants as well as foreign immigrants, but then in the mid-eighties began the numerically tremendous "new immigration." In the face of this in-flow of population, the middle classes moved steadily uptown and to the city's outskirts, away from ethnic ghettos and what the journalists described romantically as the "haunts" of vice and the poor. But the poor could neither be totally disregarded nor could middle-class people of conscience fail to put their consciences to work upon the problems of the poor. While some reformers blamed the new industrial order itself, others only perceived that something had to be done about the slums and the unfortunates who filled them. Some of this reform was primarily religious, some was economic or political, and of course some was educationally oriented.

Middle-class people, mostly women, also discovered and came in contact with the poor inside the large urban hospitals which were increasingly flooded with helpless victims of the new urban conditions. In some of the larger Eastern cities, New York and Boston for instance, public-spirited women began to introduce into the hospitals a measure of cleanliness, decency, and order, since both hospital housekeeping and the care of patients left much to be desired.

Hospitals were staffed for the most part with women, some of them drunks, many of them dirty. Few of them were, from middle-class vantage, well trained or educated. Into hospitals like Bellevue in New York, the fastidious ladies began to introduce a system, imported from England, for training nurses and staffing hospitals. Sometimes, as at Bellevue, they imported English nurses who could implement the "Nightingale system." The Bellevue school "was independent of the Hospital and subject to the direction of a Board of Lady Managers."[3] The latter had followed a key tenet of Florence Nightingale's, namely, that school and hospital were to be under separate administration; otherwise the hospital would soon dominate the school, while the school correspondingly would exert less influence upon the work of the hospital. The school and its students were to be guardians of nursing care in the hospital — banishing from its corridors and rooms the vulgar sounds and sights, the horrendous scenes, and the omnipresent dirt that traditionally held sway there.

The principal role in this working system of hospital reform belonged to one woman, who was both superintendent of the training school and chief nurse at the hospital. She taught the students (generally she was their sole nursing teacher during the early years of reform), and she supervised their work at the hospital (for they

---

[3]E. Johns and B. Pfefferkorn, *The John Hopkins Hospital School of Nursing* (Baltimore: Hopkins Press, 1954), p. 40.

manned the institution until graduated, when they left to nurse in patient's homes). The students received more medical aspects of training from special lectures by the hospital's physicians, who necessarily simplified the subject matter for their listeners.

The first superintendent of The Johns Hopkins School for Nurses announced in her inaugural speech that:

The proposed plan of study is much like that in other large schools for nurses. The first year the pupils will engage in hospital work entirely, acting as assistants in the wards and, under the instruction of appointed head nurses, being changed from time to time from one department of work to another. In connection with this practical work, they will receive theoretical teaching, given systematically in classes, and by means of lectures. In their second year, they are expected to be sufficiently taught to be able to assume more direct responsibility of patients in the hospital, and to undertake the care of patients in private families. In addition to this, a certain portion of each pupil's second year will be devoted to district nursing among the poor, in their homes, under a competent head nurse. . . .[4]

Another important feature of the Nightingale system was the careful inculcation of proper demeanor and good moral behavior. In America, these first training schools seem to have recruited heavily from small towns, attracting girls from "good" if not well-to-do families. Many had been school teachers, or at least educated in seminaries. Some recruits to the training centers became superintendents. It was typical during their careers for them to found one or more training schools, which *ad infinitum* were supposed to produce genuinely trained nurses, including some who would institute yet more schools.

The Bellevue student nurse, whose picture appeared in 1882 in a *Century Magazine* article titled "A New Profession for Women," exemplified this expansion of nursing reform. Miss Hampton, a girl from a small town in Ontario, was the daughter of a successful merchant. After a bit of schooling at a local "College Institute," she earned a low-ranking teaching certificate which enabled her to teach briefly until she followed two fellow teachers to the Bellevue School of Nursing. After her graduation, she carried the school's ideals and methods to her first superintendency at Chicago's Illinois Training School — quite like other graduates of Bellevue who were becoming heads of hospitals and schools to meet "the great demands from the large cities in different states."

At the Illinois school, Miss Hampton was confronted by problems identical to those which the Lady Managers had sought earlier to banish from Bellevue. Not long after, she was asked to head the

[4]*Ibid.*, p. 43. The words are by Miss Isabel Hampton.

30

newly founded training school at The Johns Hopkins University. When she retired because of marriage, she passed along the superintendency to a former student who had already been absorbed into the slowly expanding teaching staff. To jump ahead in our story, this second head of the Hopkins school became the first professor of nursing at Teachers College, Columbia University, where she immensely influenced the course of nursing education for some decades; while Miss Hampton — now Mrs. Robb — became the primary organizer of the entire profession until her early death.

By 1893, nurses were prepared to accept an invitation to run a special conference at Chicago's Columbian Exhibition. The mood of the conference was optimistic. Nursing had come a long way. Trained nurses had proven what rigorous schooling and high standards could do toward reconstituting hospitals and aiding physicians in their care of the sick. The conference speakers optimistically dwelt upon plans and programs.

But along with the images of progress and a roseate future, another image appeared repeatedly in speeches at the Chicago conference. The true concept of a training school had been perverted by most hospitals and their schools. What had actually happened was this: the nation's vast geographical spread, the immense mobility of its population, and the diversity of its sectarian groups had together engendered the rapid increase of hospitals — each independently financed and administered. Since the supply of trained nurses was short and finances were skimpy, and since the hospital administrators were often laymen or physicians of no great education themselves, the great majority of these newly founded hospitals disregarded Nightingale precepts. (No doubt many hospitals were unfamiliar with her precepts.) They only adopted one bending it to their own uses. The increase in the founding of hospital affiliated schools for nurses was phenomenal. But these schools did *not* give the training that Nightingale and Nightingale-inspired nurses required; rather they were designed to supply the hospitals' needs for steady help at a reasonable price. This is the most generous construction that can be put upon the rise of "hospital schools." A less generous one, which surely fitted some schools, is that through them cheap, exploitable female labor was fed into the hospitals. During the 1880's and 1890's, however, working women were available, whether exploited or not; their availability arose from such conditions as immigration, regional mobility, and the movement of families from the farm to the town and city.

The Chicago conferees—believing that training schools should *upgrade* hospitals, not supply them with tractable, exploitable, uneducated female labor — adopted plans to organize in some manner to exert proper control over the practice of nursing, and over the destiny of the profession as well. Their chief mode of organizing at first was to further the founding and development of alumnae societies at reputable schools, along with the founding of a society embracing all the superintendents of those schools. Registration and licensing of nurses would come later, but were already being mentioned. But most of all, raising standards through excellence of training was urgent — indeed was more than urgent: it was the principal weapon with which to combat hordes of uneducated and half-educated nurses.

Despite these steps and this resolve, the reform movement in nursing was to be confronted for many years, certainly up to the 1950's, with what came to be known as the problem of the "hospital schools." Although the reformers did provide and maintain control over much of the occupation's organizational framework, the market for nurses was dominated numerically by graduates from what the reformers believed were inferior schools. This belief only fortified their basic belief in the value of good training for nurses, and led directly into a movement toward higher education.

REFORM AND THE IDEA OF "PROFESSION"

Before discussing this educational trend, it is profitable to consider a question that is much related to education in nursing. The early reformer nurses believed that nursing was a profession, and apparently were successful in convincing the public of this. The question has not to do with why they were successful, but with the meaning of "profession" to the reformers. (The answer is neither simple nor at all self-evident.) It is clear enough that profession meant to them an occupation with impeccable standards — or at least they strove for such standards — along with the idea of a "calling." But that is not all that a profession meant to them. Again let us turn to Miss Hampton since she was perhaps the most influential nurse of the day and, significantly, superintendent of the first university training school. During her inaugural speech in 1889, she made no mention of nursing as a profession: only good training through careful recruitment, relatively rigorous discipline, high standards, and the best kind of teaching available.

But the idea of profession was in the air. The superintendent of The Johns Hopkins Hospital had already recommended to the Board of Trustees that "careful attention should be given to the more purely intellectual part of the nurse's training to the end that nursing may be elevated to a profession and raised as far as possible above the status of a mere trade." The Chicago conference, four years after Miss Hampton's inaugural speech, was full of talk about the profession, especially in conjunction with plans for raising standards and forming nurses' organizations. So there is no question that these nurses were determined to make of their work professional work. In what sense was it to be professional? And how were they to make it professional?

At this point in the historical narrative, we might just as well consider a curious paradox. The Hopkins training school — the first of many nursing schools affiliated in some sense with universities — was providing students to service the Hopkins hospital. At the Hopkins medical school, students took genuine university courses and earned a genuine university degree. The student nurses did neither, for the Board of Trustees never considered that the "Training School for Nurses" at Hopkins was more than merely superior training school — not a place where students got a university education.

Miss Hampton's own model of professional education and attainment was not at variance with this administrative assumption. We have seen why this should be so. She had been pointedly explicit on this matter, writing in the opening pages of her textbook, *Nursing: Its Principles and Practice,* that:

The superintendent of a training-school is under a threefold obligation: first, to the hospital where she works; secondly, to the patients who are entrusted to her care; and thirdly, to the women for whose education as nurses she is responsible. The hospital and patients should always be first considered, but not to the exclusion of what is just and right toward the pupil nurses.[5]

It is not difficult to see, either, why the great physicians at the medical school and hospital did not redirect Miss Hampton's goals. They were distinguished clinicians, who valued well-trained nurses but could scarcely conceive of a truly university trained one. A woman graduate of a university medical school was quite another matter: several good exemplars of that possibility were then alive.

The one man who could have had a different conception of nursing education was the President of the university, Daniel Coit Gilman. Under his administration, Johns Hopkins became the graduate institution that so profoundly influenced American higher education, and he was the driving force behind the establishment of a scientifically oriented medical school. In his inaugural address, he laid down some of his basic beliefs upon which he later acted, including that a medical school should be a genuine part of the university rather than under the control of the university hospital. But what

---

[5] (Philadelphia: Saunders, 1893), pp. 17-18. It is significant that she held this view despite the excellence of her students, for many were the daughters of businessmen, a few were college educated, while the fathers of others were on the Hopkins Board of Trustees.

he was fighting to establish on the American scene for medicine he did not at all imagine for nursing. Unquestionably he visualized the education and function of nurses as technical. The circumstances under which he came into close contact with nursing at Hopkins furthered this conception. When the Trustees came to open the hospital, after many years of preparation and construction, they felt "much uncertainty as to the best method of organizing the work and putting the institution into active operation. . . . It was felt by all that the undertaking was of no ordinary proportions and called for the assistance of a skilled and wise organizer."[6] The Trustees requested Gilman to do the job, and he did it, down to minute admministrative detail, that included hiring higher personnel and outlining their duties. "He selected very wisely the first principal of the Training School for Nurses and the first head nurse. He was ever after much interested in the Training School and often visited it, and on several occasions made addresses to the pupil nurses."[7]

In preparing for this monumental job of organizing a model hospital, about which he knew nothing when he undertook the enterprise, Gilman visited countless other institutions, including the most reputable training schools for nurses. Presumably, it was then that his ideas of nursing functions were formed or at least fortified, abetted by the actual administrative task that he himself had sworn to accomplish. He viewed nurses only as a means to staff his hospital. The better trained the nurses were, the better the staff would be. In addition, like every other part of Johns Hopkins itself, he anticipated that the Training School was to be an exemplary symbol to other nursing schools. The additional irony of his conception was that Gilman was the very man who did most, perhaps, to establish the idea of science in the American university, and his inaugural speech at Hopkins makes clear his determination to make graduate education relevant to the purposes of the wider community, far beyond the confines of university walls.

Was there anything else, we might well ask, which prevented Gilman from readjusting his views of nursing as a merely technical skill toward reconceptualizing nursing as a professional field: part public service and part abstract knowledge? Analogizing from American medicine, which was then in sad shape, he might have foreseen perhaps that nursing was only further behind in evolutionary development. We might hazard that Gilman, like some educational leaders of the era, looked with disfavor on higher education for women. But

6The words are those of Hurd, Superintendent of the Hospital, quoted in Fabian Franklin, *The Life of Daniel Coit Gilman* (New York: Dodd, Mead and Company, 1910), pp. 260-261.

7*Ibid.*, p. 262.

he does not seem to have held such views, although neither does he appear on the stage of history as a flaming champion of women's educational rights. Had he been, had he even visualized in less suffragette terms that a university education might be germane to the establishment and efficiency of "professional nursing," then the course of American nursing might have taken a radically different turn. But the nurses, practicing in a man's world, under the aegis or at least the eye of physicians, and confronting the immediate threat posed by a flow of poorly trained recruits through the hospital schools, could scarcely be expected to place this emphasis upon university education.

To do the early nursing "leaders" justice, we ought to remember also that the idea of professional training *qua* university training had yet to emerge clearly on the American scene. The idea had been born; it was in operation. But before the 1890's, legal training, for instance, consisted mainly of apprenticeship, and medical training either involved apprenticeship or was given in diploma mills. Many academic professions, whether in the physical or social sciences, were just being initiated, and most had not become very visible. The age of burgeoning professionalism had yet to arrive.[8] In 1915 Abraham Flexner would enumerate his famous criteria for a true profession — criteria which were already leading to the sweeping reform of medical education.[9] It would require an anthropologist writing as late as 1936 to admonish nurses that postgraduate work in nursing was being used primarily to supplement the deficiencies of weak undergraduate nursing schools, rather than constituting genuine graduate education.[10] During the closing years of the nineteenth century, the influential teachers of nursing could only see the medical profession as its model — a completely comprehensible perception since physician and nurse worked as companions in arms against disease. That the nurse looked up at the physicians, as well as across the bedside at them, is also understandable. The physicians were men, in command, and more advanced in their cumulative knowledge. Miss Hampton, addressing the Chicago conference, modestly said, "Medicine made us a profession; now we must live up to it."[11] This was

[8]Cf., B. Berelson, *Graduate Education in the U. S.* (New York: McGraw-Hill, 1960), The University Revolution, 1876-1900, pp. 109-116.

[9]"Is Social Work a Profession?" *School and Society,* Vol. 1 (1915), pp. 901-911. Flexner's famous report on medical education appeared in 1910.

[10]Esther Lucile Brown, *Nursing for the Future* (New York: Russell Sage Foundation, 1948), p. 61.

[11]Isabel Hampton Robb, *Educational Standards for Nurses* (Cleveland: E. C. Koeckert, 1907), pp. 174-175.

said despite the considerable initial opposition by many physicians to nursing reform itself.

OPEN RECRUITMENT, EDUCATION, AND EDUCATIONAL IDEOLOGY

This historical narrative has introduced several structural features which characterize American nursing today. We can better appreciate why the occupation is massive in numbers, geographically spread, and relatively open to any woman who wishes to enter. We have seen the initial blurring of administrative and teaching functions in the work of superintendents. Also, the tendency toward hierarchy of physician above and nurse below has been established. Perhaps a word should be added about why the occupation is also a woman's occupation. Traditionally, to nurse family members was the duty of women, a practice that often extended to helping other families under conditions of crisis. Also, organized nursing evolved during a period of American history when women in increasing numbers were entering the labor market at a level above factory and domestic work. Nursing, therefore, represented one of the genuine opportunities for self-support combined with some measure of associated social status.

The next structural feature to be discussed is the curious melange of educational institutions and degrees that characterizes the occupation. Anyone not familiar with schools of nursing is likely to be bewildered when he first learns about their variety. Among them there are two-year, three-year, and five-year schools. There are hospital schools and collegiate schools. There are university schools that some nurses consider genuine "university schools" and others that they do not. There are a variety of collegiate programs, as well as an odd type termed "postmasters" programs. There will soon be doctoral programs. For many years there also has been a variety of certificates awarded for special study. Of course, thankfully, no profession is a single entity at peace with itself, hence the training of recruits is never completely standardized the country over, or are training centers exact duplicates of each other; but some professions have achieved or accepted more regularization, by law and through national organization. Nursing has neither achieved this degree of centralized control nor been forced to strict educational standardization. How this general situation has come about can be illuminated through understanding something of the ideological development of nursing educators.

At the close of the nineteenth century the plight of American nursing was shared by other occupations whose most conscientious members found that they could not effectively block the entrance of undesirable candidates. Each claimant to professional title must

36

deal with the problem of recruitment: for obtaining desirable recruits and keeping out unworthy ones are means basic to controlling the actual practice of full-fledged practitioners. Some professions, in some countries during some eras, manage to secure firm control over recruitment, but the control is never perfect or always desired by all members; and, in fact, the various professions and occupations vary considerably according to degree of control exercised over candidacy. Whether a given profession gains characteristically rigorous or loose control has grave consequences for other features of "its" existence.

The avenues into the nursing of patients for pay traditionally had been open to any woman who cared to enter. Consequently, when the first generation of influential "trained nurses" began to graduate from schools affiliated with such progressive hospitals as Bellevue, Hopkins, New York Hospital, and Massachusetts General Hospital, this generation aspired only to convince hospital authorities how immensely valuable could be well-trained nurses of good character. They did not presume to unrealizable powers whereby they themselves might admit or deny license to other practitioners of nursing. Anyway most hospital authorities would not have heeded their decisions.

Since the well-trained nurse's rise to prominence was paralleled by a corresponding increase in nurses all over the nation, whom the former considered to be poorly trained and frequently downright ignorant, what options did the trained nurses visualize? What could they do? Nursing historians see no problem here: nursing "leaders" *had* to work toward raising "standards" through improving the education of nurses until collegiate schools could be founded. Eventually advanced university degrees in nursing would be obtainable. But if this interpretation is not merely an instance of *post-hoc* reasoning, it is at least an oversimplification of what transpired.

Like many trail blazers, the prominent trained nurses did not see the trail very clearly at its beginning. There is some doubt whether they even knew they were treading the trail at all until after they had made a fateful turn. What happened is that, at first, many superintendents of training schools, like Miss Hampton (Mrs. Robb) at Johns Hopkins, experimented with new courses and methods of training; then in 1898 Mrs. Robb conceived the idea that, since they were all in the business of teaching, perhaps they should learn much more about teaching from experts in pedagogy. Addressing herself to this issue before the American Society of Superintendents of Training Schools for Nurses, she argued that:

It is generally conceded by instructors in other kinds of schools that in addition to the diploma secured, it is necessary for those who intend to teach to have a further course in a school of pedagogy or in a normal school, where they may supplement the knowledge they have acquired by learning the best methods of teaching and how to apply them. Why should not this hold equally well with a woman who elects to become a teacher in a school for nurses?

Then, taking a great stride, she made explicit a distinction between practitioners in the profession and teachers of the practitioners:[12] "It is one thing to graduate as a trained nurse but another to enter upon the duties and responsibilities of a training school without a thorough and proper grounding in the managements of such work."[13]

Without pausing to examine the premises of this argument, her audience quickly reacted to its evident good sense. They appointed, at her suggestion, a committee to discover and approach the authorities of a suitable school of pedagogy. Consequently she and Adelaide Nutting, a member of her committee, visited the Dean of Teachers College at Columbia University. That institution had been selected after previous inquiries unearthed no other with a program sufficiently "practical to meet our wants." The Dean of Teachers College listened with surprise to their proposition. But he was receptive, and so the committee and he worked out a course for superintendents designed, in Mrs. Robb's words, toward achieving "uniformity in curriculum and training school methods, which would make the standing of a trained nurse practically the same from any training school," and finally perhaps supply thoroughly trained superintendents to take charge of the small hospitals and training schools.[14]

The title of the first course of study, *Hospital Economics*, accurately reflected its aim, and that title was retained for a decade. In 1907, Miss Nutting was given a chair at Teachers College. But from the very first year of affiliation with Teachers College, superintendents who successfully matriculated there were granted certificates as   qualified superintendents over training schools for nurses and over hospitals. In short, the Society of Superintendents had joined in limited partnership with a "school of pedagogy." Within

[12]And, in fact, most practitioners, except for the students who manned the hospitals went into private duty nursing. As late as 1920, there were only about 11,000 nurses working in hospitals, and 11,000 in public health, while about 120,000 were in private duty and miscellaneous branches. Isabel Stewart, *The Education of Nurses* (New York: Macmillan, 1943), pp. 128 and 199.

[13]"Hospital Economics Course, Teachers College," in her *Educational Standards for Nurses, op. cit.,* pp. 130-131 especially. The original address was delivered in 1898.

[14]*Ibid.,* "Report on Hospital Economics Course" (given at the annual convention 1899), pp. 137-140.

a few years, the early administrative focus of the program had been supplemented by "new courses dealing with the special problems of teaching in schools of nursing." These latter were directed at teachers as well as superintendents.[15]

Meanwhile those nurses who took their professional responsibilities seriously (because they were "trained") continued to be powerless to seal off the profession against a flood of undesirable recruits, who were poorly trained in the nation's rapidly multiplying training schools. In 1890, there were only thirty-five training schools; by 1900 there were 432. During the next decade, an additional 700 were founded; and from the years 1910 until 1920, yet another 600 were founded. The number of graduate nurses and students combined shot from 1500 in 1890 to 11,000 at the century's close. Ten years later this female labor force had reached 82,000, and by 1920 it soared to almost 150,000. Contributing to these phenomenal increases were several national trends. Among the most important were the movement of women into the labor market, the expansion of our population, and an increased valuation of health which resulted in the rise of the modern hospital. An additional contributor to the expansion of nursing can be detected from figures in the following table, which shows what happened when organized medicine took seriously Abraham Flexner's recommendations for improving medical education. After medicine began severely to control its recruitment—despite continued increases in the general population — someone had to bear the brunt of corresponding increases in patient population.

Such figures make vivid what those nurses who represented trained nurses were working with — or against — at the end of the nineteenth century and during the decades which followed. The major problem of the profession as they conceived it, and the initial step towards its management, had already been set forth by Mrs. Robb. The next steps, both in conception and strategy, can be traced conveniently through the writings of Miss Nutting, who, from her post at Teachers College, dominated nursing education for two decades. She sponsored her students into innumerable other schools and hospitals. She sparked educational reforms within the profession and helped to represent the profession to interested influential outsiders for many years. Her initial ideas about nursing and education, as well as the later evolution of those ideas, are most instructive. The contemporary literature makes plain that her views were shared by most in the influential core group of nurse educationalists.

At Teachers College, Miss Nutting taught that — since the main task was to help raise the standards of less progressive training

[15]M. A. Nutting, *A Sound Economic Basis for Schools of Nursing* (New York: Putnam's, 1926), p. 345.

schools through educational reform — these schools be persuaded to hire well-trained teachers. These teachers could be expected to have an impact upon the training of students. They could also help to implement the reduction of students' working hours, as well as urge upon their superiors additional measures useful for "raising standards." Hours spent on studies definitely should be lengthened; adequate classrooms, equipment, and books should be provided; classes should be given during the day, rather than after the day's grueling work; certain basic subjects, such as bacteriology, should be taught; and the student's total years of attendance at the school should be extended. Miss Nutting's suggested solution to the basic professional problem was, in brief, to integrate genuine schools into hospitals, most of which possessed only sham schools. As she remarked, one year after moving to Teachers College: There is in most hospitals "no place in this strenuous life for the machinery of a school . . . any scheme of education must, of necessity, take a second and insignificant place. A school, to fulfill its functions, cannot take such a place." Her language betrays a significant addendum of boldness over Mrs. Robb's inaugural address at Hopkins twenty years before. (By now, though, Mrs. Robb had reached similar conclusions.) In 1908 both were facing a changed world. Now the newly emerged *graduate* nursing education, whether at Teachers College or elsewhere, could be a means for getting genuine training schools into recalcitrant hospitals.

TABLE 1

Ratio of Nurses and Physicians to Population in the
United States, 1900, 1910, 1920, and 1930[16]

	1900	1910	1920	1930
Population	75,994,575	91,972,266	105,710,620	122,775,046
Graduate and Student Nurses	11,804	82,327	149,128	294,189
Physicians	132,002	151,132	144,977	153,803
Per 100,000 Population:				
Nurses	16	90	141	240
Physicians	174	164	137	125

[16]Esther Lucile Brown, *op. cit.*, p. 20.

Later, in 1916, after repeating the foregoing argument ("the entire control of training schools is, with few exceptions, vested in hospitals, but the purposes of the two institutions are not identical. On the contrary, they diverge, and widely at many points") [17] we find Miss Nutting hazarding that:

For the ideal control of schools of nursing in the future we shall, I am confident, turn more and more to the universities, just as other professional schools have done, seeking there the educational resources freely available — teachers, scientific laboratories, libraries, and other equipment. [18]

Here is a theme new to her thinking. Why did she now, in 1916, enunciate it? What was happening around her?

To begin with, several schools of nursing had become associated with universities. She could now visualize, not only gains in status that had accrued to the profession from such affiliation, but gains in "the new freedom and opportunity to develop the intellectual aspects of nursing." [19] There was an additional reason for her emphasis upon the more intellectual aspects of nursing. Approximately eight years before she became aware that a great flood of able women, who formerly would have entered nursing, were choosing to enter the many alternative occupations open to them; but in the meantime, "colleges for young women have grown and multiplied." Here is "where to look for some of the women who twenty or twenty-five years ago might have stood at the hospital training school door asking for admittance." The increased prosperity of the country, she observed, made it easier to get a college education, hence the free tuition of training schools was now far less of an inducement to enter them. Perceiving these trends, Miss Nutting's concern with most hospitals' ill-conceived university affiliated schools of nursing was correspondingly strengthened.

By 1920, she was able to celebrate the development that over fifteen schools of nursing had become affiliated with universities. She had also begun to write about specialization. For the first time, she was comprehending of what a genuine graduate education—along professional lines — consists, although her thinking on this issue was more analogical than analytical. Even medicine had yet to provide clear images of how specialized graduate education could be laid atop a full undergraduate university course of study. Furthermore,

[17] *Op. cit.,* p. 224; in a paper titled, "Some Ideals for School of Nursing," pp. 22-236.

[18] *Ibid.,* p. 225.

[19] *Ibid.,* p. 226.

the trend toward specialization was not such an assumed fact of American life that Miss Nutting might recognize how, in other established professions, the general practitioner would become a minor figure. In 1920, and for some years thereafter, she foresaw only that nurses' specialized tasks properly called for specialty training, which was best given in university schools of nursing.

How then did she integrate this conception of university schools with her major conception that the task of advanced education was to penetrate the hospital schools? (She had not budged an inch from her indictment of hospital schools.) She drew the conclusion, after setting forth her views of future professional training, that:

Significant, however, for the future of our work as this new line of advance may prove to be, we must not over estimate its present importance or dimensions, but should realize that our great efforts must for some time to come be directed toward the immediately necessary improvements in the hundreds of hospital training schools which form the bulk of our educational system.[20]

She can hardly be criticized for failing to come to grips with how to integrate specialty training and undergraduate training: the profession would confront, with internecine warfare, this issue for many years. They continue to do so to this day.

It is worth repeating that although Miss Nutting's views evolved over the three decades through which we have followed her, her basic view, as noted above, did not. Continual uncontrolled recruitment into the profession forced this view upon her and kept it a profound conviction. It even shines through her approval of the establishment of what was, in 1923, considered to be the first genuine university school of nursing at Yale. That school had been founded, following upon the famous Goldmark report, with Rockefeller Foundation money. This school was considered then the first true university school because of its independent financing and administration, and it had equal status with other professional schools at Yale. Miss Nutting had enunciated the first two requirements, years before.

The founding of this school evoked jubilation among the ranks of nurse educators.[21] Its Dean, Miss Goodrich, had been a faculty mem-

[20]*Ibid.,* p. 271. Also p. 292 (1923 speech).

[21]An historian of American nursing had portrayed what that excitement meant, and incidentally demonstrated how long it had lasted with some educators, when she wrote in 1954 about its founding. Mary M. Roberts, *American Nursing: History and Interpretation* (New York: Macmillan, 1954), p. 180.

ber at Teachers College. Her ideas hewed closely to its traditional views about the profession.[22]. Of course, she carried the Robb-Nutting battle further into enemy terrain, arguing in 1934 that "within a decade, every nursing school should be definitely associated with a college or university or be discontinued."

In summary, for the nurse educator, a basic fact about their profession was its lack of control over recruits who come in through the hospital schools. Therefore, the educator's basic strategy was to influence, and if possible exert control over, the educational policies of hospital schools. During the ensuing professional tug of war, the graduate training of nurses became firmly embedded in schools of education, from the moment that Mrs. Robb led them into Teachers College. How little even later generations could conceive of any other kind of graduate training can easily be discovered through their writings. For instance, Isabel Stewart, an outstanding nurse educator, writing in 1943, could not conceive of training for leadership in nursing "without formal preparation in a school of education." [23] Even today, few nurses receive doctorates in fields other than education, and master's degrees in education are earned with frequency. Master's programs in nursing tend to be linked more closely with education than with any other branch of the university or college, unless it be medicine itself.

At any rate, a derivative of nursing educators' efforts was the evolution of that melange of nursing degrees and programs described earlier. Perhaps a good way to picture the situation is to imagine a long army climbing a mountain. Some men are low down at its base and others are near the top. They are not climbing a single trail but scrambling up the peak from different sides. Schools of nursing have begun and developed at different locales, under different specific conditions, and at different times. Therefore their programs, their curricula, their affiliations with other educational institutions (colleges, universities, hospitals) have taken diverse forms. As Margaret Bridgeman has pointed out,[24] when the first collegiate program was offered at Cincinnati as a result of World War I's duress, the first class was already a mixed one, composed of two groups: girls

---

[22]Cf., Annie W. Goodrich, *The Social and Ethical Significance of Nursing* (New York: MacMillan, 1932). For her conceptions of university schools, see especially the papers gathered under the section titled, "The Nurse and the University," pp. 285-365. (*Op. cit.*, Roberts, pp. 515-516.) This was only two years before the Brown report which took a similarly strong stand.

[23]*Op. cit.*, pp. 342-352, and especially 342. This nurse educator, incidentally, gave the first courses at Teachers College for *qua* teachers.

[24]*Collegiate Education for Nursing* (New York: Russell Sage Foundation, 1953), pp. 48 and 54.

who had had two years of college who then received a regular hospital school training atop of those years, and girls who received their nurses' training directly after high school. The dominant collegiate pattern became two years of education at a college, to which was added a nonintegrated period of hospital-school training taught by a separate faculty of nurses.

Another prevailing pattern consisted of simultaneously giving students hospital training and college education, but using two faculties, so that in essence the two programs ran side by side but were not integrated. Similarly, when the School of Nursing at Yale started its training program, it accepted only college graduates, and to their college education it added a nursing education as taught by nurse educators: the entire program was termed a "master's program." Moreover, as each school "affiliated" with its local center of learning, whether college or university, it made such arrangements as were possible — and the arrangements were quite varied. (Many fell under the domination or control of schools of medicine, either through choice or force of circumstances.) These nursing schools were never equal partners in the parent institution with other departments or schools partly because of financial considerations and partly because nurse educators were not aware of what constituted conventional educational status. Mostly they were playing for smaller stakes, or at least more immediate ones pertaining to influence over hospital schools and over the nursing profession itself. Eventually they even won considerable control over the entire educational process within nursing, as evidenced by the national accreditation system, the strength of The National League of Nursing, and the increasing prestige of university schools of nursing.

SOME CONSEQUENCES OF AN EDUCATIONAL TRADITION

The occupation is still reaping the bitter fruits of this historical trek upward into higher education (the gains are more obvious). I shall discuss briefly only three of the most momentous: first, the level of prestige accorded nursing within universities; second, the heritage of an education or normal school mentality; and third, the augmented strain on relations between practitioners and educators.

If Gilman had instituted at Johns Hopkins a genuine School of Nursing, one comparable to the School of Medicine, nurses' education nationally might well have been modeled after the neighboring profession. But Gilman did not mark the trail into higher education nor did any of the other influential academic leaders of that celebrated innovative era. Gilman thus consigned nursing to a fateful partnership with schools of education — an act all the more ironical since this was the era when science, both theoretical and utilitarian, began to triumph within institutions of higher learning.

The movement toward scientific education drove relentlessly toward research, toward graduate education atop collegiate education, and toward the Ph.D. degree as the capstone of the graduate system. Indeed, along with that degree, research was, as Berelson remarks, "the activity that quickly became the *raison d'etre* of graduate study and still is. . . ."[25] From this scientific movement, as established in graduate education rather than in medical schools, nursing was effectively barred by its alliance with schools and departments of education. Nurses did move into graduate education, within schools of education and in masters' programs within schools of nursing, but remained quite outside the university nucleus of genuine training. After World War II, when Ph.D. training began first to increase and then later to soar,[26] nursing remained linked with the school of education.

The latter functioned primarily to feed into the nation's public schools enormous quantities of teachers and administrators. Those who wished a graduate education, with or without advanced degrees, obtained it at the university schools of education. The university schools also trained faculty for each other. Thus it is understandable why those schools, although on university campuses, were by-passed by the main surge of research-oriented, science-dominated, graduate education. Schools of education within the larger universities tended to take on the trappings of the doctoral program, even offering the Ph.D. program, but rarely was the adoption convincing to other branches of the university. There is no need to document this last assertion: the low prestige of departments and schools of education on university campuses is well known, revulsion being expressed in the familiar terms of fake degrees, ignorance of real research, foolish "methods" courses, and the ruination of true initiative. Those are all key terms, of course, which reflect esteemed values of "true" graduate education. Since the nurses who attended schools of education were pragmatically oriented toward "service," they found nothing particularly wrong with the educational fare offered them at those schools. Were they not teachers or administrators themselves? And what could they, given their own traditions, know of university graduate education?

---

[25]Bernard Berelson, *Graduate Education in the United States* (New York: McGraw-Hill, 1960), p. 12.

[26]*Ibid.*, pp. 33-34, for graphs picturing this increase. The increase was in numbers of degrees, numbers of fields giving degrees, and in degree-granting institutions.

It seems incontestable that the special goals of schools of education stamped upon many students — including the nurses — certain styles of approach to problems and to education. Probably also, those goals affected students' generalized views of the world, and what they themselves might possibly do to manage it or change it. The teaching paraphernalia of these schools of education, especially since World War I, has included a number of items familiar to everyone who has lived through our public schools. The field of education has found indispensable the use of the syllabus, whereby a course is planned in virtual entirety by the teacher before he faces pupils. The syllabus is planned around a series of topics, neatly ordered with subtopics and, if possible, moving smoothly from one to the next. Through syllabi and textbooks, which are assigned to pupils, an attempt is made "to cover everything," or as much as time permits. (In many city and state public-schools systems, proper coverage is reinforced by standard and sometimes legal measures.) The pupils' understanding of classwork and text is tested by recitation and examination. Through these devices, attention is focused upon "course content"; but as many critics have observed, pupils tend to learn that content by rote, as if it were well established for all time. Textbook, syllabus, together with classroom teaching which utilizes them closely, seem to give pupils an orderly, definitive view of subject matter and the world. The teacher, who has gone through a normal school or a school of education, may be somewhat more sophisticated than her own teaching, but in those schools she is apt to get an education not very different from the one she passes to her pupils. This tendency is often abetted by the phenomena of keeping education students confined to education courses that parallel ones taught elsewhere on the campus. Thus the graduate student in education often gets "watered-down" versions of materials taught on higher planes elswhere in the university.

The standard educational devices, and the emphasis upon curricula and course content, characteristically are supplemented by required courses in teaching methods — that is, on how to ply one's trade properly. One learns not only how to use syllabi and other devices, but also the principles of good teaching, a practice that is virtually unheard of in graduate science departments. (It is as if teachers who are self-conscious about teaching have to teach teachers-to-be, as well as teachers-already-teachers, how to teach.) Among the devices recommended, explicitly or implicitly, for improving teaching and learning are those that lead to good curriculum construction and revision. There are courses on how to do those things well. Again, this is a radical departure from the graduate departments found elsewhere in the university. Curriculum and method courses are replete with advisory or mandatory rules, procedures, and principles.

46

Assuming the above description is not altogether a caricature — although admittedly overdrawn if applied to the better schools of education — what does it suggest as to the consequences for nursing? Nursing educators introduced into their own schools the same styles of thought and the same educational devices, in imitative conviction. The transmission was made easier since they faced some of the same problems as their professors did, notably the instruction of masses of students most of whom possessed familial backgrounds insufficient to underpin that instruction. Educators' reliance upon curriculum revision and accreditation of schools only served to re-enforce nurse educators in their battle against the low standards of hospital schools. Educators' emphasis upon "principles" and "aims" found a ready response among nurses who had been trained to act but who needed rationales for acting better.

A final consequence deserves underlining: the narrow academic sphere which enclosed the nurses prevented their discovering what a great world of knowledge existed around them on the campus. The books of nurse educators are studded with references to colleagues and educators, and to an occasional educational psychologist or a philosopher who happens to have written about education; but they are almost devoid of reference to the writing of sociologists other than specialists in educational sociology. Until very recently, the whole surge of social science during this century had swept past them, except for an occasional fortuitous contact, such as with the group therapy movement. By and large, nurses were profoundly influenced only by two professions, education and medicine, and nurse educators were influenced mainly by education.

The alliance of nursing with education had the further consequence of helping to widen a gap between nurses who taught and nurses who practiced (at the bedside or in administration). To practicing nurses even today, "the educated nurse" has connotations of someone whose advanced training has taken her away from her proper place working with or near the patient. (American nurses have been criticized from time to time by foreign nurses who make an identical accusation.)

From the earliest days when trained nurses were graduated from schools like Bellevue and sent as superintendents to other hospitals, they experienced internal strains in balancing dual loyalties: to the hospital in their capacities as superintendents and to students as authorities responsible for education. A superintendent's two tasks were not always consonant. As long as she stayed in close contact with bedside nursing, the dissonance could always be kept individualized; but when collegiate and university schools began to hire faculty who had no lengthy bedside experience, or who began to draw away from work with patients via teaching — in other words, when full-time educators emerged into visibility — then differences of perspective between "service and education" were intensified. The policing or "raising of standards" functions that educators had taken upon themselves augmented the tension which is frequently found in professions where training is carried out somewhat or totally separate from the job.

THE PERVASIVE IMAGERY OF BEDSIDE NURSING

Next let us consider that particular activity which to outsiders and to nurses themselves seems at the very heart of the profession: namely, bedside nursing. This discussion should illuminate the evolution of certain relationships between nursing and medicine, which still exist, as well as underscore further relationships between nurse educators and practicing nurses.

The image of nurses at the bedside persists despite great and increasing numbers of nurses who administrate or teach in nursing schools. The persistence of this imagery has something to do with reality but also with sacred aspects of the profession. Nurses are not so different than other professionals who idealize some cluster of esteemed activities supposedly embodying the very essence of their particular profession (lawyers litigate in courts of justice, physicians give medical care). Of course, not everyone in a profession engages in such characteristic professional actions. Inevitably such a great diversity of tasks are performed in the name of any profession that its different segments do not agree upon the full range of activities which the profession ought to encompass or exactly how its work should be organized. Nevertheless, certain traditional activities appear to tap such deeply embedded sentiments that although "not all of us" are engaged in the work which historically marked us off from every other profession, that work does remain truly ours.

Current as well as older histories emphasize that the image of the ministering angel — the lady with the lamp — crossed the ocean from England where it was originated, in its modern form, by Miss Nightingale. Proper professionalized nursing care took root on American soil in the hospitals where previously, it is said, nursing care was either absent or given haphazardly by well meaning but untrained personnel. The introduction of the Nightingale concept meant that now a disciplined core of ministering angels moved efficiently, but with kindliness, around the patients. This official account is substantially correct as far as it goes; but since it derives from the writings of nursing leaders, and is focused little upon contemporary American life as it was during the early days of nursing, the account needs amplification and considerable qualification.

48

Nursing is first and foremost a woman's occupation, and this fact profoundly affected which kinds of activities were idealized as right and proper for the profession. To understand the types of women that this profession idealized and probably selected, it is necessary that something of the range of womanly types afforded by the nineteenth century be understood. It is commonly supposed today that the nineteenth-century woman was either a contented homemaker or a suffragette (with allowances for the "fallen women" of the day). Of course, such a restriction of feminine possibilities does little justice to America's complexity. As long ago as 1834, de Tocqueville remarked upon American women's alertness, their relative freedom to mix and converse with men, and upon a certain equality of the sexes peculiar to this continent. During that same decade, a major national theme, easily recognized as quite vigorous today, emerged: the young wife should subordinate herself to her husband's career, as he busily strives to climb the business ladder. Home should be a place where he returns at night to find sustaining familial roots. That equation was turned topsy-turvy by A. D. Mayo, a caustic critic of social life in the late fifties, who complained that the ambition of wives for material goods "drives their companions of the other sex into overheated exertions in business and exhausts their health and freshness . . . drives the young couple to live beyond their means and sacrifice constant comfort and true family life."[27]

The tremendous mobility afforded some families by the nation's growth unquestionably led to life styles which emphasized material well being and de-emphasized quiet home life. In the larger cities, the society woman was a conspicuous feature of the landscape. Even among the more sober of the higher orders, a fierce womanly individualism was springing up. In the South, a romanticized ideal of the lady flourished, especially after the Civil War. On the Western frontier other feminine values were esteemed: among them stoic, sturdy, work companionship as well as the gay companionship of unmarried women for unmarried men. On the frontier, also, the arrival of women acted as a steadying civilizing influence upon masculine frontier crudities (a tradition which has come down to us in movies about the school marm). Indeed, by the end of the century the American woman as national culture bearer was well established: the busy male had little time for the "finer things" in life except as he was reminded of them by his more polished wife, especially if he had "married up" which was his right if he had been successful. Meanwhile, young women were flooding the larger cities in search of jobs, adventure, and husbands. Other women whose lives held less adventure and glamour were exemplifying another facet of American

[27]*Symbols of the Capital* (New York: Thatcher and Hutchinson, 1859), p. 279.

family life: they were busily feeding and raising their children despite abandonment by their husbands. Other ladies were stoutly fighting the suffragette cause or helping to reform urban social ills.

In short, a full gaze at the range of life styles possible for women during the late nineteenth century would include a fair range of possibilities, most still extant today. These styles represented idealized clusters of values. A woman might be an aid to her husband's success story, indeed the power behind it. She might embody adventure and glamour: the prominent elements here are sex, romance, love, and fashion. She might be the civilizing influence on men and the nation: the aesthete, the art appreciator, the spiritual influence. She might be the gentle lady embodying virtues or purity, gentility, fragility, virginity, irresoluteness, and manners. She might be a companion: sharing work, conversation, mutual interest, and married conjugality. She might be the stable moral element in the family: the truly responsible person, the stronger of two partners. She might be primarily a childrearer rather than a wifely companion. She might be a religious, social, or political reformer. All these were her postive virtues, but each had its negative side. The matron could be a bore; the culture bearer might only be an aesthete, a prig, or aggressive missionary. The woman behind the success story might be hard as flint or corrupted by the social ascent. The search for adventure might end in frivolity, sin, or degradation.

Of this array of feminine virtues and vices, which ones were built into nursing and which were more or less screened out? Presumably neither the core of elite nurses nor the members of most hospital boards wished to train and hire nonselectively. Presumably also, not every kind of woman was attracted to nursing work. In general, the occupation crystallized around certain virtuous feminine themes: responsibility, motherliness, feminity, purity, service, and efficient housekeeping. To itemize these virtues is immediately to emphasize other virtues which were omitted from the idealized profession: glamour, fashion, the success theme, which scarcely received emphasis, the theme of the artistic, genuinely cultured lady, and the political (equal-rights) reformer. Such values did not enter perceptibly into the formation and development of nursing, whereas both the positive and negative aspects of mother-housekeeper values received self-conscious scrutiny. After all, nursing moved into hospitals under aegis of hospital boards cognizant of nurses' efficiency and (at least a modicum of) compassion, while nurse reformers themselves fought against various lower-class values conceived of as exemplifying disorderliness, drunkenness, uncleanliness, even sinfulness, as well as inefficiency, lack of compassion, and nonprofessionalism.

America's first trained nurse, Linda Richards, some years ago commented that in the small town where she was raised certain women were called "natural nurses," because they were naturally gifted in caring for the sick. They were called upon by neighbors in the event of family sicknesses. But every mother might act as a nurse in her own family upon occasion. Hence a combination of maternal care and maternal orderliness already existed as a model for the early professional nurses. They had also Miss Nightingale's code to build upon. Miss Nightingale insisted (according to one recent commentator) that the nurse have "method, self-sacrifice, watchful activity, love of the work, devotion of duty (that is the service of the good), the courage, the coolness of the soldier, the tenderness of the mother, the absence of the prig."[28] Besides the "service" feature, these characteristics are the very embodiment of the scrupulous housekeeper and uprighteous mother. We may translate those idealized terms into nurses as disciplined angels!

"Responsibility" meant orderliness, cleanliness, prudence, industriousness, self-discipline, and sensibility. She was to banish disorder. She was not to be frivolous, romantic, irresponsible, or flighty. The mother and housekeeper values were also closely linked: the nurse was to "nurse," care, guard over, be compassionate; she was also to manage efficiently the hospital, giving the establishment a homey, comfortable atmosphere. Her more purely feminine values embodied sensitivity and purity as well as feminine sensibleness, along with the aiding and understanding of males (patients and doctors). She lent a moral tone to the hospital. She was not to contest the physician's dominance. The service aspect of the occupation had to do not only with making nursing a regularized profession but with reforming the hospital and properly caring for patients, most of whom came from the lower classes.

We need not suppose that every young woman who became a nurse exemplified all those ideal qualities. Indeed it is the idealization itself which should interest us here, and not whether nurses actually were able to translate those ideals into behavior. Presumably some women were anything but sober, prudent, and responsible. As one nurse, in 1892, remarked: there is one group of women who enter nursing,

who, although they may not lack youth and energy, are led by motives which are only frivolous and impracticable. This sort of applicant usually starts into her training with romantic idea that nursing consists merely in smoothing the dying patient's brow, but when she discovers that it consists in smoothing his bed as well, she also finds that all sentimental rhapsody and romantic ideas are swallowed up in

[28]Lucy Seymer, "Florence Nightingale Oration No. 2, 1947"; quotation reprinted in Luella Morison, *Stepping Stones to Professional Nursing: Workbook for Student Nurses* (St. Louis: C. V. Mosby Company, 1954), pp. 52-53.

hard, practical everyday-work. These young women are black sheep in the fold of the Nursing Profession.[29]

A self-conscious propagation of nursing ideals was made more necessary by the relatively open recruitment, combined with the virtual impossibility of drumming out conspicuous failures. Also, since almost all the graduates of training schools became private duty nurses, they had to be well fortified against laxity, irresponsibility, and temptation.

Consequently, a prominent feature of books written for the young nurse was a secular sermon which set forth her proper bearing and character. Some books were frankly titled *Nursing Ethics* or *Ethics for Nursing,* but most nursing manuals, which were otherwise devoted to practical matters, began with a chapter or two on the proper nurse herself: her attributes and obligations. Quotations from some of these early manuals will convey their flavor and underscore the kinds of attributes assigned to the nurse. These attributes have not changed appreciably through the years. The nurse quoted directly above instructed her readers that, "There are three qualities the nurse must possess, in order to become efficient in her profession, namely: common sense, truthfulness and obedience." The meaning of those attributes is spelled out with various adjectives: tactful, conscientious, loyalty to physician and patient, cleanliness, sympathy for the patient, and proper deportment.[30]

Mrs. Robb herself, in *Nursing Ethics* (1900), summed up the nurse's qualifications: "Good *physical health* is the first essential. The second is *education,* which must not only be theoretical but practical; which . . . should not have lacked the study of thrift and economy. But in addition . . . she must have *culture.*" Lest we read too much of the upper-class lady into the last requirement, we should see what Mrs. Robb means by culture: "This is, as a rule, a home product that has generally been instilled into the young girl." Mrs. Robb's nurse must also be kind and courteous, slightly reserved, and she need not be handsome or pretty. "Her whole manner should suggest quiet, but at the same time a steady firmness of purpose." And again, the rhetoric of responsibility and self control: "Given these qualifications, I know of no occupation better adapted than nursing to render a woman self-reliant, of steady nerve, observant and responsible."[31]

[29]Lisbeth Price, *Nurses and Nursing* (Philadelphia: George Jacobs and Company, 1892), p. 8.

[30] *Ibid.,* pp. 11-15.

[31]*Op. cit.,* (Cleveland: E. C. Koeckert, 1914 edition), pp. 48-49.

Another textbook, *Studies in Ethics* for Nurses, first published in 1916, went through numerous editions in the 1940's. The student is advised from the opening lines that: "The training of a nurse includes two distinct parts — distinct, yet inseparable. First the technical instruction and experience required in the practical care of the sick. Second, the training in conduct, in ideals of personal living." The latter, the student is quickly warned, "will greatly influence her practical work every day of her nursing career."[32] Rather then repeat the usual attributes as emphasized in this book, I shall quote a few lines to indicate how alternative attributes — so characteristic of other American feminine ideals — are warned against:

Ambition: An eager desire for the attainment of certain objects is an important element in the making of a nurse, yet it may easily become an inordinate desire for preferment, honor, position, or power. . . . Ambition is a quality which every individual should cultivate, yet diligently keep under control.

Hence the young nurse is admonished against striving to outreach competitors. And in speaking about proper temperament, both the dominant matron and the glamour-seeking youngster are talked down.

Recent manuals use a more modern vocabulary but emphasize the same womanly virtues. Like earlier nurses, the present-day one has a strong shoulder for the patient to rest his troubles upon but, metaphorically speaking, her very bosom is absent as an object for him to gaze upon! The nurse is still to be decorous in bearing and grooming. ("Your coiffure should truly 'crown' the features of your face in an attractive manner . . . be neat, clean and well arranged" — but scarcely seductive in intent.)[33] And as much as ever, the feminine basis of the good nurse is spelled out: "At this point," remarks one author summing up the nurses' guiding attitudes and principles, "it is well to remember that a good woman is the foundation upon which the finished moral structure of a good nurse is erected."[34]

Again, let us be clear that these manuals of proper behavior do not prevent black sheep from entering the professional fold. An occupation so extensive is sufficiently capacious to attract the entire rainbow of American female types. Indeed the manuals only make evident that there is some fear that the professional ideals will not always be obtained.

[32]Charlotte Aikens (Philadelphia: W. B. Saunders, 1916), p. 7.

[33]Luella Morison, *op. cit.*, 1954, p. 60.

[34]*Ibid.*, p. 110.

During the earliest years of "organized nursing," physicians were not always convinced of the usefulness of women reared upon such ideals. Even the great Osler was skeptical at first of "the trained nurse." He is described as having been flippant and condescending until converted to an appreciation of the girls who worked at the Johns Hopkins Hospital. Since nursing histories report a certain amount of resistance from physicians to the introduction of the best in nursing, understandably the nurse reformers sought allies within the medical profession. However, the rapid introduction of trained nurses (superintendents and students) into hospitals throughout the country during the 1890-1910 period suggests that the value of a good woman — versus the old-fashioned female who used to tend the sick — caught on quite quickly. Moreover, private duty nursing increased remarkably during the same decades.

What the physicians appreciated was a combination of bedside physical care and generally efficient management. It is worth underlining that the tasks of nurses and physicians fitted together nicely. Of course their respective work followed a characteristic subordinate-superdominate pattern since, after all, nurses were women. Although the language of 1892 is archaic, seven decades later the relationships remain understandable:

There are [begins one manual on nursing] few professions — perhaps it may be said with truth, that there is NO profession — which has its limitations marked with such rigid distinctions, as that of nursing. . . . There are many reasons. . . . The chief one is this: the profession of nursing is dependent upon the medical profession; from it, in fact it has emanated . . . it is the cultured, the educated, and the womanly woman who intuitively discovers and appreciates these limitations and does not venture beyond them. Her intelligence, her experience, her knowledge amount to nothing if she forgets the one great object of her training, which is the revealing of her sphere, and teaching her how to keep it.[35]

We scarcely need read further to guess what is her sphere! But additionally, both at the hospital and in private duty nursing, the nurse's work complemented the physician's. He gave medical care; she gave physical nursing care. After his proper diagnosis, she carried out his orders. She did the hospital's housekeeping, while he visited and used the establishment. Another distinguishing characteristic of the two echelons was this: ideally at least he was concerned with "knowledge," with relatively abstract learning; whereas nurses were supposed to be interested in technical learning, abstract only to the point of usefulness in assisting the doctor.

[35]Lisbeth Price, *op. cit.*, pp. 1-2.

Yet there is little question that nurses also were conceded certain moral and spiritual jobs which either supplemented or complemented the work of physicians. Not only were nurses supposed to give physical care but the special kind of moral care so well provided by women. If the doctor was fatherly, the nurse was womanly and sometimes motherly; that is, sympathetic and compassionate. One book on nursing ethics aptly quotes a patient:

I wish to speak especially for the head nurse. She seems . . . so obliging, so sympathetic and so kind a woman. She creates a smile even if she had none. She makes a sympathy with every little complaint to her. She walks around scattering grace and peace everywhere.[36]

This early hand-in-glove fit between physician and nurse duties is not the last time in the history of American medicine that physicians' work was so nicely complemented by assisting groups. Physicians deliberately have elevated groups of technicians (X-ray assistants and laboratory assistants, for instance), founding schools for these groups, and putting their graduates, so to speak, into business; but none of these groups is expected to possess the moral maternal touch. None can claim, or has cared to claim, the bedside image; indeed, neither has the woman physician.

The mutual association of physicians and nurses began, then, with the awarding of a dual mandate to the nurses. They were to carry out delegated medical (or quasi-medical) tasks necessary for the medical care of the ill. They were also to supply the psychological and moral overtones necessary to properly accomplish those medical tasks.

During the intervening seventy or eighty years since they became the handmaidens of physicians, the medical side of nurses' work has grown enormously in complexity and range. Later I shall discuss how physicians not only abandoned valued prerogatives to nurses, taking up new ones themselves, but how through the continuous development of medical technology a variety of unforeseen tasks evolved which someone had to do — and often the nurse did them. In managing these new kinds of work, the nurses were abetted by thoughtful (or anxious) physicians who helped them work out safe and efficient methods. Nurses themselves have also been innovators, adapting medical and biological knowledge to their specific nursing jobs. Among the most self-conscious innovators in the evolution of this aspect of nursing care have been the nursing educators.

The psychological-moral side of nursing care also had undergone considerable evolution. In general, what was once regarded as a

[36]C. Aikens, *op. cit.*, pp. 188-189.

rather simple intuitive matter is now perceived as deserving careful scrutiny. Where fine moral character and common sense once served, many nurses have come to believe that perhaps the nonmedical aspects of nursing also should be taught. Attention ought to be given to the patient's psychological needs, to "the total patient," to the interpersonal relations which should exist between patient and family or patient and nurse. Since World War II, there has been a conspicuous increase within nursing journals of literature which either reflects or advocates an intensified focus upon this phase of nursing.

In this matter nurses have not received much assistance from physicians — other than the psychiatrists — since most physicians are specialists in medicine rather than in psychological or social relations. Rather, the nurses have been assisted by nonmedical experts: namely the psychotherapeutically oriented psychiatrists, the psychologists, and more recently the social scientists. Those experts have written articles for nursing journals, given talks at nursing conferences, even published a few books specifically for nurses. The adaptation of such information by nurses themselves should not be underestimated. Many have gone directly to psychiatry, psychology, or sociology for "principles" which might be applied to the care of patients. As they are not beholden to medical authority on this aspect of nursing, they have been more independent and "on their own" than with the more strictly medical side of nursing care.

It is important to note that the psychological-moral aspects of nursing care have always displayed a certain ambiguity. Whereas the medical and quasi-medical tasks have possessed a fair degree of concreteness, the psychological-social tasks were, after all, initially based upon a generalized set of feminine virtues — hardly a rock of concreteness. These virtues had somehow to be applied to the care of the sick. In a certain sense, the medical tasks required "doing," whereas the moral tasks required "being" as much as doing. Once the profession began to scrutinize the moral and psychological dimensions of nursing — began to convert the ethical-feminine qualities into informed procedures — something of the ambiguity attending those psychological dimensions began to appear. Thoughtful nurses have wrestled ever since with pinning down those elusive dimensions.[37]

Over the years, nursing journals have published articles by practicing nurses who suggest how to give better nursing care to patients

[37]For instance, as late as 1961, one well-known nursing educator attacked the problem in a paper titled "The Significance of Nursing Care." While her approach advocates a specific stance, it well illustrates how nurses have attacked their problems. See Dorothy Johnson, *American Journal of Nursing*, 61 (November, 1961), pp. 63-66.

bedridden with specific diseases, but it is the nurse educators who, especially in the last three decades, have most self-consciously introduced concepts and perspectives from the various scientific disciplines. Understandably it has been the educators who have been concerned with nursing-care-in-general (or with systematized knowledge about specialty nursing care), and it has been the educators who have authored the influential nursing care movements which periodically enter the field. A decade or so ago, the concept of "total patient" (or "the patient as person") was popular.

Careful thought should be given to the concept of the individuals under our care as persons. . . . With this concept, the nurse can better help individuals to adjust to the discomforts, inconveniences, pain, and fears associated with illness and may assist the doctor to recognize and uncover psychosomatic factors that complicate recovery.[38]

Along with "patient needs" and "total patient," communication has more recently been suggested as an addition to the psychological armamentarium. For instance, in *Communication for Nurses,* the foreword notes that the author

has made a valuable contribution to the nursing profession. This long-waited book brings the word "communication" into clear focus as it is related to the very core of nursing — meeting human needs through understanding and being understood. It is no longer considered sufficient that the nurse master technique alone.[39]

Topics listed in a chapter titled, "Develop Clinical Skills" will suggest the drift of the book: the communicating nurse will perceive the patient's private world, learn his language, his profile, interpret him, and chart his response.[40]

More recently such focus upon the patient's needs has shifted to a more explicitly psychiatric perspective, couched in the language of that discipline and informed with its emphasis upon self-knowledge as well as knowledge of the patient. ("Most of us are uncomfortable with someone who begins to cry.[41] How can we learn to handle these feelings of discomfort so that we can be useful to patients in this

[38]Florence Kempf, *The Person as a Nurse* (New York: Macmillan, 1957) , pp. 187-188; and see her "The Patient as a Patient," *Modern Hospital,* June, 1948, pp. 59-61.

[39]The foreword is by Lucille Spaulding, p. 3. The author referred to is Florence Lockerby, whose book was published in St. Louis by C. V. Mosby in 1958.

[40]*Ibid.,* pp. 89-114.

[41]Catherine Norris, "The Nurse and the Crying Patient," *American Journal of Nursing,* 57 (March, 1957).

situation?") The rise of psychiatry as an influential medical specialty has left its mark upon nursing in general, as well as upon psychiatric nursing specifically. Although as early as 1930 a few nurses were suggesting that the skills necessary for nursing mental patients could be generalized to include "the so-called difficult normal individuals,"[42] before a full-blown psychodynamic viewpoint could be absorbed by nurses perhaps the simpler approach was necessary (that is, the patient has psychological as well as biological needs). The more thorough-going psychiatric approach scrutinizes not only the patient but the nurse herself, and in the hands of some practitioners it requires a focus not only upon nurse to patient relationships but upon nurse to nurse, nurse to physician, nurse to administrators, and nurse to whomever is present including members of the patient's family. Throughout the profession today, the impact of psychiatry has been felt somewhat unevenly. Some schools have been more influenced than others, and perhaps some nursing specialties (pediatrics) have been more persuaded to a psychiatric approach than have others. Nevertheless this kind of approach is spreading rapidly throughout nursing as is evidenced by the increasing numbers of journal articles informed by a psychiatric viewpoint.

To return now to the various psychological approaches — "total patient," "communication," "psychological needs," "psychodynamic," "interpersonal relations" — each approach represents an attempt to improve the psychological and social aspects of nursing care. Each involves more or less analysis of something that was originally more or less taken for granted, but now is scrutinized for efficiency's sake. As a consequence, nurses are being offered somewhat differing prescriptions for "how to give the best nursing care possible." True, some prescriptions are believed supplementary, but others are thought sufficiently different that their proponents assert their differences. Some nurses believe that the psychological "needs" approach is old-fashioned, that the psychiatric is useful but too extreme, or that some varieties of the interpersonal-relations approach or the pediatrics nurses' "stress" approach are merely diluted psychodynamics.

One way to understand what is transpiring within the contemporary profession is to view these various approaches as historical strata: that is, some were introduced earlier and some later. The older generations of nurses tend to adhere to older viewpoints, while more recently educated (or "re-educated") nurses tend to put their faith in newer approaches. This situation causes considerable generational

---

[42]Marion Farber, "The Value of Psychiatric Nursing as a Method of Teaching Mental Hygiene Students," *American Journal of Nursing*, 30 (1930), pp. 69-75; see also Christian Beebe, "Psychiatry for the Student Nurse," *American Journal of Nursing*, 21 (1920), pp. 80-82.

conflict within the profession: however, the conflict is not merely generational. It is widely recognized that in university and collegiate schools of nursing, medical-surgical nursing is accused of lagging behind all other specialties in acceptance of an interpersonal approach. Fierce battles are occurring within medical-surgical departments where the old confronts the new. Closer inspection of the schools — and of each specialty — also suggests that even when the psychodynamic and interpersonal approaches are accepted not everyone is interpreting them identically. (And in psychiatric nursing will the guide be Freud, Sullivan, Ruesch, or Gerald Caplan?) Some of the most subtle if not the most overtly bitter fights flow from these differences, fights not only among the nursing specialists but within the ranks of single faculties. Listening to the passionate discussions within these faculties and specialties, one may discern an ongoing dialogue, whose subject from the nurses' view is nursing care but from the sociologist's view represents a continually evolving occupational ideology. Inevitably the outcome of that evolution pertains not only to relations with other health personnel and patients, but also bears upon questions of power within the profession: power to influence the direction of nursing care, nursing education, nursing specialties, and professional policy in general.

Much of the passion entering this ideological argumentation and innovation flows from *deep* commitment to the ideal of bedside nursing *per se*. Inevitably, the identity of nurses has to do with the nursing care of patients, however far removed an administrator or educator may be from the bedside. Nursing grew up around those intensely sacred crises of human life — death, illness, and birth — and so it is understandable that nursing (the very word connotes those crises) should signify something more than the efficient care of patients.

Indeed the power of the bedside imagery is such that nurses who work away from the bedside (notably administrators and educators) must justify their activities in terms of ultimate benefit to patients. Like physicians without patients, or research administrators no longer engaged in research, nurses require adequate rationale if they work away from the bedside. They require rationales not only for public legitimation of their work but also for internal justification. It is widely recognized within the profession that many nurses will not be tempted into "the responsibility of" administrative posts, because administration takes them too far away from patients. Nurses also voluntarily demote themselves to staff nursing for the same reason. With nursing teachers, something of the same situation seems to exist. The upshot is a certain blurring of work functions within the profession — an important structural feature.

AMBIGUITIES OF NURSING ADMINISTRATION

Nevertheless, it is entirely possible for nurses who work away from the bedside to believe that their work is just as important, and indeed more important, than direct patient care. As I have indicated, there is a history and an institutional framework that, for nurse educators, support this kind of belief. The same can be said for nurses who administrate. In fact, one of the ironies of the profession is that the administrators (along with the educators) have gotten most of the prestige and power, and the bedside nurses have gotten little of either.

During the early decades of organized nursing, nursing reform was focused equally upon the careful training of student nurses and upon the proper care of hospitalized patients. The second aim took priority but could not be achieved without the first. The reformer-superintendent was therefore simultaneously a teacher and an administrator of nursing care within the hospital. She was also an administrator over countless housekeeping details within the hospital. As the training-school system, mostly without its radical reformistic tendencies, swept the nation, the administrative role of the superintendent became firmly established. Later when the public health agencies were staffed with nurses, there was additional need for administrative functionaries. Finally, when the continually enlarging hospitals began to hire staff nurses (around the end of the 1920's), releasing students for relatively full-time study, a hierarchy developed within the nursing services, whose function was to supervise the lower echelons. Today we have assistant heads of service, supervisors, head nurses, and assistant head nurses, while the staff nurses themselves take a hand in supervising the practical nurses and nursing aides. Public health agencies have developed less extensive but discernible hierarchies.

From this history it is easy to see why the private duty and ordinary staff nurses had little prestige or power within the profession. Both the hospital and the public health agency made administration the route into full professional visibility and institutional power. Indeed, the mass of bedside nurses were so faceless that during the early decades they hardly appeared in the nursing journals as personages; even now they neither write nor are written about with nearly as much frequency as administrators or educators. Yet by sheer weight of numbers, they far outweigh those groups. Their voices have been heard, of course, over the decades in the continual fight to raise salaries and fees, but even there they have not usually assumed principal leadership.

The importance of administration within nursing has led to a curious, and widely recognized, situation. Most women enter nursing because they see themselves as bedside nurses. Yet they are often urged up the administrative ladder, despite their understandable reluctance to take on duties for which they were neither trained nor had conceived themselves as undertaking. Even top nursing administrators admit, sometimes in public, that they feel inadequate in administrative posts. They, and the supervisors below them, sometimes do not feel like true nurses, because they are too far from the bedside. Yet if a nurse aspires to rise in the profession or to make more money, she must choose the administrative route (this is true even for educators, who end up as departmental chairmen or deans). The situation is mitigated, however, by the relative absence of the intense career aspirations and expectations found within many masculine-dominated occupations. Nurses frequently change jobs, moving up and down the hierarchy without thought of how their "careers" may be affected. Hospitals and agencies generally do not require references or ask about the recruit's past work history. As long as she is licensed to nurse, she is eminently employable.

Beside the structurally induced tension between administrative reality and a bedside-nursing ideal, there is another structurally induced problem which currently arouses anxiety among nursing leaders. Some fear that the administration of nursing service will fall, under the rationale of increased efficieny, to business-trained (male) administrators. Unquestionably professional ire has been roused, but also there is genuine fear that the best nursing care of patients cannot be given under the administrative aegis of non-nurses. What is being reaffirmed is that nursing administration is, in the last analysis, closely linked with the imagery of bedside care even in an era when nurses are increasingly forced by institutional developments into administrative roles away from the bedside.

NURSES AND THEIR ASSISTANTS

The personnel who take the place of the hospital nurse at the bedside have a variety of titles. The most usual are "practical nurses," "vocational nurses," and "nursing assistants" (or "aides"). The latter are essentially untrained helpers, while the practical or vocational nurses have some specialized schooling. The entry of both groups into hospitals has been a rather recent development. Inevitably it followed the gradual evolution of hospitals, which initially used students as nursing manpower, then staff nurses, and finally supplemented the latter with lower-order nursing echelons. This trend in manpower was stimulated by the ever-increasing size and range of hospitals and their services.

It is well known that nurses have been ambivalent about handing over the intimate care of patients to these echelons, and nursing leaders have been very gingery about the evolution of practical nurses as a special group. The nursing profession has closely supervised the development of schools for practical nurses, and looks with disfavor upon an incipient movement among practical nurses to seek independent status. Yet nurses had to be prodded by interested laymen and governmental representatives into coopting practical nurses into their own occupational structure.[43]

A brief review of the historical and structural conditions which led to the current delicate relationships between nurses and their assisting personnel is worthwhile. A good place to begin is with the early relationships around 1900 between "trained nurses" and "untrained nurses." The former were graduates of hospital schools, a few were entering doctors' offices, but most were nursing sick patients at home. In any case, these trained nurses were the operational right arms of practicing physicians. But the untrained nurses were also paid, by sick patients, to nurse under the guidance of attending physicians. In general, the graduates of nursing schools cared for the upper strata of Americans, while the untrained women nursed at less affluent homes (and at state mental hospitals). As late as 1935, an editorial in the *American Journal of Nursing* stated that, "Over half the paid private duty care in 1929 was received by families with incomes of $5000 or more. As 71% of the families had incomes of less than $2500 in that year, it is clear that private duty nursing falls in the class of luxuries."[44] A later study by the Committee on Costs of Medical Care showed that families earning $2000 or less got only 14% as much nursing care as families earning $5000 or more, while families earning under $1200 got only 7%.[45] It should be no surprise, then, that untrained nurses far outnumbered graduates of nursing schools. (For instance, in 1900, only 11,000 of 108,000 were trained nurses.)[46]

[43]Joseph Mountin of USPHS wrote in 1944 that "The nursing profession as a whole . . . until recently has manifested very little interest in auxiliary workers" but that formal recognition and guidance by the nursing profession itself of those workers had to develop, since "either nursing is a luxury service for the rich or . . . the poor are being denied something they should have." ("Suggestions to Nurses on Post-War Adjustments," *American Journal of Nursing*, 44, pp. 321-325.) See also Mary Robert's description of how nursing was persuaded into moving into association and control over the auxiliary nursing workers in her *American Nursing* (New York: Macmillan, 1954), especially pp. 266-268, 459-463.

[44]Vol. 35, pp. 35-36.

[45]Quoted by Joseph Mountin, "Suggestions to Nurses on Post-War Adjustments," *American Journal of Nursing*, 44 (1944), pp. 321-325.

[46]See the editorial on "Trained Attendants," *American Journal of Nursing*, 3 (1903), p. 827.

In consequence, the nursing reformers were faced not only with open recruitment to hospital schools but also with masses of less-trained nursing personnel. These latter they preferred not to call nurses. Until recently, they were indexed in the *American Journal of Nursing* as "subsidiary workers" or "attendants." National emergencies, such as the two world wars, were accompanied by enormous pressure upon the profession to turn out quantities of nurse-graduates and to utilize auxiliary personnel, a pressure which added to nurse leaders' attempts to raise, and keep raising, "standards of nursing care." Throughout the years, more mundane considerations of licensure and fees have motivated the rejection of auxiliary women by less reform-minded nurses (Dr. Charles Mayo, in 1921, accused the ANA of being a closed union and, remarking upon the "white cap famine" during the preceding war, called for 100,000 sub-nurses.)[47] But despite considerations of status, money, and standards, the profession was finally persuaded — partly by outsiders and partly by its own leaders — to recognize formally the usefulness of auxiliary nurses and to permit them some claim upon the title of "nurse." Nurse educators carefully began to oversee curricula and teaching in schools for practical nurses. Nurses are deeply involved in the licensing of practical nurses. Also a distinction was quickly drawn between trained and untrained practical nurses. ("At this time it seems best to provide for permissive licensure of the practical nurse while efforts are being made to develop an adequate number. . . . Permissive licensing provisions which protect the title of licensed practical nurse at least identify for the public those persons who have met minimum qualification standards.")[48] The graduates of these schools work mainly in hospitals under the supervision of nurses. Both echelons are, in turn, assisted in hospitals by aides who ordinarily receive no training except on the job on through in-service courses. In essence, aides get no formal schooling, while students at schools of practical nursing and schools of nursing learn in isolation from each other.

Understandably there is some ideological confusion within the nursing profession as to who is doing genuine nursing and who is not. Nurses tend to think that only their own work is thoroughly professional. Yet everyone recognizes that the work of the various echelons frequently overlaps, and nurses freely admit that experienced aides and practical nurses are sometimes better at some nursing tasks than are some nurses. The confusion over who is really "nurs-

[47]See the counterattacking editorial, "Are Nurses Self Seeking?" in the *American Journal of Nursing,* 26 (1921) pp. 73-79.

[48]Anonymous, "The American Nurses's Association and Non-Professional Workers in Nursing," *American Journal of Nursing,* 55 (1955), pp. 43-45.

ing" is increased by the increased assumption of administrative and supervisory tasks by staff nurses, leaving much bedside nursing to the lower echelons. Interviews with aides reveal that they believe they "know more about the patients" than the nurses, "because we spend more time with patients." Staff nurses sometimes admit that nurses know specific patients less well, in the sense of knowing them personally, but believe their own knowledge to be much more technically and professionally informed.[49]

The foregoing ideological confusion within nursing is, it appears, a rather complex phenomenon. Some of it derives from the situation described above: namely, that nurses are anxious not to "lower standards," not to "dilute" the profession with relatively unskilled personnel; not to allow the occupation to be invaded by outsiders; and not to yield the core activity of bedside nursing to other women. Beyond this, some of the ideological confusion seems to flow from naivete about the elaborate division of labor required by any complicated occupation. Just as engineering needs a host of echelons differentiated by level of skill and training, presumably so does nursing. The example of engineering is additionally instructive, since its lowest echelons are neither denied the title of "engineer" nor refused admission to engineering associations. Only reluctantly have nursing leaders admitted, and then begun to convince the profession, that staff nurses need assisting personnel. But the proffering of full title (nurse) to assisting personnel lies somewhere in the distant future, if ever.

MEDICINE, MEDICAL TECHNOLOGY, AND NURSING

In that last regard, nursing is only following a path pioneered by the medical profession. American medicine has persistently refused its own exact title (physician) to assisting personnel. Yet physicians have required assisting personnel in great numbers and, during recent decades, in more and more medical areas. Pharmacists were used in the nineteenth-century hospital, and social workers were being hired early in the present century. Physicians have literally created whole groups of technical assistants, setting them up in business and carefully supervising (after founding) their schools. This creation of medical technicians follows closely the splitting off of medical specialties themselves. Radiologists created X-ray technicians, pathologists invented the laboratory technicians — down to the latest

---

[49]My colleagues and I have discussed this for psychiatric hospitals, A. Strauss, L. Schatzman, R. Bucher, D. Ehrlich, and M. Sabshin, *Psychiatric Ideologies and Institutions* (New York: Free Press of Glencoe, 1964).

groupings like the inhalation technician who has been fathered by anesthesiology. To none of these groups has the medical profession proffered either its own title or equal status.

One interesting question about the American medical terrain is which of the various groups (other than physicians) working there claim, or aspire to claim, an actual professional title. Some groups gained public recognition as professions before entering seriously upon medical terrain: notably the psychologists and social workers. A few groups initiated by physicians may eventually achieve general recognition as professions, but probably not many will.

The position of nursing is particularly interesting for several reasons. To begin with, the nurses successfully laid claim to professional title before most other groups appeared on the medical scene, indeed before medicine itself had cleaned house under Flexner's examining eye. Yet physicians have never given nurses anything like equal status, and unquestionably many have doubted whether nursing was a genuine profession, rather than merely an assisting occupation, and of rather low order albeit necessary. Nurses themselves reflect some confusion as to whether nursing "really" is a profession. Even nursing educators have moments of doubt, expressed in terms of puzzlement over what is nursing's central job and basic knowledge. If nursing were to rise *de novo* today, it is doubtful whether the public, and certainly the physicians, would immediately accord it the title of profession. Yet nurses received the title, and long ago. Hence the peculiar ambiguity in their relations with physicians: partly acceptance of their subordination, and partly frustration because physicians do not accord them equal status. The latter reaction is heightened by the belief that problems of illness require attack by an elaborate division of labor, within which nursing should have an honored role, while medicine should have an important but not dominant one.

A capsule, but probably not unfair, summarization of current relations between physicians and three major groups of nurses follows. First, nurses at public health agencies work with relative freedom, away from the physical presence of physicians. Indeed, nurses commonly say that they enter these agencies, rather than work at hospitals, to get away from physicians. Second, at university and collegiate schools of nursing are found those nurses who are the most unequivocal exponents of an equal-partner doctrine. These nurse educators have little immediate influence upon hospital nurses and relatively little actual contact with physicians. Yet they are best able to conceive how innovative nurses might enhance the nursing care of patients. Occasionally an educator is able to convince both floor nurses and practicing physicians of her own genuinely innovative capacities.

But physicians, as a group, generally experience great difficulty in perceiving nurses as anything other than the women with whom they work. The highly educated nurse is either not perceived at all or as nonsensically "overtrained" — to the detriment, it is said, of genuine bedside care. A third group of nurses, who work in hospitals and physicians' offices, evince a whole range of reactions to physicians, running from rage at their stupidity to adoration of the dominant male and skilled professional. But the important point is that the superordinate position of physicians as a group is almost never openly challenged by these nurses. Whatever they may think of particular physicians, their own profession is distinctly subsidiary to the main work of medicine itself.

Finally, a word should be said about important relationships between nursing and medicine that flow from technological innovation within medicine itself. One of the most striking developments in twentieth-century medicine has been the emergence of specialties. In turn, specialties split into new specialties. Principally these developments rest upon innovations of medical technology and growth of medical knowledge. As the specialties emerge, physicians engaging in specialized practice require specialized graduate training and must pass boards in their chosen specialties. These practitioners require technical assistants who are, to some degree, also specially trained. Among those assistants are the nurses. To a considerable extent, therefore, specialization within nursing has followed specialization within medicine itself. (A revealing instance was the evolution of the nurse anaesthetist, who later was displaced at the surgeon's side by the physician anaesthetist. Nurse anaesthetists now work mainly in rural or small-town hospitals.) Where the medical specialties are clear and long established, as in surgery, then the nurses tend to conceive themselves as specialists. Most hospital nurses, however, work with enough types of specialist (and types of patient) that they scarcely think of themselves as specialists at any type of nursing. The typical situation in hospitals is that nurses learn what amounts to specialty nursing from other nurses who have worked longer at that kind of nursing. Some of her knowledge may come from physicians associated with that particular medical service. Most strikingly, when new kinds of specialty services are opened (open-heart surgery services, for instance), the nurses learn how best to nurse there partly through the coaching of the chief physician or his assistants, and partly through their own innovative efforts.

Nevertheless, there is probably some discrepancy between the fact of nursing specialization and its conception by most nurses. In fact, current nursing is fairly specialized along lines which follow medical specialization. The long-established nursing specialties are, of course, fairly clearly perceived by most nurses (public health nursing, psychiatric nursing, hospital nursing). In schools of nursing, what are usually termed "clinical fields" (medical-surgical, maternal-pediatric, psychiatric, public health) are seen by some faculty members as fairly specialized fields. Beyond that degree of very general specialization, nurses seem not to perceive specialization although they readily admit that certain areas (premature-baby nursing, tuberculosis nursing) do require concrete kinds of clinical experience. But there is a distinct tendency within the profession — or so it seems to an outsider observer — to wish for a unified, uncleavaged, nonspecialized style of nursing. If I am correct in this observation, perhaps the tendency goes back to the belief that any well-trained nurse can quickly be taught to nurse any type of patient in any type of institution. Perhaps the all-purpose nurse is related to the persistence of the bedside imagery? Probably she is also related to the only gradual emergence of higher education within nursing, since even today much higher education is more the "making-up of deficiencies" in previous training than specialty training in nursing. At university schools, faculties still shrink somewhat from the idea that they might know enough to give genuine specialty training (broken down much more finely than the usual clinical fields). They wonder where nurse educators who are sufficiently "advanced" can be found to teach such specialty courses.

To return to the main thread of my argument, however, it seems inevitable that nursing specialization will increase as it follows in the wake of medical specialization. This does not mean that nurses will merely take their cues from physicians; but as long as nursing is linked subordinately with medicine, nurses will engage in less innovation, and certainly in less radical innovation than they might otherwise.

A CONCLUDING NOTE ON PROFESSIONS*

That chemists claim true professional status raises important theoretical issues for students of professions and occupations, not all of whom would agree with this claim. Some social scientists would, but not all. The decisions would rest partly upon definitional grounds; it would also be affected by assumptions made about the relationships of occupations to each other and about how professions have arisen.

Leaving this question to one side for a few pages, we may note first that social scientists emphasize two paths that those occupations claiming to be professions have traveled. The classic professions have their roots first of all in medieval universities. (Carr-Saunders quotes Bacon as noting that "I find it strange that they are all dedicated to profession, and none left free to arts and sciences at large.")** Historically, many more occupations become professional by working up from a lower status, as well as from outside to inside the universities. As Hughes so well puts it:

> The practitioners of many occupations — some new, some old — are self-consciously attempting to achieve recognition as professionals. Among them are librarians, social workers, and nurses. All these occupations, in their present form, result from new technical development, social movements and/or new social institutions. The old service or function, formerly performed by amateurs or for pay by people of little or no formal training, comes to be the lifework of a large and increasing number of people. Its basic

*This chapter was prepared by Anselm Strauss
Reprinted by permission from
THE PROFESSIONAL SCIENTIST
(with Lee Rainwater et. al.), Chicago, Aldine Pub. Co., pp. 217-229
Copyright © By Social Research Corp.

**A. M. Carr-Saunders and P. A. Wilson, "Professions," in the *Encyclopaedia of the Social Sciences,* XII, 476-81. See also *The Professions* (Oxford: Clarendon Press, 1933).

techniques are changed. Most of the new professions, or would-be professions, are practiced only in connection with an institution. Their story is thus that of the founding, proliferation or transformation of some category of institutions: schools, social agencies, hospitals, libraries, and many others. Whether the institution be new or whether it be an old one transformed, there is likely to be a struggle of the new profession with the other occupations involved (if there are any), and with the laymen who have some voice in the institution — a struggle for definition of the part of each in the functioning of the institution. . . . The first people to take formal training, when schools for the purpose are established, are likely to be people already at work in the occupation. . . . The training school itself generally starts as a vocational school, without college or university connections. . . . In time, the training schools may seek and gain connections with universities. . . . The development continues in the direction of standard terms of study, academic degrees, eventually higher degrees, research in some field or fields considered proper to the profession and the institution in which it operates, and a continuing corps of people who teach rather than practice the profession directly. At the same time, prerequisites to the professional training will be multiplied . . . The standardized schooling and training become . . . effectively the license to work at the occupation. These developments inevitably bring a campaign to separate the sheep from the goats, to set up categories of truly professional and of less-than professional people.*

Assuredly this is a well-trod path taken by many would-be professions.

Attention has been focused upon these two paths to claimed professionalism and diverted us from more recent phenomena, such as is represented by chemistry's emergence from university departments into the professional arena. It is important to scrutinize this newer kind of claimant to professional status because the conditions under which the claim is made are different; so also are the attendant consequences and problems. Neither the classic claimants nor the up-from-the-ranks aspirants are entirely comparable to the new scientific professionals. As noted earlier, chemistry led the way out of the universities; but, especially since the end of the war, an increasing number of sciences have been self-consciously preparing their no-

*E. C. Hughes, *Men and Their Work*, pp. 133-35. In an early article Hughes suggested the following classification of the division of labor: missions, professions and near professions, enterprises, arts, trades, and jobs. See "Personality Types and the Division of Labor" in Hughes, *op. cit.*, pp. 23-41.

vitiates for positions outside their universities. Psychologists openly call their discipline a profession, while one of the most eminent of sociological theorists has written of "Some Problems Confronting Sociology as a Profession."* And when a professor of physics wryly comments (as has been reported to us) that, although physics departments train students to strive for the highest scientific goals, students are later sent out to do things that they were taught not to respect, then physicists are also on the road to claiming professionalization, a trend that one can safely predict will be completed within a decade.

There would appear to be several reasons why increasing numbers of scientists —university professors among them — are so easily able to conceive of themselves as professionals, chief among which is the massive introduction of excellently trained scientists into industry and government. As long as university departments graduate only those students who follow primarily in the footsteps of their teachers, there is no question of professionalization. The graduate is a scientist — or, more accurately, a scientist and a professor. Of course, in some fields, sociology for instance, it has long been customary to grant Master's degrees to students who either were judged incapable of obtaining the coveted doctoral degree or themselves chose to end graduate work at the lower level. These terminal students disappear into non-academic settings, their exact whereabouts remaining obscure to their former professors, who, in the main, are uninterested in their careers. Professors in pure-science disciplines typically are interested in teaching future colleagues, not in turning out personnel for non-academic settings. But when it becomes apparent that the universities are functioning parts of a division of labor that includes training of reputable scientists for diverse locales, then it becomes increasingly difficult for university scientists to deny their own roles in the area. Although most basic research does remain securely anchored within the university departments, excellent research is increasingly carried out in non-academic locales, and it becomes easier for all members of the discipline to feel true colleagueship. The entire trend is abetted by the mobility that frequently exists, as in chemistry, between academic and non-academic locales, not only with careers crisscrossing, but with academicians being called upon to consult frequently in those non-academic settings. (This leads to such paradoxes as are found in physics, where it is easier for a theorist than for an experimentalist to do effective consulting during the summer months.) It is no hindrance to permeability of institutional boundaries, either, when non-academics stand ready — as they do, for instance, in physics —

*Talcott Parsons, *American Sociological Review*, XXIV (1959), 547-59.

to utilize or check upon the latest discoveries coming from the universities.

The trend is also affected by what has been happening in, and to, the university departments. In those disciplines that have received considerable financial support from the government and the foundations, university departments not only have expanded and proliferated but have taken on discernibly different institutional characteristics — principally, the associated institutes and the presence upon the campus of a "secondary faculty" composed of researchers without academic status. Frequently the size of research projects requires subsidiary personnel, either graduate students or lower-echelon technicians. The presence on the campus of fully trained, and indeed eminent, research scientists without academic portfolio is a postwar phenomenon, one inevitably fateful for the very structure of the modern university.

We might note the following vivid example of the scientific revolution upon campuses. Not long ago the central administration of a great research university circulated among administrative heads a draft proposal suggesting that certain changes be made in the status of "non-faculty" people, known at this specific university as "Non-Faculty Professional Research Personnel." That title was to be shortened by dropping "Non-Faculty." Moreover, such professionals were to be distinguished from "Non- Academic Employees" — such as laboratory technicians or others who did not actually engage in original research — and graduate students were not to be eligible for the professional title or the accompanying salary. Also those men currently titled "Junior Research" personnel would now be called "Postgraduate Research" personnel, since the old title might be felt unbecoming to men who held doctoral degrees. Thus one is afforded a graphic instance of a great university's confronting, although scarcely yet solving, a thorny institutional problem, a problem paralleled in some ways by what is happening to the customary division of labor within those large industrial concerns that rely heavily upon scientific personnel.

Such trends within the universities have been accompanied by significant changes in the scientific departments themselves. Some faculty have been hired who are specifically interested in applied science, who may have been hired explicitly for that reason. Their presence occasionally has caused cleavage along applied versus theoretical dimensions, as in psychology departments. Even when men have not been hired for their special interest in applied areas, the curriculum has been affected by an awareness that some students are being trained for applied research, or at least for research in non-academic settings.

The evolution of non-research universities into moderately good, or even excellent, research institutions has been more subtle. Within such institutions, departments sometimes have specialized deliberately in carefully chosen areas of research (sometimes closely allied to industrial or applied work), thereby hoping to establish reputations quickly.

Such changes in university and departmental structure, we reason, have tended to heighten awareness of a division of labor that binds university, government, and industry together. Aiding this fusion also, no doubt, are the numbers of high-ranking scientists who consult either with or within government agencies, plus the concern, in some social science disciplines at least, with the importance of keeping the discipline ably represented in the highest reaches of foundations and government research agencies. All such trends impel the discipline toward professionalization.

Those professional schools long since associated with universities, as well as the more recently associated ones, have, not unexpectedly, been affected by some of the same trends. Medical schools, for instance, are moving steadily toward research emphasis and toward hiring greater proportions of research men, whether they be physicians or Ph.D's, whether faculty or "non-faculty." One pharmacology school with which we are acquainted has not a single non-Ph.D. on its faculty; and one prominent school of social work has awarded more prestige and power to social scientists on its staff than to its other faculty. As was noted in an earlier chapter, there is a distinct trend among professional schools both toward graduate education and toward granting doctoral — if not Ph.D. — degrees. There are implications in such trends for the division of professional practice and professional research; but this is offset by traditional emphases within the professional school that join school and practitioner in common cause.

To return now to our main theme: Why are increasing numbers of scientists so easily able to conceive of themselves as belonging to professions? To all the reasons discussed above can be added an unwillingness to settle simply for the title of "scientist" (or "chemist" or "psychologist"). As the discipline emerges from the University, increasing numbers of its members appropriate the title to which higher social prestige is attached. That appropriation is made easier by the many groups that have already played at this earnest game as well as by the wonderfully vague dimension of the notion of "profession" itself.*

*Howard S. Becker has noted such points in his "The Nature of a Profession," to appear in the forthcoming yearbook of the National Society for the Study of Education, entitled *Education for the Professions*.

Even when social scientists discuss professions, they use definitions not so very different, although sometimes more elaborate, than those found in the dictionary and in common usage; and when their interest as professionals is aroused, they, too, write articles wherein professional status is claimed or denied. Such articles by men of all occupations are numberless, eloquent testimony to the exhortatory and evaluative propensities of aspiring professionals (a few written by chemists have been noted in this book.) When professionals attempt to make explicit what they mean by a profession, either quoting someone else's definition or coining variations of their own, then the meaning of professionalization gets entwined in a rhetoric by which men stake claims for prestige. Scientists stake these claims too, not being content with the more neutral title of their own specific discipline. The very license to practice one's trade (the clinical psychologists, for instance) may turn upon recognition of professional status — and the license may be opposed by already established professionals.

The major thrust toward appropriation of the professional title, toward recognition of the discipline as a profession, presumably comes from men located outside the college and university campuses. Nevertheless, it is essential that the professionalization of a discipline be legitimized by the men at the universities. Not only do they have major prestige, but adequate training programs cannot be organized entirely separate from the universities.

Legitimization is far easier than for occupations that come to the universities from the outside. Nevertheless, as the postwar history of psychology has demonstrated, tensions develop when academicians are reluctant to legitimize the work of colleagues outside the universities — unless they themselves can retain secure control over the training and work.* (And at a recent important conference psychologists went on record as favoring control by psychology departments over the hiring of psychologists within other segments of their respective universities, such as medical and business schools.) Strains develop also within the discipline during the earlier phases of professionalization because some academicians resist the process, or at least fear that the scientific aspects will be harmed.** Whether chem-

---

*Some psychoanalysts have been wary of academic affiliation for their specialty because of the dangers of losing control either to non-analytically trained psychiatrists or to non-psychiatrists; yet an academic affiliation can be viewed as giving a certain respectability and offering wider possibilities for the training of the next generations. See B. Bandler's presidential address to the American Psychoanalytic Association, "The American Psychoanalytic Association, 1960," *Journal of the American Psychoanalytic Association,* VIII (1960), 389-406.

**See the essay, "Professional and Career Problems of Sociology," by E. C. Hughes, *op. cit.,* pp. 57-68. Within the same discipline, the drive toward professionalism can be seen in such papers as T. Parsons, *op. cit.*

istry experienced such tensions during its earlier professionalization we do not know, but it seems likely.‡

In physics, which is just entering upon professionalization, such strains seem minimal, if present at all. The graduate students who enter the aircraft and other industries are scarcely regarded at the great universities as equal to physicists who remain on the campus or who join such institutions as Bell Laboratories. Yet the future can be glimpsed when professors begin speculating, in however desultory a fashion, whether two kinds of doctoral degrees should not be granted to their students: one for graduates going into industry and the other for more highly trained men.

Conceivably, when a discipline begins moving out of the universities into the outside community, the universities might lose control. But both the necessity for legitimization from the universities and the desire of the faculties to retain considerable control over professionalization appear to result in assigning to the universities a secure position of power and prestige within the division of labor that tightly binds together university, industry, and government — and, in some areas, hospitals, clinics, agencies, and private practitioners as well.

Industry and government abet the universities' position, sometimes wittingly and sometimes unwittingly. After the last war, one large chemical corporation sought to build a division that would concentrate upon basic research, but the conditions for basic investigation are in many corporations too fragile, too easily disturbed, to offer researchers genuine competition as a workplace when compared with the universities. Recently, too, the university as a competitor for talent has been rediscovered by physicists (and presumably by others), who now recognize that more money is to be made by remaining outside industry than by working within it — by consultant fees from industry to complement their basic university salaries.

But, of course, industry and government have also come directly to the universities in search of solutions to their problems, or at

‡The British physicist and historian of science, J. D. Bernal, writing about the nineteenth century says: "Nor were the scientists, in general, eager to intervene in industry. Throughout the century there was a growing separation of scientist from the manufacturers. The intimate, personal and family connections that had existed between science and industry in the later eighteenth century gradually diminished. This separation was quite as much due to the success of science as to that of industry. As the century progressed, science began to play a larger and larger part in the universities and government teaching establishments, first in France, then in Germany and Britain, lastly in Russia and the United States. The talented amateurs . . . gave way to the professors." But in industrial advance, "even at the end of the century the major innovations were still coming from a race of inventors without a university background." Bernal, *Science and Industry in the Nineteenth Century* (London: Routledge and Kegan Paul, 1953), pp. 150-51.

least for partnerships in research. There is a fairly clear recognition that the governmental institutes that do basic research in physics and chemistry will be located on or near campuses, while the applied work can be done at places like Oak Ridge and Los Alamos. One military agency recently awarded money to four universities for building and staffing research centers. The recent move toward awarding "career investigatorships" may soon blossom into tenure positions supported by non-university funds.

The time between basic discoveries — usually made within the universities either in experimentation or in theory — and their application in industry has been growing steadily shorter. The larger diversified corporations that recognize the necessity for long-range thinking about markets are increasingly doing their best to shorten that span still further. IBM, for instance, has one of its research divisions located almost on the Columbia University campus, its men in communication with the academicians. Some firms, like Varian, started by faculty from Stanford University, hire men directly from that campus, use its faculty as consultants, and generally work closely with that university. As *Fortune* recently reported, in an article based on interviews with twenty "Egg-head Millionaires,"

> . . . the biggest clusters of rich young scientists are around several universities: the Boston group, many of whom work on the famous Route 123, are there because they have close ties to the Massachusetts Institute of Technology; most of the San Francisco group are bound to Stanford or the University of California at Berkeley. These new millionaires are attached to the university by several considerations. Most of them are in the business of making a sophisticated instrument or component, and need a steady supply of technical brain power. Proximity to a university gives them access to new ideas in their fields, and to bright graduate students, and allows company staffs to participate in seminars and discussions that may directly affect next year's sales. A number of the young millionaires are established authorities in their fields — and are interested in staying close to other authorities. Besides, universities provide the kind of community they like, and in which they feel at home. Of the young men interviewed . . . eight had done undergraduate or advanced work at M.I.T. or Stanford.*

While such firms owe their very existence and impetus to research done at the universities, presumably the administrators of even the larger, more established corporations will become increasingly aware

*"The Egghead Millionaires," *Fortune*, LXII (1960), 172-78.

that, unless their firms work in close conjunction with the universities, they will run a danger of falling behind their competitors.

We cannot emphasize too much that professionalization of the sciences necessarily differs from that of crafts and trades and businesslike occupations. An adequate view of professions, in our opinion, would include several related perspectives. One is that there are at least three separate streams of professionalization, as discussed in this chapter: namely, the medieval origin of certain classical professions, the later and continuing movement of lower-order occupations into professional status, and the relatively recent emergence of scientific disciplines to professional stature. Another perspective is that professions be regarded less as rather stable communities of colleagues and more as temporary resting places within a historical stream of events — at which resting places men can be observed loosely organized under common title for certain common causes. Such organizations of occupational effort comprise less a community than extensive coalitions, which in some areas of effort, at least, frequently run the risk of fragmentation and even dissolution.

A third perspective is that there be sharper focus upon the relationships among specific professions and occupations. For instance, when medicine moved inside the modern hospital and began to utilize its amazing technological apparatus, it moved into alliance with — some say dominance over — a number of other occupations, some of which the physicians themselves, in effect, initiated (e.g., X-ray technicians). But none of these occupations and professions can be understood properly without viewing them in historical relationships with certain others. Law and accounting vis-a-vis each other and business provides another illustration of what is meant. Another excellent example is the relation of psychology to psychiatry, for psychology represents a scientific discipline rooted in the universities but with men engaged in private practice as well as employed by large establishments. Psychology's clinical wing has been shaped not only by battles with university faculties but also by its drive for recognized status, as in therapy and practice. The latter development has affected psychology departments, which could not afford to ignore either the strength of the clinical movement or its drive toward professionalization.

As applied to chemistry, the perspectives noted above not only raise some questions untouched upon in this book but, more important, raise some about the future of chemistry as an assumed profession. Under the impact of specialization, how long will the symbolization of chemists manage to bind them into one single unit (or as we have termed it, an extensive coalition)? As new branches of chemistry and allied sciences emerge, what will be the professional relationship?

Since no one can forsee with any great accuracy the forms to be taken by our great research universities, how will changes on campus affect chemistry professors, and thus the entire profession? How will the very structure of professional relationships within chemistry be affected in the foreseeable future as chemists gain increasing power in industrial corporations and governmental agencies? How will new institutions affect the work and careers as well as the identities of chemists? If the trend in the nation's labor force continues toward a greatly increased technical and scientific personnel, what will be the implications for chemistry's current technician-researcher-administrator relationships? What will be the outcome of the increase in layers of technicians and administrators in enlarging research hierarchies? And as the scientific revolution proceeds, will scientists still require the sense of belonging to a profession, or will they require other insignia or identity? In short, how will the *meanings,* as well as the forms, of professionalization, as scientists know them today, undergo radical change?

PART II

CAREERS

CAREERS, PERSONALITY, AND
ADULT SOCIALIZATION[1]

(With Howard S. Becker)

In contradistinction to other disciplines, the sociological approach
to the study of personality and personality change views the person
as a member of a social structure. Usually the emphasis is upon
some cross-section in his life: on the way he fills his status, on the
consequent conflicts in role and his dilemmas. When the focus is
more developmental, then concepts like career carry the import of
movement through structures. Much writing on career, of course,
pertains more to patterned sequences of passage than to the persons.
A fairly comprehensive statement about careers as related both to
institutions and to persons would be useful in furthering research.
We shall restrict our discussion to careers in work organizations and
occupations, for purposes of economy.

CAREER FLOW

Organizations built around some particular kind of work or situation at work tend to be characterized by recurring patterns of tension
and of problems. Thus in occupations whose central feature is performance of a service for outside clients, one chronic source of tension
is the effort of members to control their work life themselves while

1 Everett C. Hughes, of the University of Chicago, has undoubtedly
done more than any other sociologist in this country to focus attention
and research on occupational careers. Several of our illustrations, will
be drawn from work done under his direction, and our thinking owes
much to his writing and conversation.

Reprinted by permission from
AMERICAN JOURNAL OF SOCIOLOGY
Vol. LXII, November 1956, pp. 253-63
Copyright © 1956 by The University of Chicago

in contact with outsiders. In production organizations somewhat similar tensions arise from the workers' efforts to maintain relative autonomy over job conditions.

Whatever the typical problems of an occupation, the pattern of associated problems will vary with one's position. Some positions will be easier, some more difficult; some will afford more prestige, some less; some will pay better than others. In general, the personnel move from less to more desirable positions, and the flow is usually, but not necessarily, related to age. The pure case is the bureaucracy as described by Mannheim, in which seniority and an age-related increase in skill and responsibility automatically push men in the desired direction and within a single organization.[2]

An ideally simple model of flow up through an organization is something like the following: recruits enter at the bottom in positions of least prestige and move up through the ranks as they gain in age, skill, and experience. Allowing for some attrition due to death, sickness, and dismissal or resignation, all remain in the organization until retirement. Most would advance to top ranks. A few reach the summit of administration. Yet even in bureaucracies, which perhaps come closest to this model, the very highest posts often go not to those who have come up through the ranks but to "irregulars" — people with certain kinds of experiences or qualifications not necessarily acquired by long years of official service. In other ways, too, the model is oversimple: posts at any rank may be filled from the outside; people get "frozen" at various levels and do not rise. Moreover, career movements may be not only up but down or sideways, as in moving from one department to another at approximately the same rank.

The flow of personnel through an organization should be seen, also, as a number of streams; that is, there may be several routes to the posts of high prestige and responsibility. These may be thought of as escalators. An institution invests time, money, and energy in the training of its recruits and members which it cannot afford to let go to waste. Hence just being on the spot often means that one is bound to advance. In some careers, even a small gain in experience gives one a great advantage over the beginner. The mere fact of advancing age or of having been through certain kinds of situations or training saves many an employee from languishing in lower positions. This is what the phrase "seasoning" refers to — the acquiring of requisite knowledge and skills, skills that cannot always be clearly specified even by those who have them. However, the escalator will carry one from opportunities as well as to them. After a certain

2Karl Mannheim, *Essays on the Sociology of Knowledge,* ed. Paul Kecskemeti (New York: Oxford University Press, 1953) pp. 247-49.

amount of time and money have been spent upon one's education for the job, it is not always easy to get off one escalator and on another. Immediate superiors will block transfer. Sponsors will reproach one for disloyalty. Sometimes a man's special training and experience will be thought to have spoiled him for a particular post.

RECRUITMENT AND REPLACEMENT

Recruitment is typically regarded as occurring only at the beginning of a career, where the occupationally uncommitted are bid for, or as something which happens only when there is deliberate effort to get people to commit themselves. But establishments must recruit for all positions; whenever personnel are needed, they must be found and often trained. Many higher positions, as in bureaucracies, appear to recruit automatically from aspirants at next lower levels. This is only appearance; the recruitment mechanisms are standardized and work well. Professors, for example, are drawn regularly from lower ranks, and the system works passably in most academic fields. But in schools of engineering young instructors are likely to be drained off into industry and not be on hand for promotion. Recruitment is never really automatic but depends upon developing in the recruit certain occupational or organizational commitments which correspond to regularized career routes.

Positions in organizations are being vacated continually through death and retirement, promotion and demotion. Replacements may be drawn from the outside ("an outside man") or from within the organization. Most often positions are filled by someone promoted from below or shifted from another department without gaining in prestige. When career routes are well laid out, higher positions are routinely filled from aspirants at the next lower level. However, in most organizations many career routes are not rigidly laid out: a man may jump from one career over to another to fill the organization's need. When this happens, the "insider-outsider" may be envied by those who have come up by the more orthodox routes; and his associates on his original route may regard him as a turncoat. This may be true even if he is not the first to have made the change, as in the jump from scholar to dean or doctor to hospital administrator. Even when replacement from outside the organization is routine for certain positions, friction may result if the newcomer has come up by an irregular route — as when a college president is chosen from outside the usual circle of feeding occupations. A candidate whose background is too irregular is likely to be eliminated unless just this irregularity makes him particularly valuable. The advantage of "new blood" versus "inbreeding" may be the justification. A good sponsor can widen the limits within which the new kind of candidate is judged, by asking that certain of his qualities be weighed against others; as Hall says, "the question is not whether the applicant possesses a specific trait . . . but whether these traits can be assimilated by the specific institutions."[3]

Even when fairly regular routes are followed, the speed of advancement may not be rigidly prescribed. Irregularity may be due in part to unexpected needs for replacement because a number of older men retire in quick succession or because an older man leaves and a younger one happens to be conveniently present. On the other hand, in some career lines there may be room for a certain amount of manipulation of "the system." One such method is to remain physically mobile, especially early in the career, thus taking advantage of several institutions' vacancies.

THE LIMITS OF REPLACEMENT AND RECRUITMENT

Not all positions within an organization recruit from an equally wide range. Aside from the fact that different occupations may be represented in one establishment, some positions require training so specific that recruits can be drawn only from particular schools or firms. Certain positions are merely way stations and recruit only from aspirants directly below. Some may draw only from the outside, and the orbit is always relevant to both careers and organization. One important question, then, about any organization is the limits within which positions recruit incumbents. Another is the limits of the recruitment in relation to certain variables — age of the organization, its relations with clients, type of generalized work functions, and the like.

One can also identify crucial contingencies for careers in pre-occupational life by noting the general or probable limits within which recruiting is carried on and the forces by which they are maintained. For example, it is clear that a position can be filled, at least at first, only from among those who know of it. Thus physiologists cannot be recruited during high school, for scarcely any youngster then knows what a physiologist is or does. By the same token, however, there are at least generally formulated notions of the "artist," so that recruitment into the world of art often begins in high school.[4] This is paradoxical, since the steps and paths later in the artist's career are less definite than in the physiologist's. The range and

[3]Oswald Hall, "The Stages in a Medical Career," *American Journal of Sociology*, LIII (March, 1948), 332.

[4]Cf. Strauss's unpublished studies of careers in art and Howard S. Becker and James Carper, "The Development of Identification with an Occupation," *American Journal of Sociology*, LXI (January, 1956), 289-98.

diffusion of a public stereotype are crucial in determining the number and variety of young people from whom a particular occupation can recruit, and the unequal distribution of information about careers limits the possibilities of some occupations.

There are problems attending the systematic restriction or recruiting. Some kinds of persons, for occupationally irrelevant reasons (formally, anyway), may not be considered for some positions at all. Medical schools restrict recruiting in this way: openly, on grounds of "personality assessments," and covertly on ethnicity. Italians, Jews, and Negroes who do become doctors face differential recruitment into the formal and informal hierarchies of influence, power, and prestige in the medical world. Similar mechanisms operate at the top and bottom of industrial organizations.[5]

Another problem is that of "waste." Some recruits in institutions which recruit pretty widely do not remain. Public caseworkers in cities are recruited from holders of Bachelor's degrees, but most do not remain caseworkers. From the welfare agency's point of view this is waste. From other perspectives this is not waste, for they may exploit the job and its opportunities for private ends. Many who attend school while supposedly visiting clients may be able to transfer to new escalators because of the acquisition, for instance, of a Master's degree. Others actually build up small businesses during this "free time." The only permanent recruits, those who do not constitute waste, are those who fail at such endeavors.[6] Unless an organization actually finds useful a constant turnover of some sector of its personnel, it is faced with the problem of creating organizational loyalties and — at higher levels anyhow — satisfactory careers or the illusion of them, within the organization.

TRAINING AND SCHOOLS

Schooling occurs most conspicuously during the early stages of a career and is an essential part of getting people committed to careers and prepared to fill positions. Both processes may, or may not, be going on simultaneously. However, movement from one kind

[5]Cf. Hall, *op. cit.;* David Solomon, "Career Contingencies of Chicago Physicians" (unpublished Ph.D. thesis, University of Chicago, 1952); Everett C. Hughes, *French Canada in Transition* (Chicago: University of Chicago Press, 1943), pp. 52-53; Melville Dalton, "Informal Factors in Career Achievement," *American Journal of Sociology,* LVI (March, 1951), 407-15; and Orvis Collins, "Ethnic Behavior in Industry: Sponsorship and Rejection in a New England Factory," *American Journal of Sociology,* LI (January, 1946), 293-98.

[6]Cf. unpublished M. A. report of Earl Bogdanoff and Arnold Glass, "The Sociology of the Public Case Worker in an Urban Area" (University of Chicago (1954).

of job or position or another virtually always necessitates some sort of learning — sometimes before and sometimes on the job, sometimes through informal channels and sometimes at school. This means that schools may exist within the framework of an organization. In-service training is not only for jobs on lower levels but also for higher positions. Universities and special schools are attended by students who are not merely preparing for careers but getting degrees or taking special courses in order to move faster and higher. In some routes there is virtual blockage of mobility because the top of the ladder is not very high; in order to rise higher, one must return to school to prepare for ascending by another route. Thus the registered nurse may have to return to school to become a nursing educator, administrator, or even supervisor. Sometimes the aspirant may study on his own, and this may be effective unless he must present a diploma to prove he deserves promotion.

The more subtle connections are between promotion and informal training. Certain positions preclude the acquiring of certain skills or information, but others foster it. It is possible to freeze a man at given levels or to move him faster, unbeknownst to him. Thus a sponsor, anticipating a need for certain requirements in his candidate, may arrange for critical experiences to come his way. Medical students are aware that if they obtain internships in certain kinds of hospitals they will be exposed to certain kinds of learning: the proper internship is crucial to many kinds of medical careers. But learning may depend upon circumstances which the candidate cannot control and of which he may not even be aware. Thus Goldstein has pointed out that nurses learn more from doctors at hospitals not attached to a medical school; elsewhere the medical students become the beneficiaries of the doctors' teaching.[7] Quite often who teaches whom and what is connected with matters of convenience as well as with prestige. It is said, for instance, that registered nurses are jealous of their prerogatives and will not transmit certain skills to practical nurses. Nevertheless, the nurse is often happy to allow her aides to relieve her of certain other jobs and will pass along the necessary skills; and the doctor in his turn may do the same with his nurses.

The connection between informal learning and group allegiance should not be minimized. Until a newcomer has been accepted, he will not be taught crucial trade secrets. Conversely, such learning may block mobility, since to be mobile is to abandon standards, violate friendships, and even injure one's self-regard. Within some training institutions students are exposed to different and sometimes

[7]Rhoda Goldstein, "The Professional Nurse in the Hospital Bureaucracy" (unpublished Ph.D. thesis, University of Chicago, 1954).

antithetical work ideologies — as with commercial and fine artists — which results in sharp and sometimes lasting internal conflicts of loyalty.

Roy's work on industrial organization furnishes a subtle instance of secrecy and loyalty in training.[8] The workers in Roy's machine shop refused to enlighten him concerning ways of making money on difficult piecework jobs until given evidence that he could be trusted in undercover skirmishes with management. Such systematic withholding of training may mean that an individual can qualify for promotion by performance only by shifting group loyalties, and that disqualifies him in some other sense. Training hinders as well as helps. It may incapacitate one for certain duties as well as train him for them. Roy's discussion of the managerial "logic of efficiency" makes this clear: workers, not trained in this logic, tend to see short cuts to higher production more quickly than managers, who think in terms of sentimental dogmas of efficiency.[9]

Certain transmittable skills, information, and qualities facilitate movement, and it behooves the candidate to discover and distinguish what is genuinely relevant in his training. The student of careers must also be sensitized to discover what training is essential or highly important to the passage from one status to another.

RECRUITING FOR UNDESIRABLE POSITIONS

A most difficult kind of recruiting is for positions which no one wants. Ordinary incentives do not work, for these are positions without prestige, without future, without financial reward. Yet they are filled. How, and by whom? Most obviously, they are filled by failures (the crews of gandy dancers who repair railroad tracks are made up of skid-row bums), to whom they are almost the only means of survival. Most positions filled by failures are not openly regarded as such; special rhetorics deal with misfortune and make their ignominious fate more palatable for the failures themselves and those around them.[10]

Of course, failure is a matter of perspective. Many positions represent failure to some but not to others. For the middle-class white, becoming a caseworker in a public welfare agency may mean failure;

[8]Donald Roy, "Quota Restriction and Goldbricking in a Machine Shop," *American Journal of Sociology,* LVII (March, 1952), 427-42.

[9]Donald Roy, "Efficiency and the 'Fix': Informal Intergroup Relations in a Piecework Machine Shop," *American Journal of Sociology,* LX (November, 1954), 255-66.

[10]Cf. Erving Goffman, "On Cooling the Mark Out: Some Aspects of Adaptation to Failure," *Psychiatry,* XV (November, 1952), 451-63.

but for the Negro from the lower-middle class the job may be a real prize. The permanent positions in such agencies tend to be occupied by whites who have failed to reach anything better and, in larger numbers, by Negroes who have succeeded in arriving this far.[11] Likewise, some recruitment into generally undesirable jobs is from the ranks of the disaffected who care little for generally accepted values. The jazz musicians who play in Chicago's Clark Street dives make little money, endure bad working conditions, but desire the freedom to play as they could not in better-paying places.[12]

Recruits to undesirable postions also come from the ranks of the transients, who, because they feel that they are on their way to something different and better, can afford temporarily to do something *infra dig*. Many organizations rely primarily on transients — such are the taxi companies and some of the mail-order houses. Among the permanent incumbents of undesirable positions are those, also, who came in temporarily but whose brighter prospects did not materialize, they thus fall into the "failure" group.

Still another group is typified by the taxi dancer, whose career Cressey has described. The taxi dancer starts at the top, from which the only movement possible is down or out. She enters the profession young and goodlooking and draws the best customers in the house, but, as age and hard work take their toll, she ends with the worst clients or becomes a streetwalker.[13] Here the worst positions are filled by individuals who start high and so are committed to a career that ends badly — a more common pattern of life, probably, than is generally recognized.

Within business and industrial organizations, not everyone who attempts to move upward succeeds. Men are assigned to positions prematurely, sponsors drop proteges, and miscalculations are made about the abilities of promising persons. Problems for the organization arise from those contingencies. Incompetent persons must be moved into positions where they cannot do serious damage, others of limited ability can still be useful if wisely placed. Aside from outright firing, various methods of "cooling out" the failures can be adopted, among them honorific promotion, banishment "to the sticks," shunting to other departments, frank demotion, bribing out of the organization, and down-grading through departmental mergers. The use of particular methods is related to the structure of the or-

[11]Bogdanoff and Glass, *op. cit.*

[12]Howard S. Becker, "The Professional Dance Musician and His Audience," *American Journal of Sociology*, LVII (September, 1951), 136-44.

[13]Paul G. Cressey, *The Taxi-Dance Hall* (Chicago: University of Chicago Press, 1932), pp. 84-106.

ganization; and these, in turn, have consequences both for failure and for the organization.[14]

ATTACHMENT AND SEVERANCE

Leaders of organizations sometimes complain that their personnel will not take responsibility or that some men (the wrong ones) are too ambitious. This complaint reflects a dual problem which confronts every organization. Since all positions must be filled, some men must be properly motivated to take certain positions and stay in them for a period, while others must be motivated to move onward and generally upward. The American emphasis on mobility should not lead us to assume that everyone wants to rise to the highest levels or to rise quickly. Aside from this, both formal mechanisms and informal influences bind incumbents, at least temporarily, to certain positions. Even the ambitious may be willing to remain in a given post, provided that it offers important contacts or the chance to learn certain skills and undergo certain experiences. Part of the bargain in staying in given positions is the promise that they lead somewhere. When career lines are fairly regularly laid out, positions lead definitely somewhere and at a regulated pace. One of the less obvious functions of the sponsor is to alert his favorites to the sequence and its timing, rendering them more ready to accept undesirable assignments and to refrain from champing at the bit when it might be awkward for the organization.

To certain jobs, in the course of time, come such honor and glory that the incumbents will be satisfied to remain there permanently, giving up aspirations to move upward. This is particularly true when allegiance to colleagues, built on informal relations and conflict with other ranks, is intense and runs counter to allegiance to the institution. But individuals are also attached to positions by virtue of having done particularly well at them; they often take great satisfaction in their competence at certain techniques and develop self-conceptions around them.

All this makes the world of organizations go around, but it also poses certain problems, both institutional and personal. The stability of institutions is predicated upon the proper preparation of aspirants for the next steps and upon institutional aid in transmuting motives and allegiances. While it is convenient to have some personnel relatively immobile, others must be induced to cut previous ties, to balance rewards in favor of moving, and even to take risks for long-run gains. If we do not treat mobility as normal, and thus regard attach-

[14]Norman Martin and Anselm Strauss, "Patterns of Mobility within Industrial Organizations," *Journal of Business*, XXIX (April, 1956), 101-10.

ment to a position as abnormal, we are then free to ask how individuals are induced to move along. It is done by devices such as sponsorship, by planned sequences of positions and skills, sometimes tied to age; by rewards, monetary and otherwise, and, negatively, by ridicule and the denial of responsibility to the lower ranks. There is, of course, many a slip in the inducing of mobility. Chicago public school teachers illustrate this point. They move from schools in the slums to middle-class neighborhoods. The few who prefer to remain in the tougher slum schools have settled in too snugly to feel capable of facing the risks of moving to "better" schools.[15] Their deviant course illuminates the more usual patterns of the Chicago teacher's career.

TIMING IN STATUS PASSAGE

Even when paths in a career are regular and smooth, there always arise problems of pacing and timing. While, ideally, successors and predecessors should move in and out of offices at equal speeds, they do not and cannot. Those asked to move on or along or upward may be willing but must make actual and symbolic preparations; meanwhile, the successor waits impatiently. Transition periods are a necessity, for a man often invests heavily of himself in a position, comes to possess it as it possesses him, and suffers in leaving it. If the full ritual of leavetaking is not allowed, the man may not pass fully into his new status. On the other hand, the institution has devices to make him forget, to plunge him into the new office, to woo and win him with the new gratifications, and, at the same time, to force him to abandon the old. When each status is conceived as the logical and temporal extension of the one previous, then severance is not so disturbing. Nevertheless, if a man must face his old associates in unaccustomed roles, problems of loyalty arise. Hence a period of tolerance after formal admission to the new status is almost a necessity. It is rationalized in phrases like "it takes time" and "we all make mistakes when starting, until . . . ."

But, on the other hand, those new to office may be too zealous. They often commit the indelicate error of taking too literally their formal promotion of certification, when actually intervening steps must be traversed before the attainment of full prerogatives. The passage may involve trials and tests of loyalty, as well as the simple accumulation of information and skill. The overeager are kept in line by various controlling devices: a new assistant professor discovers that it will be "just a little while" before the curriculum can be arranged so that he can teach his favorite courses. Even a new superior

[15]Howard S. Becker, "The Career of the Chicago Public Schoolteacher," *American Journal of Sociology*, LVII (March, 1952), 470-77.

has to face the resentment or the cautiousness of established personnel and may, if sensitive, pace his "moving in on them" until he has passed unspoken tests.

When subordinates are raised to the ranks of their superiors, an especially delicate situation is created. Equality is neither created by that official act, nor, even if it were, can it come about without a certain awkwardness. Patterns of response must be rearranged by both parties, and strong self-control must be exerted so that acts are appropriate. Slips are inevitable, for, although the new status may be fully granted, the proper identities may at times be forgotten, to everyone's embarrassment. Eventually, the former subordinate may come to command or take precedence over someone to whom he once looked for advice and guidance. When colleagues who were formerly sponsors and sponsored disagree over some important issue, recrimination may become overt and betrayal explicit. It is understandable why those who have been promoted often prefer, or are advised, to take office in another organization, however much they wish to remain at home.

MULTIPLE ROUTES AND SWITCHING

Theoretically, a man may leave one escalator and board another, instead of following the regular route. Such switching is more visible during the schooling, or pre-occupational, phases of careers. Frequently students change their line of endeavor but remain roughly within the same field; this is one way for less desirable and less well-known specialties to obtain recruits. Certain kinds of training, such as the legal, provide bases for moving early and easily into a wide variety of careers. In all careers, there doubtless are some points at which switching to another career is relatively easy. In general, while commitment to a given career automatically closes paths, the skills and information thereby acquired open up other routes and new goals. One may not, of course, perceive the alternatives or may dismiss them as risky or otherwise undesirable.

When a number of persons have changed escalators at about the same stage in their careers, then there is the beginning of a new career. This is one way by which career lines become instituted. Sometimes the innovation occurs at the top ranks of older careers; when all honors are exhausted, the incumbent himself may look for new worlds to conquer. Or he may seem like a good risk to an organization looking for personnel with interestingly different qualifications. Such new phases of career are much more than honorific and may indeed be an essential inducement to what becomes pioneering.

Excitement and dangers are intimately tied up with switching careers. For example, some careers are fairly specific in goal but diffuse in operational means: the "fine artist" may be committed to artistic ideals but seize upon whatever jobs are at hand to help him toward creative goals. When he takes a job in order to live, he thereby risks committing himself to an alternative occupational career; and artists and writers do, indeed, get weaned away from the exercise of their art in just this way. Some people never set foot on a work escalator but move from low job to low job. Often they seek better conditions of work or a little more money rather than chances to climb institutional or occupational ladders. Many offers of opportunities to rise are spurned by part-time or slightly committed recruits, often because the latter are engaged in pursuing alternative routes while holding the job, perhaps a full-time one providing means of livelihood. This has important and, no doubt, subtle effects upon institutional functioning. When careers are in danger of being brought to an abrupt end — as with airplane pilots — then, before retirement, other kinds of careers may be prepared for or entered. This precaution is very necessary. When generalized mobility is an aim, specific routes may be chosen for convenience sake. One is careful not to develop the usual motivation and allegiances. This enables one to get off an escalator and to move over to another with a minimum of psychological strain.

Considerable switching takes place within a single institution or a single occupational world and is rationalized in institutional and occupational terms, both by the candidates and by their colleagues. A significant consequence of this, undoubtedly, is subtle psychological strain, since the new positions and those preceding are both somewhat alike and different.

CLIMATIC PERIODS

Even well-worn routes have stretches of maximum opportunity and danger. The critical passage in some careers lies near the beginning. This is especially so when the occupation or institution strongly controls recruitment; once chosen, prestige and deference automatically accrue. In another kind of career the critical time comes at the end and sometimes very abruptly. In occupations which depend upon great physical skill, the later phases of a career are especially hazardous. It is also requisite in some careers that one choose the proper successor to carry on, lest one's work be partly in vain. The symbolic last step of moving out may be quite as important as any that preceded it.

Appropriate or strategic timing is called for, to meet opportunity and danger, but the timing becomes vital at different periods in different kinds of careers. A few, such as the careers of virtuoso musical performers, begin so early in life that the opportunity to engage in music may have passed long before they learn of it. Some of the more subtle judgments of timing are required when a person wishes to shift from one escalator to another. Richard Wohl, of the University of Chicago, in an unpublished paper has suggested that modeling is a step which women may take in preparation for upward mobility through marriage; but models may marry before they know the ropes, and so marry too low; or they may marry too long after their prime, and so marry less well than they might. Doubtless organizations and occupations profit from mistakes of strategic timing, both to recruit and then to retain their members.

During the most crucial periods of any career, a man suffers greater psychological stress than during other periods. This is perhaps less so if he is not aware of his opportunities and dangers — for then the contingencies are over before they can be grasped or coped with: but probably it is more usual to be aware, or to made so by colleagues and seniors, of the nature of imminent or current crises. Fortunately, together with such definitions there exist rationales to guide action. The character of the critical junctures and the ways in which they are handled may irrevocably decide a man's fate.

INTERDEPENDENCE OF CAREERS

Institutions, at any given moment, contain people at different stages in their careers. Some have already "arrived," others are still on their way up, still others just entering. Movements and changes at each level are in various ways dependent on those occurring at other levels.

Such interdependence is to be found in the phenomenon of sponsorship, where individuals move up in a work organization through the activities of older and more-well-established men. Hall[16] has given a classic description of sponsorship in medicine. The younger doctor of the proper class and acceptable ethnic origin is absorbed, on the recommendation of a member, into the informal "inner fraternity" which controls hospital appointments and which is influential in the formation and maintenance of a clientele. The perpetuation of this coterie depends on a steady flow of suitable recruits. As the members age, retire, or die off, those who remain face a problem of recruiting younger men to do the less honorific and remunerative work, such as clinical work, that their group performs. Otherwise they themselves must do work inappropriate to their position or give place to others who covet their power and influence.

[16]Hall, *op. cit.*

To the individual in the inner fraternity, a protege eases the transition into retirement. The younger man gradually assumes the load which the sponsor can no longer comfortably carry, allowing the older man to retire gracefully, without that sudden cutting-down of work which frightens away patients, who leap to the conclusion that he is too old to perform capably.

In general, this is the problem of retiring with honor, of leaving a life's work with a sense that one will be missed. The demand may arise that a great man's work be carried on, although it may no longer be considered important or desirable by his successors. If the old man's prestige is great enough, the men below may have to orient themselves and their work as he suggests, for fear of offending him or of profaning his heritage. The identities of the younger men are thus shaped by the older man's passage from the pinnacle to retirement.

This interdependence of career may cross occupational lines within organizations, as in the case of the young physician who receives a significant part of his training from the older and more experienced nurses in the hospital; and those at the same level in an institution are equally involved in one another's identities. Sometimes budding careers within work worlds are interdependent in quite unsuspected ways. Consider the young painter or craftsman who must make his initial successes in enterprises founded by equally young art dealers, who, because they run their galleries on a shoestring, can afford the frivolity of exhibiting the works of an unknown. The very ability to take such risk provides the dealer a possible opportunity to discover a genius.

One way of uncovering the interdependence of careers is to ask: Who are the important *others* at various stages of the career, the persons significantly involved in the formation of one's own identity? These will vary with stages; at one point one's age mates are crucial, perhaps as competitors, while at another the actions of superiors are the most important. The inter-locking of careers results in influential images of similarity and contrariety. In so far as the significant others shift and vary by the phases of a career, identities change in patterned and not altogether unpredictable ways.

THE CHANGING WORK WORLD

The occupations and organizations within which careers are made change in structure and direction of activity, expand or contract, transform purposes. Old functions and positions disappear, and new ones arise. These constitute potential locations for a new and sometimes wide range of people, for they are not incrusted with traditions and customs concerning their incumbents. They open up new kinds of careers to persons making their work lives within the institution and thus the possibility of variation in long-established types of career. An individual once clearly destined for a particular position suddenly finds himself confronted with an option; what was once a settled matter has split into a set of alternatives between which he must now choose. Different identities emerge as people in the organization take cognizance of this novel set of facts. The positions turn into recognized social entities, and some persons begin to reorient their ambitions. The gradual emergence of a new specialty typically creates this kind of situation within occupations.

Such occupational and institutional changes, of course, present opportunity for both success and failure. The enterprising grasp eagerly at new openings, making the most of them or attempting to; while others sit tight as long as they can. During such times the complexities of one's career are further compounded by what is happening to others with whom he is significantly involved. The ordinary lines of sponsorship in institutions are weakened or broken because those in positions to sponsor are occupied with matters more immediately germane to their own careers. Lower ranks feel the consequences of unusual pressures generated in the ranks above. People become peculiarly vulnerable to unaccustomed demands for loyalty and alliance which spring from the unforeseen changes in the organization. Paths to mobility become indistinct and less fixed, which has an effect on personal commitments and identities. Less able to tie themselves tightly to any one career, because such careers do not present themselves as clearly, men become more experimental and open-minded or more worried and apprehensive.

CAREERS AND PERSONAL IDENTITY

A frame of reference for studying careers is, at the same time, a frame for studying personal identities. Freudian and other psychiatric formulations of personality development probably overstress childhood experiences. Their systematic accounts end more or less with adolescence, later events being regarded as the elaboration of, or variations on, earlier occurrences. Yet central to any account of adult identity is the relation of change in identity to change in social position; for it is characteristic of adult life to afford and force frequent and momentous passages from status to status. Hence members of structures that change, riders on escalators that carry them up, along, and down, to unexpected places and to novel experiences even when in some sense foreseen, must gain, maintain, and regain a sense of personal identity. Identity "is never gained nor maintained once and for all."[17] Stabilities in the organization of behavior

[17]Erik H. Erikson, *Childhood and Society* (New York: W. W. Norton & Co., 1950), p. 57.

and of self-regard are inextricably dependent upon stabilities of social structure. Likewise, change ("development") is shaped by those patterned transactions which accompany career movement. The crises and turning points of life are not entirely institutionalized, but their occurrence and the terms which define and help to solve them are illuminated when seen in the context of career lines. In so far as some populations do not have careers in the sense that professional and business people have them, then the focus of attention ought still to be positional passage, but with domestic, age, and other escalators to the forefront. This done, it may turn out that the model sketched here must undergo revision.

SOME ASPECTS OF RECRUITMENT INTO
THE VISUAL ARTS[1]

I.

"Surprisingly little is known about occupational choice in our own or any other mobile society."[2] This summary judgment was made recently in a survey of occupations and professions by an astute and knowledgeable social scientist. The study of how people chose occupations or careers can be approached from two different, though obviously related, points of view. One is from the perspective of the person who does the choosing. The other is from the angle of vision of the occupation which must attract good youngsters; educate and train them; retain them; and replace them when they retire or, for some reason, leave the field. No matter how smoothly the course of recruitment and training runs, it is always beset by knotty problems: some specific to the particular field, and many of more general scope. It is my hope that in the solution of some of these persistent and important problems, the social scientist will not be conceived as an outsider, a meddler, but as a useful resource; for balancing his lesser knowledge of particular fields is his comparative and valuable knowledge of many occupations and professions.

Because of my own interest in art and artists, I have found it congenial to ask the kinds of questions about recruitment in the visual arts that are currently being asked about medicine, law, nursing, and other lines of endeavor. My research is by no means conclusive for it concerns the students of only one art school, although a very fine, and I trust representative, one. Nevertheless I accepted the invitation to give a paper today with alacrity, for it allows me to suggest what might be done in conjunction with the interests and methods of social scientists.

[1]A paper delivered at the Midwestern College Art Conference, Indiana University, October 28-30, 1954.

[2]Theodore Caplow, *Sociology of Work*, Minneapolis: U. of Minnesota, 1954, p. 214.

About seventy students matriculating at the School of the Art Institute of Chicago were interviewed, the number being divided equally among those majoring in commercial art, art education and fine art. The students were drawn from each grade level, from many sections of the city and region, and from various friendship groups. The questions bearing upon their occupational choice were part of a two hour interview covering experiences prior to and after coming to the school. The School has a student body of around 800, mainly drawn from Chicago, from Illinois and from surrounding states. Probably the majority of Chicago's fine artists, and many of its art teachers, have attended the School. The emphasis at this institution is upon high artistic standards and upon basic art.

II.

In some countries, during some eras, there has been fairly tight control in the arts both of the numbers of recruits and the course of their careers. This certainly is not characteristic of the United States today, for we are in a period when the market for visual arts — and for other arts as well — is rapidly and vastly expanding.

This expansion, combined with a relative absence of any central-ized occupational control, suggests that the world of art — fine and commercial — must recruit in a rather generous if not excessive fashion. The picture of recruitment in excess of demand is perhaps particularly striking for another art world, that of drama — the pull of Broadway and Hollywood has so often been portrayed — but probably it is not less characteristic of music and visual arts. There is in fact no dearth of critics of this situation: these either bemoan excess of supply over demand (accusing art teachers and adminis-trators of deliberately fostering it or at least of ignoring the situa-tion), or argue in opposite key that much more demand is needed to meet the abundant and excellent supply. A third type of critic, usually one with a commercial job, maintains that the market can absorb any amount of supply, since it is just a matter of the idealistic artist readjusting his activity and his product to fit the market, or through enterprise discovering the specific outlets for this particular style.

The over-generous attraction of potential artists is taken care of in manifold ways, for art worlds appear to have certain resources for allocating people to jobs wholly or partially non-productive of art products for a market. A number of persons with artistic train-ing get positions in museums and other organizations, including the art-sections of department stores. A great many more become teach-ers who directly or indirectly help to atttract future teachers, or in-struct future artists. Probably the majority of art teachers, however, function to enlighten and recruit the more general consumer audience: as teachers of youngsters or hobbyists, or as popularizers in one capacity or another of art. Presumably also considerable numbers of former art students, especially married women, neither exhibit nor sell very often, maintaining more of an amateur than professional status, becoming also through their training part of the larger consumer art public. Add to this, critics, art salesmen, and any number of subsidiary artistic jobs.

Unlike certain occupations, art worlds need not under-recruit for purposes of controlling a valuable skill, with its accompanying monetary rewards, prestige and honor. Much of the rather "open" recruitment in art is reflected in the various gentle practices and policies of many of the American schools. Probably few applicants are refused admittance. Students occasionally drop out of school of their own accord, but rarely are flunked out as in law or engineering schools. There are few or no crucial tests or other hurdles that a student must pass to remain in school. Grades mainly seem to function to yield encouragement or prestige, but seem not to be utilized to keep down enrollment or to force repetitions of course work. And anyone who has the time and money can go to any number of commercial art schools.

III.

Because recruitment to the art world is neither tightly limited nor carefully controlled, we should not be led to assume that artists somehow just drift into art. There exist whole social paraphernalia for getting persons committed to their artistic identities: that the machinery is not very visible to them does not of course make it any less real.

The chief mechanism for pumping a flow of talent into art today is the public school system — aided by the art schools and often abetted, albeit unwittingly, by the family. This is true among other reasons because nowadays artists do not appear to come from very high or very low social classes. An artistic career is not generally initiated by an education at prep school or elite college — neither do persons of low economic standing usually become artists by emulating models found in their communities (as boxers do). Parents of various strata introduce their offspring to art stressing humanistic, hobbyist and other values; but probably not many parents conceive of the visual arts as a propitious locale on which to fight and battle for class and occupational success. No evidence exists in our interviews that any parent (except one) very directly influenced entry into art — not withstanding the plausible suggestion made by David Riesman that since, in common with other fields, art has become glamorized in recent years, one might expect to find parents urging children to pursue artistic rainbows.[3] Attendance at galleries and museums, with or without parents, plays no discernable part in recruitment; and, in fact, a rare art student reports having any art "in his background." Neither does he, when first he comes to art school, generally know artists of any kind except his public school art teachers; nor is he acquainted with art history, or with much if any biographical writing about famous artists.

The public school art teachers begin to function quite early in the art career, generally in grammar school. Impoverished or misguided though their teaching sometimes may be, they may introduce the youngster to the satisfactions and delights of drawing and painting. The art classes serve to keep interest alive throughout the school years: while the teacher bestows approval upon the child — through gestures, singling him out for special honors, placing his work in public view, or assigning him honorific tasks like the decoration of blackboards.

In high school he continues taking art classes and often has an opportunity to major in art. The teachers may begin to suggest that he go to art school — a step that otherwise would not occur to some — and may procure information and even scholarships for their proteges. The high school milieu sometimes affords additional prestige, for the child may win a school or city prize, even a national one, or receive acclaim by decorating stage sets, or drawing for the school paper.

The art schools make contact with and reach down into the public schools in various ways. Their graduates teach the children. Talented students are given scholarships all through the school years to special children's classes and many attend at their own expense with encouragement from their teachers. Art schools and associations sponsor prize-winning contests and give scholarships. Without this bounty many from poorer families could not receive parental consent to continue schooling, and others might instead get jobs, enter other occupations or go to college. By the time he leaves high school, if he is not yet sure of his bent, the future artist may enter through a way station: the summer school or the night school, whose teachers function to build confidence and encourage the promising.

The youngster who is processed through this recruiting machinery perceives only that he has some artistic talent. Although his family may be indifferent to his painting and drawing, more often they too

[3]David Riesman, *Individualism Reconsidered,* Free Press, 1954, pp. 215-16.

take note of his abilities. It makes little difference that parents, teachers, or other students may evaluate him too highly: his capacities for artistic production are confirmed, and that very confirmation sets him apart in some sense from his peers. Occupational choice is not closely linked, as it may be in some fields, with a high-school friendship group going forward almost as a unit.

This appreciation of his own talent does not automatically prepare the youngster to become a professional artist: far from it. Initially, all it signifies is an orientation toward art as something that is "fun." Presumably many talented children never learn to take art seriously. In the conversion from avocation to vocation, the art teacher is an indispensable agent for he may indicate some of the vocational possibilities of art. Rarely does a student report that a schoolmate, parent, or relative brought home to him any such possibility. The teachers do not seem to function as models for occupational emulation; nor do they build into the student a sense of occupational dedication. Of the intricacies of the world into which he is about to enter, the teachers reveal rather little; although they may cue him to some specialties that he will encounter. We might predict that the public schools will function increasingly to start the student along the path of occupational specialization, particularly in the larger, better, more advanced urban and suburban schools. (*School Arts* in April, 1954, reported "A High School Art Career Program" in operation in Albuquerque, and included a photo showing students grouped in front of a number of signs, each sign bearing the name of an art specialty.)

IV.

The prerequisite that art be conceived as a serious adult pursuit is necessary but not sufficient for an artistic commitment, because strong alternative vocational paths may exist. College with its social life beckons the economically well-to-do. Professions and occupations of various kinds carry promise of security and prestige, particularly if high school grades are excellent or good. For some poorer adolescents, family finances do not permit further schooling and some have already worked at jobs that appear to have a future.

In the final decision, the role of the family is crucial. Parents may discourage art as a career or job, urging or pressuring the youngster to college or into work that will pay. Because strong dedication to art as an ideal and a style of life generally seems to develop in art school — if it develops at all — parental restraint can be particularly potent before entry into art school. Although before entry into art school, students occasionally decided upon art despite considerable family disapproval, inseparable rifts or severe rejections by either party appeared not to occur because of such decisions.

On the positive side, parents exert little influence in inducing entry into art. Pressure for an art career is virtually non-existent, and guidance in this direction is weak. But the significant fact about these parents is that generally they do not have very many, or strong, alternative courses to suggest or impose. Rather, the children educate their parents to the vocational opportunities. Because the offspring possesses artistic ability — sometimes additionally certified to by the prizes and scholarships — and because he may bring to bear the weight of counselling at high school, his parents appear to assume that some degree of financial security lies at the end of art school. Many students who decide later to be fine artists, at the time of entry assume that they will earn money through commercial art or art teaching, and this promise is concrete enough to satisfy parents. If money has already been brought in through commercial art jobs, then the future seems all the more assured. Sometimes a girl's family goes along with her plans because she is expected to marry eventually — and meanwhile she will learn a useful trade and at worst will have something to occupy her spare time. We may sum up the important parental role, without greatly oversimplifying the matter, by saying that: if parents are vague about vocational opportunities, even though wishing material success for their child, then his entry into art is made easy; but if they strongly oppose an artistic career or hold out attractive alternatives to it, then his matriculation in art school is unlikely.

V.

How, then, are the alternatives perceived and scrutinized by the youngsters themselves? There is of course the possibility of going to college. This was an unappealing alternative to many, either because they did not enjoy schoolwork or because they felt themselves inadequate at it. (You would have perhaps a different picture if you studied students in college art departments — but perhaps not.)

Like others of their age, virtually all had had some occupational experience, particularly at part-time or summer jobs in factory, store and office. This demonstrated to them either that they cared less for this work than for their art, or worst yet they conceived an immense dislike for the work which may then come to represent the entire distasteful or boring or meaningless or hateful world of "business." This brief or very partial contact with business thus acts to seal off job and career alternatives very different than those to which actually they have been exposed. Those who enter art school expecting to specialize in commercial art more often enjoy their contact with business and are attracted to it, but have also worked at commercial art jobs and find these more interesting or lucrative; so their work experience has a more positive influence upon occupational decision. (Indeed it is probable that some persons still get drawn directly into commercial art jobs and never receive formal training. A few of our students had started along this route, but decided they could advance further by first attending art classes.) Other students also have had a fling at commercial art and dislike or do not care for the work but are sufficiently fond of art in general, and dislike business enough in general, to wish to do something with their art other than doing commercial art: "teach or something." Occasionally, too, recruits come late to art, after running afoul of failure or disappointment at college or business; or getting a revealing vision of what lies ahead for themselves in business by looking around at their older office mates. (Where recourse to art would mean denial of considerable obligation to others or much investment in time and money, probably there is little late-coming into art: thus I ran across no one who had dropped out of a family business or a pre-professional course). Each of these types of work experience — good, bad, and indifferent — should be thought of as crucial to committing oneself to art. In a literal sense, these experiences are part and parcel of many artists' careers, albeit they occur before any actual commitment to pursue art as vocation.

This has bearing upon the approximate age at which vocational decision is made. Enrollment at the Art Institute is concentrated in the years eighteen to twenty-two. Among those students who were interviewed, the decision to go into art rarely if ever occured during grammar school, and seldom before the second year of high school, with most students making their decision during the last two years. By the third year of high school, students are being urged to stake out occupational courses, to declare themselves publicly as to their futures; and in many schools a barrage of essays, tests, consultations and counselings forces them to confront their post-graduate destinies. During the same years, the future art student is gaining confirmation of his artistic abilities — often through the very teachers who are dinning in an occupational message; and, in addition, part-time commercial art work brings home to some the career possibilities, while yet others are recoiling from disheartening job experiences.

Given these circumstances, the decision to enter art hardly calls for much soul searching or anxious weighing of occupational alternatives. Neither does the decision necessarily rest on anything more than the recognition that art can be turned to some purpose. Unlike those who persuade themselves, or are dissuaded, to put aside their childish play upon stepping into adulthood, the prospective artist is able to justify his continued artistic activity on grounds other than sheer enjoyment. Teachers, scholarships, the existence of art schools and their publicity, and the immediate and forceful fact of one's own artistic ability: all contribute toward building an expectation that a living can be made at art.

Generally speaking, material aspirations at entrance to art school are not great; one is not impressed by driving ambitions or high expectations. Students majoring in commercial art, as might be anticipated, place more emphasis upon making money and materialistic ends: and presumably students attending the more usual kinds of commercial schools might place even greater stress upon those ends. However, one is struck by a relatively "short escalator of expected mobility"[4] particularly as many students, commercial or otherwise, come from families of little or moderate income.

The expectation of earning a living at art does not mean that the youngster has any clear idea of how this is to be accomplished. Even those who have done some commercial art work may be uncertain as to what kind of commercial specialty they should pursue. As for the others: some anticipate becoming art teachers; some assume they will discover a specialty during their training and welcome the further schooling as a moratorium on immediate occupational decision; and some, particularly the girls, seem relatively unconcerned with specific occupational decision. The terms of committing self to continuing in art thus are properly vague or general — job security, career, and liking art best — reflecting both the students' fairly prosaic objectives and their as yet undifferentiated knowledge of the art world.

Art school represents for them, variously: technical training for future job or career; getting a degree and training that will lead to teaching; obtaining further technical training at doing something which one enjoys doing. Art school is not a beacon whose contemplation has excited them for years, not something they have built up great expectations of attending. They move into it mainly as one more step in schooling although, once the decision has been made, sometimes with excitement.

In their concept of art there is as yet little or no ingredient of calling or dedication, and the sense of self-destiny that often accompanies these: this sense, at least in the students interviewed, develops during the first two years of art school — if it develops at all. The capacious limits of the art world certainly allow for many types of artists: and the dedicated artist, extolled in biographies and art books, is possibly very much in the minority, at

4A phrase coined by R. Richard Wohl, of the University of Chicago.

least in our era. From the nature of the recruitment process, it is plain why such a conception of calling should generally be absent when the decision to become an artist is first made. That process should also help explain why there are probably so many drop-outs after school — through marriage, economic disappointment, and entering other occupations — as well as post-school discoveries of work where training in art is required, although not quite as envisioned beforehand.

PSYCHIATRISTS IN A PRIVATE HOSPITAL*

The Setting at PPI

The locale now changes. We leave the old-fashioned hospital to enter a genuinely modern institution within which increasing numbers of patients are receiving psychiatric care. On psychiatric services within general hospitals throughout the nation, new treatments for the mentally ill are being explored. Such exploration is especially necessary because *hospital* practice of psychiatry is relatively new, in contrast to other medical specialties, which have made excellent medical care virtually synonomous with care in hospitals. Psychiatrists have scarcely begun to work with hospital personnel, to adapt their office styles to hospital settings and their theories and techniques to the kinds of patient that nowadays agree more readily to relatively brief hospitalization than to extensive office therapy. This exploration of style and techniques on the psychiatric services of general hospitals unquestionably will affect how hospital psychiatry will be practiced a decade hence. These hospitals are therefore important experimental locales — if only because they bring metropolitan physicians together with middle- and low-income metropolitan patients.

In the next chapters, we focus upon the *dramatis personae* of the psychiatric wing of one such general hospital. They include the physician, the nurses and the aides: Each echelon will be discussed in a separate chapter. We shall wish to know of each echelon who its members are, how they came to the hospital, of what their work consists, the meaning of the work to them, how they regard their coworkers, and of course how their ideologies — if any — affect all these issues. After these matters have been explored, the interactions among these various personnel will be scrutinized in detail.

*Reprinted by permission from
PSYCHIATRIC IDEOLOGIES AND INSTITUTIONS
(with L. Schatzman, R. Bucher, D. Ehrlich and M. Sabshin), N. Y.,
The Free Press, pp. 179-205.
Copyright © 1964 by the Free Press

A few words of description of PPI and its relation to the main hospital are necessary. Michael Reese Hospital was founded in the late nineteenth century by Chicago's Jewish community. It has since achieved a national reputation for its clinical care and more recently for its research staff. Its psychiatric service was initiated by Dr. Roy Grinker in 1936. By 1951, a carefully designed separate building, called PPI, had been erected. Visitors to PPI are sometimes amazed at what some call its lavish appearance; as one staff member, his face wreathed in smiles, said to us: "Some people think it looks too much like a Miami hotel and that our walls are too clean for a psychiatric hospital!" PPI has five wards: The largest houses about thirty patients and the remaining four about twelve each (about eighty patients in all). Together the wards constitute a system, with one relatively open ward, one quite closed, and three intermediate. Each ward has a first-year resident who acts as "resident administrator" and a "co-ordinator" who is either a third-year resident or a young attending man. Each ward, of course, has a head nurse and a complement of nursing personnel, including aides. PPI is designed for relatively quick turnover: Average length of stay is about forty days for private patients and ninety for service patients. Many of these patients are readmissions. (During 1959, the readmission rate was 30%.) As at Michael Reese proper, the attending men are predominantly Jewish, but patients are drawn from a wide population base, including the Negro community. Among the most important structural features of PPI is that it houses the private patients of attending physicians. We turn first to an examination of the careers, ideologies, and styles of these attending men. In later chapters, other aspects of their practices at PPI will be examined, particularly as those practices affect and are affected by the views and actions of patients and personnel.

The Psychiatrists

It is symbolic that PPI was founded and is still presided over by a physician who was at first a noted neurologist and who later, after analysis with Freud, initiated a psychiatric service of notably analytic orientation. PPI's attending staff was, and is, composed of both somatically oriented physicians and men whose affiliations are with the Chicago Psychoanalytic Institute. Although PPI's national and local image is that of an analytically oriented institution and although residents are drawn there principally because of that image, the dual ideology of its attending staff has nevertheless impressed upon us from our first days at PPI. The administrators told us of their nonanalytic men; the residents spoke of the "shock boys"; the daily census showed a preponderance of patients treated by these physicians. It became apparent that the somatic men are, if nothing else, one financial mainstay of the hospital. Another early observation was the comparative youth of the attending physicians: We were told that many were ex-residents and that a substantial proportion was studying at the Chicago Psychoanalytic Institute.

Early in the study, we posed two general questions about the attending staff:

1. What is the meaning of hospital practice to these practitioners in terms of their professional careers?

2. How do they utilize the hospital setting for treatment of their patients?

Data bearing upon these questions were gathered principally through partially structured interviews, which were carried out after extensive ward observation and informal talks with attending men. The interviewing took place in our offices, and almost all agreed to have their interviews taped. We interviewed twenty physicians, including most of those who utilized the hospital with greatest frequency. None refused an interview. We explained that we wished to know about their professional careers and their use of the hospital. Almost without exception, the men spoke fluently about those topics. Special pains were taken to learn how they treated specific patients.

We shall report the answers to the two questions we posed. These answers are especially pertinent to the current psychiatric scene, for they are relevant to the kinds of physicians that are drawn to hospitals like PPI, to why they bother with hospital practice at all, to the likely lengths of their stays in such practice, and to their conceptions of a hospital setting in relation to the treatment of patients. The answers are also related to what happens in the hospital to various staff personnel — and to patients. In later chapters, some of these consequences will be described and analyzed.

The Somaticists[1]

THE MEANING OF HOSPITAL PRACTICE

When it was founded, PPI included several attending physicians whose practices predated psychoanalysis in Chicago. Such men are still important to the hospital because they bring in a substantial

[1]On our questionnaire, this group of somaticists had mean scores of 4.4 for somatotherapy (4.0 is "high"), 2.9 for psychotherapy (4.5 is "high"), and 3.2 for sociotherapy (4.0 is "high"). The somaticists at PPI correspond roughly to the D-O psychiatrists of New Haven described by A. B. Hollingshead and F. C. Redlich in *Social Class and Mental Illness* (New York: John Wiley & Sons, Inc., 1958), pp. 155-61. The D-O group, however, probably included some who were more eclectic than somatic.

number of patients. Although differences exist among them, for our purposes their similarities are more interesting. Seven of these men practice regularly at PPI. They have entered psychiatry through two routes: neurology training (five men) and state-hospital experience (two men).

When the psychoanalytic movement began to affect the Chicago scene three decades ago, these men did not remain untouched. One man entered psychiatry through a state hospital that was, at that time, an experimental ground for Chicago analysts. He was later graduated from the Analytic Institute and now heads PPI's EST program. He receives referrals from physicians because he is known to be medically oriented and from analysts who prefer not to administer EST* themselves. A second man underwent analysis after first practicing neurology. He claims to utilize an analytic orientation, but he has not actually received any formal training in analysis. These men cannot escape the growing analytic influence in Chicago and at the hospital, but they do not consider themselves members of the Institute circle.

Although these somaticists do receive some referrals by analysts, their patients are principally referred by internists and general practitioners. In this respect, they are more closely linked with the medical profession generally, partly as a deliberate tactic and partly as a result of greater association with physicians. This link is also related to the suspicion with which psychoanalysis is viewed by many physicians. For the general medical community, the somaticists unquestionably represent a more medical approach than do the psychoanalysts.

It is also important to understand their relationship to neurology. As noted, five of these psychiatrists have received neurological training. But neurology has declined as a medical specialty, and for some years virtually no Chicago neurologist has been able to practice it full time. As we examined the careers of these five men, we found a gradual substitution of psychiatric for neurological practice. One man turned completely to psychiatric practice. Another, a nationally known neurologist, runs the main hospital's neurological service. He has many neurological patients but cannot make a comfortable living solely from them. Two other physicians whose practices still include neurological patients also find it necessary to supplement them with psychiatric patients.

These men are entering their fifties and sixties, and their practices are well established. In the main they have (as Hollingshead and Redlich found among New Haven's D-O psychiatrists[2]) what can

2*Ibid.*
*Electric Shock Treatment.

110

be termed bulk practices. That is, they can treat substantial numbers of patients precisely because they tend to limit the length of their therapy sessions and because they generally believe in less extended periods of treatment than do psychotherapeutically oriented physicians.

For their kind of practice, a hospital is very important, if not a virtual necessity, since many of their referrals require immediate hospitalization. Indeed these referrals are made because of their hospital connections. In their kinds of practice, they have always used hospitals. They tend to prescribe a fair amount of EST for certain patients — particularly for elderly depressed patients — and the hospital is a convenient, safe place to give such treatment. These physicians have the reputation among the nurses of being "busy men": One reason is that they seem to dash in and out of the wards as if on tightly budgeted schedules — which, in fact, they are. In addition to their considerable office loads, members of this very small group of practitioners regularly treat a large percentage of PPI's patients: On any ordinary day, the somaticist is likely to visit three or four hospitalized patients at PPI and occasionally as many as six or seven (and maybe even additional ones elsewhere). Of course, sometimes his quota may fall to only one or two. As a group, then, the somaticists' proportion of the total hospital census is likely to be substantial. For these men the hospital has probably much the same meaning it has for busy internists, whose practices are similarly divided between office and hospital.

But to let the matter rest there would be to miss some exceedingly important aspects of the role of the psychiatric hospital in their professional lives. To begin with, these psychiatrists enjoy a status at the hospital that is related to the large proportion of patients whom they bring there. They also contribute to the link between PPI and the main hospital by taking referrals from internists and by their own use of special medical services, as well as because one psychiatrist heads the main hospital's neurological section. He also is the major teacher of neurology to PPI's residents. Another psychiatrist heads PPI's EST service and instructs residents in this type of treatment. All these roles, one can be sure, afford appropriate gratifications.

Despite their ages, their relatively stable practices and their general importance to the hospital, the somaticists find themselves in a somewhat defensive position in relation to the psychiatric hospital. The latter faithfully mirrors the increasing prestige of psychoanalysis within the metropolitan community, and this development has affected the atmosphere within which these psychiatrists must carry on their activities. Both to the residents and the nurses, neurology appears to bear less and less relationship to psychiatry. EST is regarded by many hospital personnel as necessary perhaps but certainly not in such great amounts and for so many patients. Waves of anti-EST feeling have swept the hospital from time to time during the last decade. Open criticism by residents and oblique criticism by nurses have been expressed toward "nondynamically oriented therapy." Under the stimulus of such criticism, the somaticists have formulated a clearly verbalized defense based on judgments that some psychiatrists wait for patients' money virtually to vanish before prescribing EST; that young psychiatrists scornful of EST learn better after some months in practice; and that some analysts who talk in public against EST privately refer cases for EST.

This defensive position is further rendered vulnerable by PPI's recent recruitment of attending men. Although nonanalytically oriented psychiatrists are continually entering the metropolitan community, the situation is quite different at PPI itself. PPI recruits its newest attending men mainly from among its own residents, along with occasional graduates from the local universities. Almost all are analytically oriented. They do not have the kinds of neurological or nonanalytical orientation represented among the somaticists. The forces of the latter are thus not being replenished, either by sponsorship or by renewed administrative effort. Their "true colleagues" are not among PPI's recruits but among others like themselves who practice elsewhere, and among certain internists. Even when they assist in training PPI's residents, it is always in teaching EST and neurology. Sometimes the residents are grateful for the knowledge and technique, but generally they display little enthusiasm for this learning. The somaticists can therefore scarcely feel very important in PPI's educational program.

To the extent that they are not recruiting their younger counterparts, their future positions at PPI are safely predictable. Within a decade, two men will retire. It is unlikely that the remainder will be dropped from the list of invited attending physicians. (Such a pruning process did occur a few years ago when several organically oriented physicians were dropped from the list.) On the other hand, it is improbable that younger psychiatrists without training or interest in psychodynamics will be added as attending physicians. Hence PPI's newer men will continue to be psychotherapeutically oriented. Recently some somaticists have found it necessary to treat patients elsewhere because PPI had a full census and a considerable waiting list. As this hospital moves toward an increasingly full census and toward an increased average length of patient stay—both the partial results of a relatively affluent metropolitan population and Blue Cross insurance — this hospital becomes a less desirable place in which to practice somatic psychiatry. PPI's current plans, however, call for an expanded bed capacity within a few years. When that goal is reached there will be less competition for beds — but the additional space is unlikely to lead to the invitation of new somatically oriented staff.

But one must view the hospital practices of somaticists in a broader metropolitan perspective. Even if forced out of PPI, they will not lack for beds or prestige. There are other psychiatric hospitals, and there will surely be more. Neurology will not regain its former status, but biologically oriented psychiatrists are not going to disappear. In the interviews, we detected no note of despair about the future — only occasional querulousness about the trends at this specific hospital. For their views of the future, the somaticists find ample support in the continued use of EST by psychiatrists — even by former PPI residents — and in the probable muting of analytic influence during the coming years. Doubtless their optimism is buttressed by the absence of severe crisis that characterizes their own professional lives. In any event, their styles of practice require them to use hospitals. We can foresee no cessation in their hospital practices in the decades to come. And as long as psychiatry remains eclectic, these physicians need not feel driven to practicing within hospitals of low prestige.

The Somaticists' Organization of Treatment

When organizing treatment for a patient, each psychiatrist at PPI must take into account the hospital's rules, resources, and drawbacks. He must also aim for a specific therapeutic goal: whether merely to prepare the patient sufficiently to face the outside world, to alleviate obvious symptoms, or to use the hospital visit as the first step in an extended course of therapy. Which goal he chooses depends on both his ideology and his assessment of the patient — but also his goals depend upon the types of patient he hospitalizes.

The somaticists at PPI treat mainly "depressive reactives," "psychotics," and "schizophrenics" of various types. They are hospitalized either because their behavior temporarily renders them unsuitable to remain in society or because they can be more easily treated within the hospital. Almost none has been treated previously at the doctors' offices, although they may have initially visited there. The principal therapeutic goal is to return these patients to the outside world as quickly as possible in a condition to cope with it somewhat better. The somaticist settles for minimal functioning and expects little, if any, change in personality. For these hospital patients, in contrast to office visitors, the psychiatrist dares hope only for symptomatic cure or for a generally better, although sometimes only temporary, handling of life's daily round. Meanwhile hospitalization puts maximum distance between the patient and his stressful environment, allows treatment to be efficiently organized, and permits time for diagnosis if necessary.

These doctors pride themselves upon how speedily they move their patients out of the hospital: Indeed, this speed is a central feature of their treatment. They emphasized the value of this feature when talking to us. They believe that more analytically oriented psychiatrists labor with slower psychotherapeutic methods — when patients can be treated more quickly. They criticize the analysts for allowing patients to run through insurance money and claim that the doctor's duty is to effect relatively quick recovery. Since many of their patients possess limited finances, this consideration buttresses the preference for short hospital stays.

In addition, they have little faith that prolonged hospital stays help patients. The hospital is not regarded as having special curative or instrumental powers: It is merely a locale where specific treatments like EST or supportive therapy can be administered, and where the patient can temporarily be shielded from society — and *vice versa*. If the patient wishes continued therapy in office visits, so much the better, providing genuine benefit can be expected from such visits.

Let us visualize, then, the somatically oriented psychiatrist who brings his patient to the hospital: Where will he request that his patient be placed? In what kind of ward? His criteria for initial placement are two. A primary consideration is the patient's condition. If his behavior is quite bizarre, noisy, or in other ways difficult to control, then the proper place is in a relatively closed unit. The psychiatrist, in effect, accepts the hospital's conventional map, as the administration itself typically conceives it. But a second criterion for initial placement rests upon the consideration that one specific ward has the best arrangements for giving EST: Many patients are treated principally by that means. Furthermore, each somaticist believes he has customarily good working relationships with the personnel of that ward.

Somaticists' patients are therefore found clustered on 3EW or on one other relatively closed ward. If patients are initially judged too "difficult" for these two wards, then the psychiatrist will request transfers to them after the patients' behavior has become more appropriate. They rarely use 2E, a more open ward. Sometimes they use 2N, the most open ward, as a locale from which patients finally will return home — and occasionally for patients who need only slightly different environments from their own homes plus supportive therapy.

In his favorite unit, the somaticist counts upon reliable routine nursing care for his patients, including medication when ordered. He also counts upon its staff to arrange efficiently for various diagnostic tests given at the main hospital. Indeed he has come over the years to rely upon an efficient secretary who is attached to both wards. She saves him much valuable time in dealing with the main hospital and expedites administrative details that otherwise he himself would have to handle or delegate to head nurses.

Toward his patients, his approach is distinctly medical. He is more likely to order medical tests than are most psychotherapeutically oriented men. He tends to utilize nurses in rather traditional medical fashions. He regards their functions as chiefly managerial and nursing-care. He likes to brief his nurses or give them orders with a minimum of verbal interchange. As he is rather uninterested in utilizing nurses as auxiliary to his own therapy, his picture of the nursing staff is relatively undifferentiated: He does not make fine distinctions among those who are good in certain kinds of therapy and those who are good for other kinds, those who are especially effective with certain kinds of patient and those who are not.

Since he does not believe nurses and aides are especially important therapeutic agents, he is neither particularly sensitive to their possible interference with his own therapeutic relations nor particularly apt to become annoyed or angry at the staff's psychological ineptitude — as long as the staff does not unduly disturb his patient or make the patient's environment unpleasant. In fact, if he is not entirely impervious to covert criticism of his treatment of particular patients by members of the staff, he is at least relatively protected from it by his ideological assumption that his therapy alone contributes to the patient's improvement. He is relatively oblivious to the surges of feeling that periodically run through the hospital staff, surges to which psychotherapeutically oriented psychiatrists are sensitive and with which they attempt to cope. The somaticists do not experience the full weight of this collective mood, and entire areas of conflict with the staff are therefore avoided in somatic hospital practice.

By the same token, the somaticist rarely, if ever, realizes that sometimes the staff organizes its own supplementary therapy around his patient because it believes his patient is receiving poor therapy. He can neither approve nor condemn this additional nursing effort.

Occasionally he may even be brought up short against a high court of judgment, as when the nurses complain to the central administration that he is ordering EST for a very young patient. From time to time, the administration supports the complainants, and the psychiatrist must bend to the decision, having no recourse other than to withdraw his patient from the hospital.

Another aspect of his treatment ideology, however, leads him to believe that whatever the staff wishes to do by way of psychotherapy may actually be useful, for it contributes to keeping the staff happy while not actually interferring with his own program. The staff's actions may even make a patient's stay happier and more pleasant. One of these somaticists is therefore distinctly permissive; he tells those who show initiative to do with his patient what they think best, whether therapy or management is involved. His somatic colleagues tend to play along with the nurses, discussing patients when asked and probably giving the idea, whether intentionally or not, that everyone is important to the total therapeutic set. They reason essentially that nurses merely contribute toward making the patient's environment more tolerable or supportive.

Sometimes the somaticist runs afoul of the staff's managerial problems. The nurses may wish to transfer a patient to a more controlling ward because she is no longer appropriate to their own. If the somaticist regards this transfer as inconvenient — and this kind of psychiatrist is on a tight time schedule — then he may bargain for another day or two on the original unit; he may even raise loud objections. More often, he is likely to abide by the staff's decision, since the transfer usually does not much inconvenience him or disturb his treatment of the patient. Sometimes too he faces the consequence of PPI's notably heterogeneous patient population. His patient, for instance, may complain that she does not wish to remain on 3EW because many noisy young people are there; generally, however, he regards the composition of any given ward as not very relevant to the patient's progress but only to her comfort and pleasure.

These psychiatrists bend every effort to remain medical men in their styles of practice. They utilize the hospital and its staff in fairly traditional ways. They believe that they are well served by the institution, for it is rather well organized to serve them, and they can take routine advantage of it — routine because they scarcely need be especially clever in their use of the hospital nor especially innovative in taking advantage of its resources. As a result, they are open to sharp criticism by other attending men and by the staff, but this criticism scarcely shakes their convictions about how a hospital can effectively be utilized.

The Psychotherapists[3]

THE MEANINGS OF HOSPITAL PRACTICE

Most attending men who regularly treat patients at this hospital are ex-residents who have been graduated from its training program. While the somaticists are wedded to the institution, the ex-residents are engaged only temporarily in hospital practice. Most are merely passing through the very early stages of long careers, stages during which their initial practices are split between office and hospital. Later they will, for reasons to be spelled out, virtually cease to have hospital practices.

This group of men numbered about twenty-five at the time of our study. It consisted of all the recent residents, except those serving in the armed forces and one who has become an administrator at PPI. There is good reason for the young psychiatrist to treat some of his patients at the hospital. Most of his early referrals are patients deemed in need of hospitalization. Like the somaticist, he frequently first meets his patients only after their actual hospitalization. His former supervisors and his friends among the ex-residents refer patients whom they are too busy to see or do not wish to treat. Since most hospitalized referrals do not wish to continue in therapy at his office, the young psychiatrist can expect to develop his office practice very slowly *via* this path.

He gradually reduces the number of his hospital visits as his office referrals increase or as his office schedule becomes tighter because patients persist in longer therapy. He may also suddenly find his list of hospitalized patients dropping to virtually nothing because they are all discharged at approximately the same time. Then, too, if he receives a few office referrals, he will have correspondingly less time for hospital work. In such ways, he begins to withdraw from the hospital.

Yet while he is visiting hospitalized patients, the hospital serves him well. Many ex-residents have told us that the early months of practice are a lonely time: The hospital serves to counteract this isolation, affording a locale where they can meet and pass pleasant conversational moments with colleagues and residents. The hospital is also a locale where professional, albeit informal, advice can be had for more puzzling cases.

Once launched into practice, ex-residents are led further and further away from part-time hospital practice. In past years, a majority

[3]The mean questionnaire scores for our men were 4.4 for phychotherapy (4.5 is "high"), 3.2 for sociotherapy (4.0 is "high"), and 2.8 for somatotherapy (4.0 is "high"). This group corresponds to the New Haven A-P psychiatrists (see *ibid.*).

has entered upon the institutional ladder that leads, by the end of residency or soon after, to the Chicago Psychoanalytic Institute. Such young men have decreasing amounts of time to spend with patients, for the Institute eats up time. (It also has eaten up money, since a training analysis is required before candidacy.) The young psychiatrist begins to discover that office practice is more economical or at least requires less commuting. If he moves to the suburbs, his time becomes even more valuable and the hospital correspondingly less convenient. Besides, he often frankly admits that a hospital practice is something of a drag upon him physically: A hospitalized patient is more likely to phone at night, and hospital personnel can raise bothersome problems. The kinds of referral that he was pleased to get earlier, no longer please him so much. The further he progresses in analytic training, the more he is apt to be attracted, for purely intellectual reasons, by the types of patient seen in office practice.

There is a more important reason for young psychotherapists' abandonment of hospital practices: They have never intended to treat hospital patients past their early careers. With rare exceptions, they entered residency anticipating office practice. Although the first year of residency plunges them into administrative duties and has them treating hospitalized patients under supervision, few residents become permanently interested in administration or in hospitalized patients. Even during that first year, their attention is focused more upon supervision than upon hospitalized patients. During the next two years, they treat mainly clinic patients. After residency, they recognize that a few years must pass until they can manage a wholly office practice. Many also look forward to attending the Analytic Institute and developing concurrently a more psychodynamic practice. Such time as can be spared from practice they may devote to supervising residents, thus following the established pattern of a practitioner who also teaches. Even those ex-residents who do not go on to the Institute or to a more analytic practice conceive of practice mainly as composed of office patients.

Nevertheless, counterpressures and inducements do prevent a few from quickly or completely abandoning the hospital. From time to time, an older psychotherapist will treat a patient there — frequently an office patient who has come to need hospitalization. An occasional ex-resident does part-time research at PPI and finds it convenient to carry a few hospital patients also. In addition, PPI's associate director, who administered the residency program during the period of our research, has attempted to further residents' interest in hospital administration; partly by teaching classes in social psychiatry and also by encouraging residents, as well as recent graduates, to become coordinators of PPI's wards.

118

Whatever impact such programming may have had on the residents' therapeutic notions, it has had only minor impact on their career styles. Hospital administration does not yet command high prestige, and, to follow in the footsteps of PPI's present administrators, one must also possess genuine commitment to research. A psychoanalytic career carries much prestige in Chicago, as elsewhere, and there seems to be no decline of this prestige among these young physicians. Such careers will afford them relatively comfortable livings (although we would be hard put to make an accurate judgment of the relative weights of money and prestige — nor do we care to try). There is also no question that — given the supervision and training the PPI residents receive and despite *milieu*, transactional, and psychoanalytically emphases in the curriculum — the residents are prepared to be psychoanalytically oriented. Most do become analysts, in fact, or at least psychotherapists.

What this orientation means for the hospital, as now constituted, is that it affords a ready supply of young attending men who regularly treat patients there. Each young generation serves its period, often much enjoying its continued contact with the hospital and personnel and the intellectual and emotional pleasures of treating hospitalized patients. When at last these young physicians prepare to leave the hospital scene, another generation stands eager to take their places — for a time.

Speculation about the futures of these men is not too hazardous. Those who become full-fledged analysts probably will never return to any hospital practice. They will follow the more traditional path of supplementing an office practice with supervisory, committee, and occasionally teaching and research activities. For future PPI graduates, other contingencies exist. If the hospital becomes larger, more interest in administration may be generated, possibly abetted by the generally increasing prestige of hospital practice and administration throughout the metropolitan area. Much more likely is that residents may increasingly join the middle group of psychiatrists who are analytically oriented but not actually analysts. These psychotherapists may become interested in schizophrenics and psychotics, and such interests will lead them to remain associated with hospitals where those types of patient can be treated. But such careers belong to the future: Today's PPI resident is destined for private office practice after a brief apprenticeship divided between office and hospital.

THE ORGANIZATION OF TREATMENT

Like the somaticists, these men must take into account the hospital itself in organizing individualized treatments for patients. The hospital, with its rules and regulations, its resources and its possibilities, constitutes a framework within which they must work. But they also operate in an ideological framework, generally if loosely referred to as "a psychodynamic approach." During their training they have become committed to it, largely through the supervision of analysts (or analysts in training) and through conferences, seminars, and classes.

These two frameworks together result in a typical operational procedure. With few exceptions and despite some differences in therapeutic philosophy, most ex-residents regard the hospital as if it were a *set* of differentiated therapeutic environments. They utilize and manipulate the environments into which they place patients. These environments, along with face-to-face therapy, constitute the psychotherapist's main weapons. In order to prevent the reader from assuming that such an environmental emphasis signifies the practice of *milieu* therapy, we hasten to explain what these men actually do with their patients.

The hospital, it will be recalled, consists of five wards that vary, in terms of the central administration's conception, from the most open to the most closed. The psychotherapist recognizes the administration's map and on occasion utilizes it. But the administrative map is not a therapeutic map: The latter is a chart of the hospital's interior space according to the therapeutic consequences that may follow from placing patients upon various wards. The hospital's interior space is not pictured in the same way by each psychiatrist, but all do picture various wards according to *therapeutic* qualities and possibilities.

Here are some examples of those therapeutic dimensions. Wards can be viewed as locales in which varying amounts of "contact" are given a patient by the personnel; where he can receive varying amounts of stimulation from other patients; where he can experience varying degrees of external control over his own behavior; or where he can be confronted by varying necessities to exert control over his own behavior. Wards are locales where varying amounts of deliberately induced regression — prescribed by the psychiatrist — can be "tolerated" by the staff. There are some units in which a patient cannot get enough "support" and one large unit in which he can be "lost" in a crowd of other patients. Being lost, of course, may be therapeutically beneficial or not, depending upon the nature of the patient's condition. Conversely, there are wards that are conducive to the formation of intimate relationships among patients.

Where do the images of such therapeutic dimensions come from? In part, they derive from the psychiatrist's perceptions of certain common-sense features of the wards. Some wards, for instance, actually have high censuses of patients; some are of considerable physical size; some possess high ratios of personnel to patients; some have male aides; some tend to have more youngsters, while others tend to have numerous old people. But the therapeutic dimensions also derive, without question, from each psychiatrist's personal experiences — beginning early in residency — with treating patients upon certain wards. Through empirical experience he has discovered that certain wards seem beneficial, ineffective, or injurious for certain kinds of patient. He may also have discovered that certain wards are of dubious benefit for most of his patients, and therefore scarcely uses them.

Although some psychotherapists tend to map the hospital according to a rather limited set of therapeutic dimensions, we have actually seen them operate with somewhat different dimensions for each patient or at least for each type of patient. Consequently it is more accurate to say that each has a different map of the hospital for each of his patients. He will try to have his patient placed initially on a certain ward according to what he judges that patient needs most, whether it be "contact," confrontation with "reality," or something else. Of course, more than one therapeutic dimension may be simultaneously relevant to his treatment. (Actually, although the therapist may request that his patient be assigned initially to a given ward, the disposition depends on the ROD's judgment at the time of admission. The ROD* tends to go along with the request if it seems reasonable and if a bed is available. Often neither condition obtains.)

In other words, the psychotherapist takes into account only, or primarily, those aspects of the wards that appear relevant to his patient's condition. In so doing, he purposely ignores aspects important for treating other patients. This way of relating patients and wards places a premium upon the psychiatrist's ability to grasp the therapeutic possibilities of various wards. Even the most unimaginative pronounce given wards as useful, or not, for given kinds of treatment. The more ingenious the psychiatrist, the more therapeutic possibilities he is able to divine. With further experience, he may learn to imagine yet others. Each time that he brings in a different kind of patient, new therapeutic possibilities are likely to be revealed.

When such a psychiatrist has been successful in placing his patient upon a given ward, he has completed a considered action. He has had in mind how the environment may and may not affect his patient. But he may go further: He can attempt to control that setting to maximize its beneficial effects. He attempts to do so in

*The resident on duty.

121

two principal ways. First, he leaves "orders" that promote certain desirable possibilities for his patient. He may leave either written or verbal orders that his patient be treated with consistent firmness; be given "lots of contact"; or be forced to "confront reality" by certain treatments. A second technique for shaping the environment involves the psychiatrist's mangement of his patient's privileges. By expanding or contracting these privileges, the psychiatrist can transform the ward into different kinds of *milieu* for his patient. Thus a ward can be made relatively open by giving the patient opportunities to walk around the hospital or to visit friends on other wards. The patient may be cut off from communication with his family or allowed extensive telephone privileges. Even the most closed ward can be rendered relatively open for a patient by manipulating his privileges. Probably every attending man, regardless of his psychiatric ideology, attempts to manage the environments of his patients through proper orders and privileges, but the psychotherapeutically oriented shape those environments according to therapeutic design.

Actually, the matter is much more complicated for at least two further reasons. Since most patients whom the psychotherapists treat at the hospital have not previously been treated in their offices, the therapists must frequently spend days or weeks observing patients — either directly, or indirectly through nursing reports — in order to judge what is wrong and what would be appropriate treatment. A certain amount of trial and error, manipulation of order and privileges, and selective placement upon various wards may therefore take place. Another complication is that, after a therapeutic program has been decided upon, the patient's progress or retrogression usually calls for a reshaping of the therapeutic environment. For instance, when the patient has responded well to "firm control" by the nursing staff, the *milieu* can be made more "permissive" because the patient has developed "internalized controls."

This changing relationship of patient and environment is indeed a very important matter. It is important that one understand that the psychiatrist has a notion of "phasing" that has less to do with the patient's outward behavior than with his internal changes. (In later chapters, we shall discuss what happens when the nursing staff views a patient's phasing differently from his psychiatrist.) When a patient leaves one stage and enters another, the therapist has alternative options: He may reshape the *milieu* for his patient, or he may transfer him to a more appropriate ward. A patient who has "pulled himself together" sufficiently to have regained control over himself may either be allowed additional privileges or be transferred to more open and freer wards progressively until he leaves the hospital. Whether the psychiatrist chooses to transfer his patient or to reshape the ward setting, he is taking the *milieu* into account therapeutically.

Where then does psychotherapy fit into his treatment? One must keep in mind the wide spectrum of patients whom these physicians are called upon to hospitalize. Some patients are so bizarre, so sick, that psychiatrists rely upon ward settings more than upon their own face-to-face contacts with them. But at the other extreme, a patient may receive more benefit from some type of psychotherapy than from experiences on the ward. In any event, as we shall see in later chapters, the perceived relations between ward and psychotherapy are often very subtle. To take only one instance: A psychiatrist may place his patient on a given ward because he believes it possesses certain qualities; he may gather from nursing notes and conversation with the head nurse how his patient is responding to the *milieu;* he may further check this information through his therapeutic sessions; he may recognize certain processes taking place as a result of those sessions; he may pass on certain information and leave certain orders as a result of the sessions — and thus attempt to reshape his patient's environment.

On general ideological grounds, these physicians would insist to a man that psychotherapy is far more important than ward setting. They would deny that they are *milieu*therapists. They believe that there can be no basic change in a patient without adequate psychotherapy. But what is true in theory is not entirely relevant to their kinds of hospital practice. Few of their patients continue in office therapy after hospitalization. Nor are they really expected, although frequently advised or urged, to continue. For most hospitalized patients, the psychotherapists, like the somaticists, are willing to settle for less lofty aims. The principal aim is to get the patient back to society sufficiently improved to function better than previously. Hopefully the patient need not later return to the hospital, but perhaps he will. For these chronic or less "treatable" patients, the psychiatrist is often willing to admit that the hospital environment is more important than face-to-face therapy — or equally important or indistinguishable in impact — since each aspect of the total treatment is relevant.

This style of hospital practice can be visualized as if it were an elaborate game of chess: The therapist seeks to gauge his patient's therapeutic movement and relates that movement to various therapeutic strategies of his own; whether in shaping the environment, in transferring the patient from one environment to another, or in managing his therapeutic sessions with the patient. The analogy with the chess game, of course, is most striking when the therapist moves his patient around the hospital according to some over-all therapeutic plan.

Not that he fails to do certain conventional things: He may handle some patients very much as do the somaticists. For instance, he may use drugs, shock treatment, and a minimum of "talking" therapy for elderly depressives. Yet he tends to order less EST and relies less on drugs than do the somaticists. He tends to try psychotherapy, including ward strategy, with most patients before relying on EST. He is accused, by somaticists, of a disposition to let patients run through Blue Cross money without substantial improvement. Whether that is true or not, these psychiatrists are certainly less concerned to get patients speedily home. They have no firm philosophy that the quickest treatment is the best treatment, although, as we have said, with some patients they reach this conclusion; but in general they have more faith in longer psychotherapy and somewhat lengthier stays in the hospital.

This kind of hospital practice necessarily casts the psychotherapist into dramatic roles. He finds himself unable strategically to use the hospital without becoming a diplomat. Except in his simplest maneuvers, he cannot take ward settings for granted or merely utilize routine nursing care. Of course he frequently does, but to the extent that he wishes to control his patient's environment with more subtlety, he must make arrangements and have understandings with the nursing personnel that involve diplomatic negotiation. While somaticists must also negotiate, the psychotherapists must do much more of it because they cannot so easily rely on stable understandings and routine arrangements. To control what goes on around their patients they must negotiate, dicker, and "play ball," as well as order, caution, advise, and express wishes.

These therapists do not, however, necessarily have an unduly high regard for nurses and aides, nor do they attribute to such personnel great psychiatric understanding or capacity for comprehending treatment. The psychotherapists vary in the specific ways they handle nurses. Some spend much time talking with nurses; some display higher regard for them; some pay little or no attention to aides; some give more direction to the personnel in deportment toward the patient. Some are certainly good at this diplomatic game they must play with the nursing staff, but others are rather inept or perhaps too busy with burgeoning office practices to care. Whatever the variations in their handling of nurses, they share a single view of the *psychiatric* nurse: Some are better than others but mainly because of "intuition" or some gift for spontaneous understanding of certain patients, rather than because of genuine intellectual understanding. What is true of nurses is even more true of aides, who are classified as better or worse on grounds of interest in and concern with patients and because of native emotional capacities (they are maternal, warm, and so forth). Unquestionably, much that happens in the hospital and to patients stems from this view of the nursing personnel, in conjunction with the personnel's failure to recognize that not merely some, but virtually all, the psychiatrists share this view.

When organizing his patient's treatment, the psychotherapist must cope with certain inherent institutional problems discussed earlier in this chapter. He may reason that his patient belongs most properly on 2W, but if 2W is full his patient may have to be housed on 3EW. Later he may calculate that his patient should be transferred to a less restricted ward — but simultaneously the 3EW staff may discover that it cannot tolerate his patient. The psychiatrist may then find his patient actually transferred to a more closed unit. Then he is likely to complain that PPI, with its fast-moving turnover, cannot handle lengthier periods of therapy; that, although its personnel can be permissive with patients, they cannot maintain "a firm line"; that PPI would be a better hospital if his patients were not exposed to the talk of EST patients; that PPI's rules and regulations are designed more for keeping order than for true therapy. But it is striking that this group of psychiatrists generally finds the hospital rather a good locale for its practice. These men criticize and carp, and they have trouble with the staff and administration from time to time, yet their criticism of the hospital is neither acrid nor severe. They do not have clear conceptions of how a more nearly ideal hospital would operate. On the whole PPI suits their styles of hospital practice. If this attitude were not evident from interviews with them, we might have guessed it anyhow, for not one ex-resident has chosen to practice elsewhere in preference to PPI.

One final question about this style of practice requires an answer: How did these therapists learn to use the hospital as they do, since the chess game in which they are engaged is not simply a logical outcome of psychodynamic training and supervision? (We shall shortly see that not all psychotherapists do practice psychiatry this way.) The answer is not difficult to find. From the moment that the young physician steps into PPI's floors during his first week of residency, he hears of and sees the supposed therapeutic deficiencies and virtues of the various wards. He becomes aware of how very differently the attending men use the wards, whether for good or ill. As administrator of a ward, he finds himself in the midst of these conflicting views. He also has experience of the wards as a supervised resident, for he treats hospitalized service patients for three years. He finds himself maneuvering his patients around the hospital, just as ex-residents do. As important as anything else, however, is the absence of any clear alternative model for practicing at the hospital. He rejects what he believes is the somaticists' use of the hospital. (He typically enters residency with a bias against EST and is not supervised by somaticists.) The more idiosyncratic uses of the hospital, which will be described later, the resident does not recognize at all. To the extent that he enters into conversation with the few therapists who use the hospital differently, he notices specific strategies with particular patients, but he does not recognize that those strategies flow from models different from his own. This blindness is all the more noteworthy since some of his supervisors have never practiced in this kind of hospital, and some have not treated hospitalized patients for several years. All in all, the whole weight of the resident's training and experience biases him toward combining psychotherapy and ward strategy.

A few ex-residents use the hospital quite differently because — like some attending men trained elsewhere — they possess strong alternative models for organization of hospital treatment. It is significant that a few attending men who were trained elsewhere organize treatment exactly as do the ex-residents — mainly because they entered practice with no strong commitments to alternative models of hospital treatment. We turn now to the careers and hospital strategies of psychotherapeutically oriented men who fall into neither group of psychiatrists already discussed.

THE INDIVIDUALISTIC PSYCHOTHERAPISTS

There are approximately five such physicians who hospitalize patients regularly at PPI. Each displays an individualistic therapeutic stance, although each is psychotherapeutically oriented. All but one are psychoanalysts either in training or in fact.

The Hospital as an Enemy of Effective Psychotherapy

The first man whom we shall discuss was not trained at PPI. He is an analyst-in-training. To his referred patients, he says, " 'If you get overwhelmed and can't cope with it, why don't you come into the hospital; but if you cope . . . why don't we see how staying out will work?' I then leave the choice to them. I see them two or three times subsequently and if it is too overwhelming, I let them come in." The hospital is a less stressful locale for these patients. "As soon as they are able to meet the stress outside . . . out they go." Or they go into therapeutic sessions at his office. In short, hospitalization is only a stop gap period in which anxious, panicky, depressed, and other acutely distressed patients are temporarily separated from a stressful world.

During the period of grace, this psychiatrist tries to work precisely as if the patient were visiting his office for frequent psychotherapy. Unfortunately, PPI is far from ideal for that purpose: From his point of view, most of the hospital's physical structure and personnel actually obstruct his usual therapeutic aims. He therefore ordinarily requests that his patients be placed upon PPI's most open unit (2N) because that locale is least likely to have an adverse effect on his therapy. It is, he maintains, the least obstructive environment within PPI, for it is a comparatively open unit with a head nurse who has a permissive philosophy. If a patient seems too disturbed to the ROD responsible for new admissions, then our psychiatrist will compromise by requesting initial placement upon as open a unit as he reckons will be allowed. At the point when he thinks transfer to 2N will be acceptable, he requests the transfer.

All in all, he thinks that PPI is ridden with rules and is not permissive enough for patients. He regards its personnel as too easily upset by the "acting out" of patients and therefore as too quick to slap restrictions upon them and to transfer them to closed units. Indeed, patients "often get so involved in the relationship within the hospital, before you can get them settled and untangled from it, and start to work . . . with their therapeutic problems." The more restrictive the environment and the more tense the personnel, the more likely it is that a patient will get caught in nontherapeutic relationships — and the more likely he is to get into difficulties with staff members. Patients "on strictly controlled units end up in lots more problems with the hospital."

This therapist also has a psychodynamic rationale for his antipathy toward all units except the most open one. He has noticed that on:

> an open unit patients tend to pull together very tightly and quickly. You turn over to them as many ego functions as they possibly can handle — and many can handle much more than we give them credit for. They feel more secure and less panicky. For example, a person who feels helpless, weak, overwhelmed, when you put him in a closed type of environment it stimulates those feelings; and to reality-test all of this is sometimes an extremely long job — it may take you two or three years. The hospital stay isn't long enough to do this, so you always intensify the stimulation of paranoid, destructive, hostile feelings.

His basic strategy, therefore, is to minimize the destructive impact of the hospital environment by locating patients upon the most open units possible. Then the *milieux* can function to allow them some relief from the outside world.

Meanwhile the physician attempts to establish therapeutic relationships during face-to-face sessions. When the environment intrudes into that process, then he attempts to turn that intrusion to good purpose. For instance, the patient may complain about certain personnel or practices of the hospital.

> So you often end up with the problem, particularly with very perceptive patients, of pointing out that there's a certain neurotic distortion in the hospital structure; and say, "Yes, that is true. This [staff] person has such a problem, but this is reality. The problem for you is how you can cope with this." The patient may, for instance, come into the therapy session with a complaint that other patients got medicines from the nurses — but that he did not. The therapist will say, "How did this make you feel, when did it happen?" And so on. . . . The more sensitive patients . . . will say that they think this was deliberate. [I say] "How are you going to cope with it, let's see what it stirs up in you."

With such tactics, the therapist makes use of disturbances caused by the environment. As a correlative move, he must eliminate identification of himself with the hospital: "I have to disentangle myself and just say 'this is it. This is what you and I both have to cope with.' "

How does such a therapist regard the nursing personnel? Although he views most personnel as too restrictive, he recognizes that the more time he spends with them, the less likely they will be to eject his patient from their units. Occasionally he takes pains to talk about his patients with the nurses in order to lessen the possibility of such ejection. On the whole, he regards the personnel as distinctly peripheral to his own psychotherapy; he uses their relationships with his patient, whether stormy or not, mainly as material for the therapeutic sessions.

Although he occasionally places patients upon closed units, he definitely does not see the hospital as a set of potentially beneficial therapeutic environments. He sees the hospital environment in essentially two ways. It is a container that helps to separate patients from stressful home *milieux*. It is also a potentially antitherapeutic factor that may work against his therapy. He therefore seeks to neutralize the *milieu* as far as possible, and what cannot be neutralized is utilized as material for psychotherapy itself.

Such a conception of therapeutic practice within a hospital unquestionably has consequences for the therapist himself. Frequently he finds himself operating in enemy territory, at war, although not necessarily overtly, with the hospital and its personnel. Yet he does not enjoy this state of war. There is a further long-run consequence:

Although interested in schizophrenic patients and intellectually challenged by them, he finds himself gradually more disinclined to take on patients who need hospitalization. He is discovering that he derives similar satisfactions from activities other than treating hospitalized patients. To say that the hospital is defeating him would be to make too strong a judgment; it is safer to say that his and the hospital's approaches are sufficiently far apart to cause frequent strain for both him and the staff.

It is relevant that he believes psychiatry's greatest strides during the next decade will probably result from collaboration between the social sciences and psychiatry. He expects more basic discoveries to come from such a collaboration than from the further development of psychoanalysis, yet he himself has no personal interest in social psychiatry. His opinion is relevant both to his career and to his modes of practicing psychiatry in the hospital. What he is saying is that, although he appreciates abstractly the value of social psychiatry, it is not his meat. His own research and clinical interests do not include deep concern with environmental influences.

THE HOSPITAL AS A *Milieu* FOR EFFECTIVE INVOLVEMENT

A second psychiatrist, also an analyst-in-training, utilizes the hospital in quite a different manner from either his psychotherapeutic colleagues or the somaticists. What he seeks for his hospitalized patients is a locale in which both they and everyone around them can become deeply and therapeutically "involved" with one another. Although intense involvement is not so important for senile or depressive patients, he believes, it is essential to therapy for hospitalized schizophrenics. This therapist finds his real challenge in treating the latter.

His picture of the ideal hospital is one with full-time physicians and assisting personnel. A busy physician, dashing in and out of the hospital, has no time to build the necessary relationships either with patients or staff; nor can he build a ward structure within which optimal involvement will develop. Ideally, the staff psychiatrist — who would give psychotherapy to the patients — would share with all patients certain communications received during individual therapy sessions. In short, in an ideal hospital, a rich texture of communal therapeutic relationships would prevail.

But the real hospital within which he practices cannot supply this kind of *milieu* or can supply it only imperfectly. He finds that PPI's personnel are unable to become genuinely involved, especially with "acting-out" patients. He asserts that the hospital is best organized for the care of short-term cases, those who merely receive shock treatments or who can recover quickly from acute phases of illness. The hospital is inadequate for patients whose illnesses require lengthy stays: Its regulations and personnel are not up to the task.

Since this therapist cannot dream an ideal hospital into being, he has developed certain techniques for coping with an imperfect one. Like many other physicians, he pictures the ward system as a continuum between permissiveness and control. He tends to place patients on the most permissive wards possible and to further that permissiveness by allowing ample, if not maximum privileges. He hopes — almost literally prays — that his patients will draw staff members, as well as other patients, into therapeutic involvement. The latter's involvement is, if anything, more important than the staff's, although failure of the staff to become involved can be very destructive, especially since it frequently results in transfers to other wards.

No matter how often the staff has disappointed him by its inability to become involved, he continues to hope. If either a staff member or a patient becomes effectively involved with his patient, he capitalizes upon this involvement. He encourages it, speaks to the head nurse about it, and opposes transfer that would sever the therapeutic relationship. He will even oppose a transfer when the staff thinks his patient is well enough for a more open unit, since the existing therapeutic relationship seems more important than the mere openness of the ward.

Staff members sometimes become effectively involved, he believes, less because they are psychiatrically sophisticated than because they are unafraid, unanxious, and can leave themselves open to this kind of therapeutic relationship. He reasons that it is quite likely than an aide will be as effective in this respect as a nurse. In fact, he has given up coaching the nurses, although at one time he spent considerable time attempting to teach his version of good treatment. He has also ceased to fight furiously against transfers if no effective involvements have developed, since the wards are unlikely to become therapeutic worlds for his patients.

Because this psychiatrist is oriented psychotherapeutically, he believes that therapy sessions go hand in hand with the beneficial effects of properly organized *milieux*. He emphasizes his own psychotherapeutic efforts but also the patient's relationship with significant others. For this reason, he frequently attempts to reach the relatives of office patients and, if necessary, involves them in treatment with other therapists. To him, an ideally organized hospital would not differ radically from an ideally organized world for office patients: It would employ both effective psychotherapy and effectively developed involvements.

But it is difficult to treat schizophrenics without hospitalization. Because this therapist is greatly challenged by such schizophrenics, he is reluctant to surrender merely because PPI often frustrates his efforts. It should be evident that opposing forces play upon him — both encouraging and discouraging his continuation in hospital practice.

We may hazard certain predictions about this man's future relations with hospitals. He may of course, continue along his psychoanalytical path, abandoning his hospital practice. He may continue his current stormy relationship with PPI. He may use other hospitals that better approximate his ideal institution. Or he may even eventually run a hospital himself or at least share in administration. At the moment he is sufficiently challenged by schizophrenics to endure much on their account.

The Trusted Nurse Provides an "Intramural Setting" For Analytic Therapy

Another psychoanalyst considers psychotherapy to be the main instrument for helping hospitalized patients. But the hospital setting can interfere with psychotherapy unless one exerts control over it. He places his patients, if possible, in the hands of a particular head nurse for whom he has respect and with whom he has long had a general understanding. He attempts to keep his patient away from nurses whom he neither respects nor trusts. But good nurses and aides can be useful for supplementing his own therapy — for instance, by giving motherly warmth to his patient. Since many whom he treats at the hospital are very sick schizophrenics, he feels obliged to visit them frequently. Fortunately, this visiting tends to intensify the personnel's involvement with his patient: "The amount of involvement that you can have the auxiliary personnel get into depends in large measure on your own therapeutic investment."

On occasion, he must fight the administration to get a patient placed upon 2N, whose nurse he admires, but he is generally successful. Sometimes, certain ward characteristics seem important: for instance, the number of patients, if his patient does not "do well in crowds." But he sees the hospital's interior space mainly in terms of how co-operative the nurses are and how good an "intramural setting" each nurse provides for his own form of psychotherapy. His concern "has always been to try and establish within the hospital an intramural setting for analytic therapy . . . analytically oriented psychotherapy — or whatever you want to call it."

Naturally he encounters difficulties. His favorite nurse recently retired. Occasionally a patient causes much trouble, and then a threatened transfer becomes a problem. He pictures a more ideal setting for his type of therapy — and his type of patient: "If I could rub Aladdin's lamp and be permitted to wish only in terms of this hospital, I would wish that it were two buildings." One building would house patients who need treatment for acute psychoses and severe depressions, that is, who require pharmacological or electric shock treatment. The second building "would have a staff of full-time people who divide the responsibility of therapy and administration"; that is, personnel who know and trust one another. At PPI, the physician can neither be there for most emergencies nor give his patient a sense of continuous contact ("the sense of a person is lacking"). In an ideal hospital, physicians would be — and would feel — more a part of the establishment. What he really wishes, he says, is a psychoanalytic institute whose residency program is partly in an ideal hospital and partly in a hospital like PPI, the whole institutional setting — training, teaching, hospital, and practice — "welded into some kind of organizational whole."

The Hospital as an Over-all Therapeutic Support to Psychotherapy

The next psychiatrist has worked with hospitalized patients during his entire career: His early training (not at PPI) was in both neurology and psychiatry; later he added considerable psychoanalytic training. He has an office practice, but his more genuine intellectual interests lie with hospitalized patients. Since he is fascinated by work with acute schizophrenics, he brings many to the hospital. Because of his neurological training, referrals to him include some whom he hospitalizes for diagnosis of suspected organic defects. But it is his treatment of schizophrenics that makes his use of the hospital so different from that of his colleagues.

The primary element in his treatment is the therapeutic relationships between himself and his patients. But the over-all hospital setting is important as a facilitative agent: It "facilitates the psychotherapeutic program." How?

There are a number of displaced reactions to important people. And the manner in which the patient is treated by the ward personnel is, of course, interpreted in terms of the patient's past experiences. The manner in which copatients are treated is also part of the hospital experiences. The manner in which other patients can say what this patient may not be able to say — and how the personnel deals with them — is also part of the facilitative process in the hospital program. So although the psychotherapeutic session supposedly focalizes, concentrates, the main current of the therapeutic relationships, it is sustained and fed by the patient's relationships, especially on the unit with fellow patients and with the personnel. Further, since the setting of the hospital promotes the emergence of dependent relationships (which might have been denied on the outside), the various personnel lend themselves to satisfying or not satisfying these needs.

This therapist does not visualize the hospital's interior space as sharply differentiated. He tends to see wards along a continuum of "control." He will place a patient who needs overt control on 3N, for instance; yet on the whole he tends not to distinguish among the wards ('there are some categorical qualities, but I don't really feel there's too much difference"). Consequently he does not consider ward differences a "potent therapeutic factor." He believes that one need not "manipulate the patient and his environment too much." Rather, the "over-all therapeutic atmosphere of the hospital" is far more important than that of any specific ward. He feels "comfortable" at PPI, or he would practice elsewhere.

His perspective on the nursing personnel arises from these general considerations. Nurses have administrative tasks, and if their interest is aroused they may become involved with certain patients. But he does not attempt to utilize nurses as a direct therapeutic agent. Initially he offers only minimal commentary — then if nurses are interested enough to ask, he will generalize broadly about his patient's dynamics. Neither implicity nor explicitly does he attempt to involve the nurses in "the therapeutic situation," because he wishes to communicate that they and he have distinct (though sometimes overlapping) tasks. He expects that his patients will form therapeutic relationships with personnel and other patients. If the personnel cannot tolerate a particular patient and demand a transfer, he will spend time with them and will call a staff conference. If these tactics fail, however, he will usually suffer transfer graciously — since he believes that the hospital itself is generally therapeutic, rather than any specific ward. Furthermore, to win over the nursing personnel, he depends principally upon his own intense interest in difficult patients; this interest causes personnel to tolerate such patients longer than they otherwise might.

SUMMARY OF THE INDIVIDUALISTIC STYLES

These men share a common lively interest in acutely schizophrenic hospitalized patients, and on this point they differ from the majority of their analytically trained colleagues in Chicago, most of whom either prefer office practice or drop their hospital cases as they grow older. With the exception of the first psychiatrist, none is likely to abandon hospital practice soon. But the differences among these therapists are worth highlighting. In the process, certain other similarities should also emerge.[4]

Only the first psychiatrist places total emphasis upon his own therapeutic interactions with his patients. To him, the hospital environment appears either neutral or antitherapeutic — mainly the latter. He believes that the most neutral environment at PPI is its most open unit. To maintain control over the environment, he must both negotiate with the unit's personnel and do his utmost to keep his patient on that unit. Otherwise, he believes the hospital environment is irrelevant to the therapeutic process — except for cases of destructive purposes, that is, neutralized and made constructive by the psychotherapist.

The second psychiatrist considers the primary agents of therapy to be two: his own psychotherapy and the involvement of other patients and staff with his patient. How is the latter to be achieved in a hospital whose environment is otherwise antitherapeutic? The desired involvement is a matter of pure chance because the hospital is not organized for promoting it. But once involvement occurs, the therapist capitalizes upon it. He does his best to block transfer from the unit in question. He encourages and supports such therapeutic relationships. In his own practice of psychotherapy there is purposeful interplay between what goes on during the ward hours and what goes on during the therapy session. In an ideal hospital, the therapist himself would be part of the system of "personal involvement."

A third psychiatrist emphasizes the psychotherapeutic sessions but reasons that hospital personnel can serve as therapeutic agents in minor ways if they are interested enough in his patients. He therefore attempts to place his patients with a trusted head nurse. With proper understanding and a bit of luck, the patient will not be transferred from her unit. There occurs an interplay between the psychiatrists therapeutic practice and the staff's therapeutic actions, although the former is primary. If the patient is transferred or if the therapist can find no suitable head nurse, then he relies on psychotherapy alone. PPI then provides less an antitherapeutic than a nontherapeutic setting.

The fourth psychiatrist considers his own therapeutic relationships as primary, although they can be supplemented by relationships established by his patient with significant others upon the wards. He believes that the latter relationships inevitably develop regardless of

4Their mean scores on our questionnaire were: 4.8 for psychotherapy (4.5 is "high"), 3.8 for sociotherapy (4.0 is "high"), and 2.1 for somatotherapy. The pattern of individual distributions was highly individualistic, for instance, one man scored 4.6, 4.9, 1.4; another scored 3.1, 5.1, 2.0; and another 3.7, 4.6, 2.1.

the patients locations within the hospital, for he regards the hospital itself as generally therapeutic. The psychiatrist encourages such relationships, and prefers them to continue — but if transfer threatens, he is not too upset, for he believes that similar relationships will develop elsewhere.

Clearly the first two psychiatrists tend to focus upon the antitherapeutic potentials of the hospital fearing the effects both upon the patients and upon their own therapeutic relationships with them. The other two psychiatrists do not so sharply dichotomize the hospital's potential and are therefore less likely to war, overtly or covertly, with the hospital personnel. The second and the fourth men, however, place more weight upon ward relationships and especially upon those that develop among patients. The third psychiatrist also gives some weight to his patient's relationships with personnel but does not emphasize relationships with other patients. The second man, although he does focus upon the hospital's potentially negative effects, focuses more strongly upon the amazingly beneficial impact of a truly therapeutic *milieu*. Only he among this aggregate of psychiatrists prizes the *milieu* so strongly. Conversely, only the first man underplays the *milieu's* positive effects, scarcely recognizing any positive interplay between his own therapeutic relations and his patient's relationships with others. None of these men thinks of the ward as usually a potent therapeutic agent; and characteristically none does much maneuvering of patients from ward to ward — unlike most of their psychotherapeutically oriented colleagues at PPI.

One final question: Do the styles of these men represent merely the narrow adaptations of one basic psychotherapeutic position to the urgent requirements of this particular hospital? We may not assume that the four styles exhaust the range manifested by psychotherapeutically (or psychoanalytically) oriented men across the nation. We can assume only that the four styles represent a fair sample of the variation possible within the spectrum of the psychotherapeutic orientation — although how much variation is possible one cannot tell without investigation. For our purposes, a most important point is that psychotherapeutically oriented therapists may emphasize rather different elements of the total orientation and build their main strategies about those emphases. Probably they do so in their office practices as well as in the hospital. During interviews with *all* the attending men, we were struck by the passionate or firm convictions displayed concerning the proper ways to treat hospitalized patients. Who is right and who is wrong in their estimates is not the issue here, but how these convictions affect the actions and styles of the various physicians in this hospital.

Since most information reported in this chapter was gathered from interviews with physicians, it is pertinent now to ask whether or not it is general knowledge throughout the hospital.

The basic distinction between PPI's somatic group and its nonsomaticists is widely recognized: There are those who use a great deal of EST, and those who do not. All but the newest personnel understand this crude distinction and have a fair grasp of the first group's general styles; of its careers, however, only the central administration and a few residents are usually aware.

With regard to psychotherapeutically oriented physicians, the situation is more complicated. All but the newest nurses and aides recognize that many are ex-residents and generally understand that they use drugs or shock less and tend to work more closely with personnel. Yet there is much more about these men that is not understood. Few nurses and aides really understand, for example, why these young men are practicing at PPI or the relation of such practice to budding careers. Again, everyone understands that these men generally spend more time talking or doing more "therapy" with patients than do the EST physicians, but even central administration has not recognized the chessboard strategy so characteristic of these therapists. More important, the nurses and aides do not genuinely comprehend — and this point is pertinent to our chapter on nurses — how their own nursing efforts are regarded; they attribute to themselves far more important therapeutic functions than do these physicians.

It is safe to say that none of the hospital staff recognizes that the men whom we have termed "individualists" are any different from most psychotherapists. Their identities are indistinct because they share characteristics with the other psychotherapists, spending much time with patients and giving very little EST. Several are highly regarded because they treat difficult patients with apparent skill and one can learn from them. When the nursing personnel run into trouble with any of these physicians, they think about him in relation to specific patients — not recognizing that the trouble arises principally from his mode of practice. As one head nurse spiritedly remarked:

> I've always had more difficulties with him than with some other doctors. Remember Johnny Scott — with him Dr. Sloan told me just to hold him on your lap! He really meant it! But it wasn't realistic. He never quite understood Johnny's outbursts until he got in on it — the way he'd hit people. "It's your unit," Dr. Sloan would say, "it's a disturbed unit, isn't it; that's what you are here for. You're

not the kind of nurse that can hold him on your lap?" And Johnny yelling things like "F— you."

When certain physicians are recognized as difficult to work with on case after case, the difficulty is described principally in terms of broken rules. One head nurse said:

> Dr. Livy is a good example of someone who we have trouble with. It seems that everyone of his patients that comes in, there has to be some kind of special exception made for. . . . Dr. James likes to make special exceptions for his patients. . . . Another is Dr. Purdy: Almost everyone of his patients get special individual attention or special treatment of some sort.

In speaking of Dr. James, the first individualist we discussed, she recognizes that "he tends to put them on more open units when probably they would do better on a more closed unit," but she scarcely recognizes why he follows this practice. Even those residents who have had opportunities to exchange therapeutic views with these physicians do not understand how differently they tend to use the hospital. Probably the central administrators do not recognize this difference either, although they certainly do recognize sometimes that a given physician is employing a special therapy for a given patient. Sometimes the administrators believe that one of these men is using the hospital for a specific patient as it cannot efficiently be used.

Some of the interaction between physicians and hospital personnel turns upon the kind and amount of comprehension that personnel have of the physician's therapeutic styles. We leave to the next chapters detailed considerations of that comprehension, adding only that those psychotherapists most highly regarded and liked are those who seem to have — to quote one nurse — "a good idea of how the hospital functions." That is, they do not "break the regulations" (upset the ordinary expectations of ward personnel) too much, and they do "make us feel as if the work we are doing really contributes to what they're doing . . . and they let us know what is going on with their patients."

PATTERNS OF MOBILITY WITHIN INDUSTRIAL ORGANIZATIONS*

(with Norman H. Martin)

The organizational structure of an industrial enterprise has dual and interrelated functions. From the standpoint of management, it provides for an orderly hierarchy of responsibility and authority — a division of work rationally planned to meet the objectives of efficient operation. Vertical and horizontal movement of personnel through the various positions making up the organization is executed so as to make certain that competent men get in the right places at the right time. From the standpoint of the individual member, on the other hand, organization provides a stable set of expectations as to how they, as well as others, should act. Of equal importance, it provides a number of channels through which mobile individuals can move to realize personal objectives.[1]

This paper centers specifically upon the mobility aspects of industrial organization — upon the patterned movements of personnel within companies. It aims at developing a frame of reference for the interpretation and understanding of the phenomena of mobility within organizations.[2]

[1] This point of view has received considerable attention (see Chester I. Barnard, *The Functions of the Executive* [Cambridge: Harvard University Press, 1947]).

[2] A considerable literature on occupational mobility has developed within recent years. Perhaps the most comprehensive general work on this subject is W. Lloyd Warner and James C. Abegglen, *Occupational Mobility in American Business and Industry* (Minneapolis: University of Minnesota Press, 1955). Two other works may be cited: Oswald Hall, "The Informal Organization of Medical Practice in an American City: Case study of a Profession" (unpublished Ph.D. dissertation, Department of Sociology, University of Chicago, 1944), and Howard S. Becker, "Role and Career: "Problems of the Chicago Public School Teacher" (unpublished Ph.D. dissertation, Department of Sociology, University of Chicago, 1952).

*Reprinted by permission from
JOURNAL OF BUSINESS
Vol. 29, 1956, pp. 101-110.
Copyright © 1956, The University of Chicago

THE DEVELOPMENT OF CAREER LINES

Over time, the paths of movement of personnel through the system of positions making up a company's organizational structure tend to become more or less stabilized. Patterns of vertical and horizontal movement evolve, to form various types of career lines which terminate at various levels of the management hierarchy. These career lines, which are somewhat analogous to the trunks and branches of trees, provide escalators for mobile individuals.

The majority of these lines are minor and terminate at lower executive levels; others move beyond these positions and branch off into middle management; a few major lines lead to the top. A typical career line consists of a series of vertical and horizontal movements from position to position, i.e., vertical movement from section leader to department head within a given division; horizontal movement from department head to department head in different divisions; following this, vertical movement to division head; and so on. Ideally, horizontal mobility — the movement of an individual laterally along a given level of management — gives that person breadth of experience. Vertical mobility, of course, is movement of an individual up or down in the management hierarchy and consists of shifts from one level of responsibility to another.

Within the total complex of positions, certain ones operate as critical junctures or testing points. The performance of the individual at these crucial points determines the type of career line along which he will move — whether he moves on along a line to intermediate or higher management, horizontally to other line or staff jobs, or terminates his career at the level involved.

Typically, these turning points are quasi-training positions. For example, in the production division of one large company, the positions of assistant division manager and plant superintendent serve this function. Management can directly observe the individual being considered for higher management. They can determine his capacity to handle complex human relationships, to assume the initiative in unstructured situations, to handle responsibility, and to be adept at long-range decision-making — all of which are characteristic situations confronting higher management. If his performance is judged to be satisfactory, he moves into a line of progression leading to higher management; if it is somewhat less than satisfactory, he may be moved horizontally for further testing and training, or he may be moved into the next highest position, to remain there for the duration of his career.

At any given level in the executive hierarchy alternative channels of potential movement are present. In some instances these channels are multiple; the individual may move in any one of several directions — vertically or horizontally. In other instances the alternatives are more restricted and may even be closed. They are dead ends. This frequently happens in highly specialized types of jobs. In the case of those positions which function as critical turning points, numerous alternative paths of movement exist. This is necessary so that management can protect itself in cases where they have mistakenly judged the competence of an individual.

In order to make certain that competent and trained individuals move into the right places at the right time, more or less exact and differential training is provided at the various positions. At certain levels this takes the form of highly technical training in specific functions and areas; at others it is oriented toward the development of breadth of experience. This focus is related to a number of variables: the technological requirements of the industry, the type of organization, and the mobility structure.

For example, in one organization with a complex technology and division of labor, the pattern of movement of mobile personnel through lower levels of management is primarily vertical. Little horizontal movement occurs. Training is highly specialized. A primary concern of the management is to make certain that its first-line supervision is technically specialized. Interdepartmental coordination consequently becomes a primary function and the responsibility of middle management.

In contrast, another organization with a relatively simple technology has developed a mobility pattern in which a high degree of horizontal mobility exists at the lower executive levels. The aim of training here is to achieve a variety of experience in first-level supervision and, by so doing, to localize responsibility for coordination well down in the management hierarchy. Its organizational structure is relatively flat. In both instances, therefore, a relationship holds between mobility structure, technology, organization philosophy, and type of training. It becomes a major problem in management to achieve the right blending of these components.

The speed at which individuals move along specific career lines tends to follow fairly identifiable timetables. Acceptable age ranges are identifiable for the various strata. While these age ranges are not usually defined explicitly, they nonetheless exist in terms of some of the criteria used by management in determining who moves and who does not. A given individual being considered for advancement may, for example, be passed over because he is "too old" or, less frequently, "too young." If an individual does not move out of a given position and into another by a certain age, there will be a high probability that he will never move farther. He will, in a sense, have his mobility terminated at that level.

The existence of these career timetables enables individuals to assess their mobility prospects and even to predict their chances of advancement to higher levels. A person who does not progress in accordance with these age timetables may know, therefore, that his potential for higher levels of management has been judged unfavorably.

In general, individuals who ultimately reach higher levels in the management hierarchy tend to move rapidly along specific career lines leading to the top. Warner and Abegglen in their studies of occupational mobility in American business and industry note: "Within fifteen years of becoming self-supporting, more than half of the men studied were major executives and a quarter were minor executives."[3]

In order to facilitate the progression of men into higher executive levels and still achieve requisite competence, a skipping of levels may frequently be observed. An individual moves in an orderly manner from one position to the next and from level to level up to a point. He then moves around a given layer of management to a higher position in the hierarchy. In this manner relatively young men assume top-management responsibilities.

Horizontal and vertical movements, therefore, mesh and mutually support each other. On the one hand, horizontal movement may be thought of as being in the service of the vertical in the sense that a company is concerned with training and educating people and testing potential executives. They are also finding terminal places for mediocrity and taking care of those who were misjudged or who faded out. Gaps created by unforeseen circumstances must be filled by trained individuals with a minimum of delay, trouble spots taken care of by shifting versatile men along the line. On the other hand, although perhaps in a more minor sense, we may conceptualize the vertical system as being in the service of the horizontal. It is essential that the executive positions in all the various divisions of a company be staffed by competent and trained personnel. Major and minor career lines exist. These lines siphon off executives into the various levels and divisions. Thus there must be more or less permanent works managers and division superintendents; likewise there must be general foremen and plant superintendents. These people come from off the major vertical ladder — either on their way up or on their way off; others move directly into these positions via subsidiary and more minor career lines. From

[3]Warner and Abegglen, *op. cit.*, pp. 116-117.

142

the standpoint of the student of organization, all these interlocking horizontal and vertical movements add up to an organized system.

At this point it may be well to cite a concrete illustration of some of the already made points. Our example is a large, multi-plant industry engaged in the production of automobile parts. Movement of personnel through the lower levels of the management hierarchy is almost exclusively vertical. Little or no horizontal mobility exists at these lower levels. When it does occur, it tends to be limited to movement within one plant and between departments and is an indicator of unsatisfactory performance.[4] The position of general foreman (the top position at foremen levels) is the initial juncture or crossroads for mobile personnel. Individuals whose performance is highly satisfactory move on into superintendencies or may even jump beyond into higher positions. Those judged to be less competent may be shifted horizontally or may stay where they are.

Considerable horizontal movement of personnel occurs at the middle-management levels. Indeed here, in contrast to lower levels, failure to move horizontally is an indicator of only mediocre performance. This horizontal mobility occurs not only within the various departments and divisions of a single plant but also between plants. It brings about breadth of experience and also enables management to judge the potential of the men and to decide whether they should be moved into branch lines terminating in middle management or into career channels leading to top executive positions. This level is therefore a second critical juncture. At the higher executive levels the pattern of movement again tends to be primarily vertical.

Identifiable timetables of progression exist. Individuals must have moved through the foreman ranks and be ready for middle management at latest by the time they are around thirty-five years of age. Otherwise they tend to remain in lower-management positions. Between the ages of thirty and forty, they perform at middle-management levels and are seasoned, as it were, by a variety of experience. Upward movements out of this level must generally occur before the individual reaches forty or, at a maximum, forty-five.

In the company being discussed the main career line to the top centers in the largest of the plants. Most top executives have re-

---

[4]The situation is analogous to that frequently encountered in officer candidate schools during World War II. A candidate about whom there was some doubt as to capacity was given a series of trials in various positions. Horizontal mobility was an indicator of possible failure.

ceived the bulk of their training here. From the standpoint of the mobile individual it becomes imperative that sooner or later he get into the career lines of that plant. The characteristics of this career line, therefore, are quite specific: movement up is relatively rapid and clearly defined; youthful age limits circumscribe times by which movement must be made; horizontal mobility at certain crucial junctures is well planned to insure adequate training and testing; the final sequence of positions centers within the largest of the several plants.

In addition to this main career line, branch-off lines lead to middle-management positions. Movements along these lines are not so rapid as that characterizing those who move higher. At some point or other along the career line a faltering or a stumbling occurred, with the result that extra horizontal mobility was necessary. Sometimes these men were held at a given position well beyond the critical age range; at other times they were blocked by competitors who were more powerfully sponsored. On the other hand, some of these careers lines are purely local. Movement is confined to one of the smaller plants.

THE MOBILITY STRUCTURE FROM THE STANDPOINT OF THE INDIVIDUAL

From the standpoint of the mobile individual — the person ambitious to move ahead and up — the established patterns of movement in an organization present avenues of advancement. The perceptive individual can, for the most part, determine the channels through which he must move in order to realize his personal ambitions. Cues by which he can assess his own position and his potential for future advancement exist in a variety of forms.

One fundamental cue is the pattern of advancement already established — the complex of vertical and horizontal movements leading to specific levels of management. This, coupled with the timetables setting the ages at which movement must take place, enables him to judge his own progress. Given a stable organization, he can frequently do this with considerable accuracy.

Other cues are more subtle. At times it is difficult to determine whether a movement is a promotion or a demotion. This is especially true when we realize that too much horizontal mobility may actually act as a demotion unless it is coupled with ultimate vertical movement. The individual is growing older, and his mobility potential thereby becomes more limited because of the existence of timetables of advancement. In some industries this is so clearly realized that young executives refuse to accept more than one or two horizontal movements.

A similar comment is applicable to movements into staff positions. These positions are frequently filled by individuals who have not "made the grade" in the line. Such personnel, however, are mixed with others who are definitely competent and are there for clear reasons of function. It requires considerable discernment on the part of the mobile individual to determine the category into which he falls.

From the standpoint of pure tactics, the mobile individual would do well to become attached to a sponsor — an individual in a superior position who can pull him along. Over and beyond this, he must also acquire the ways of behavior acceptable to higher management. This means that he must, in a sense, secede from the ways of thinking and behavior of the management level in which he holds membership and adopt, instead, the norms and orientation of the level to which he aspires. A sort of "anticipatory socialization" must occur; the values of the higher group are taken as a fundamental frame of reference by the mobile person. This process, however, is not without its difficulties. Merton brilliantly characterizes the difficulty as follows:

> What the individual experiences as estrangement from a group of which he is a member tends to be experienced by his associates as repudiation of the group, and this ordinarily evokes a hostile response. As social relations between the individual and the rest of the group deteriorate, the norms of the group becomes less binding for him. For since he is progressively seceding from the group and being penalized by it, he is the less likely to experience rewards for adherence to the group's norms. Once initiated, this process seems to move toward a cumulative detachment from the group, in terms of attitudes and values as well as in terms of social relations. And to the degree that he orients himself toward out-group values, perhaps affirming them verbally and expressing them in action, he only widens the gap and reinforces the hostility between himself and his in-group associates. Through the interplay of dissociation and progressive alienation from the group values, he may become doubly motivated to orient himself toward the values of another group and to affiliate himself with it. There then remains the distinct question of the objective possibility of affiliating himself with his reference group. If the possibility is negligible or absent, then the alienated individual becomes socially rootless. But if the social system realistically allows for such change in group affiliations, then the individual

estranged from the one group has all the more motivation to belong to the other.[5]

SPONSORSHIP

Progression of individuals along given career lines is not only a result of technical competence and of being available and trained at the right time. A major influence determining who moves and how far is the action of a sponsor. In many instances, and especially at higher levels, this is almost a necessary condition for mobility.

The relationship of sponsor and protege tends to be a reciprocal one of mutual benefit and occurs for a variety of reasons: the protege may complement his superior by being strong in an area of activity where his sponsor is weak; he may serve in a role as detail man, adviser, or confidant. Regardless of reasons, when the sponsor rises, the protege moves with him. From the standpoint of the protege, therefore, he benefits by being pulled up in the hierarchy.

A given sponsor may have a cluster of proteges surrounding him. Ties of loyalty as well as need compel him to push for advancing "his men" as he moves up. As a result, top-management echelons of many companies are made up of interlocking cliques — certain powerful sponsors and their adherents. The mobility patterns in any organization are, therefore, to a considerable extent influenced by the phenomenon of sponsorship.[6]

Such arrangements are not without merit. From the standpoint of efficiency, it is possible for work to get done in an easy manner. Many smoothly working teams of executives evolve. Solidarity is high; common values and styles of action make for consistent behavior. On the negative side, however, the play of "internal politics" can create conflicts and anxiety. Executives who are not members of the cliques may be short-circuited and even undermined. Organizational efficiency may suffer. Serious problems develop when proteges lost their sponsors either because they are dropped or because the sponsor himself loses power because of shifts within the organization. The organization is then faced with the problem of working with individuals who no longer have a place within the scheme of things.

[5]Robert K. Merton and Alice S. Kitt, "Reference Group Theory and Social Mobility," in *Class, Status, and Power: A Reader in Social Stratification,* ed. Reinhard Bendix and Seymour M. Lipset (Glencoe: Free Press, 1953), pp. 409-10.

[6]Two excellent articles may be pointed out: Everett C. Hughes, "Queries concerning Industry and Society Growing Out of Study of Ethnic Relations in Industry," and Orvis Collins, "Ethnic Behavior in Industry: Sponsorship and Rejection in a New England Factory," in *Human Relations in Administration,* ed. Robert Dubin (New York: Prentice-Hall, Inc., 1951), pp. 240-49.

The existence of systems of sponsorship and resultant problems have been well documented in the histories of large companies. The history of the Ford Motor Company — and this is by no means an isolated example — clearly spells out processes of sponsorship and the results of powerful sponsors leaving the company. Harry Bennett, one of the recent powers in that organization, makes the succinct comment, "Well, Edsel and I had this much in common: When he went, he left a lot of 'orphans' in the plant; and when I left, so did I."[7]

To cite another example: The vice-president in charge of sales of a large industrial concern resigned his position for personal reasons. During the course of his career, he had sponsored several individuals into positions as department sales managers. While these managers were competent enough and remained in their positions, it soon became apparent that the new vice-president was not going to move them higher into zone and district positions. Their techniques of operation did not fit into his philosophy and strategies. Other individuals were promoted around them. Their reactions varied: one became passive and did only the minimum work required; another began to build a little empire of his own, communicating with associates and higher management only when required; others became hostile and aggressive. In brief, they became problems for management.

It would appear that the organizational structure of any concern is a result of the interplay of several factors. Ideally, such a structure should be the result of rational planning and should be developed in accordance with an over-all theory of management and policy. Actually, however, other factors, e.g., individual personalities, play a decisive role. Executives become concerned with developing their own positions and extending their power; positions are created; power struggles evolve. While this is not a universal phenomenon, it is of sufficient generality to be reckoned with. It comes directly to the fore in the activities of sponsors. Here the power structure is superimposed upon the rationally conceived organization. Career lines are frequently affected, causing changes which have an impact both upon management objectives of achieving an orderly and effective system of executive development and upon the mobility aspirations of conscientious and ambitious personnel.[8]

[7]Harry Bennett, *We Never Called Him Henry* (New York: Gold Medal Books, Fawcett Publications, Inc., 1951), p. 166.

[8]It is not intended that a moral judgment of good or bad be made here. Our intention is simply to point out the existence of power structures in many concerns and to indicate their impact, an impact that should be taken into account by management.

The meshing of horizontal and vertical movements of personnel is not always perfect. Individuals are moved into positions prematurely, sponsors drop proteges, and miscalculations are made. Problems are therefore created which must be dealt with. Incompetent individuals have to be moved into positions where they cannot do serious damage but where their experiences can still be used; frustrated mobility drives must be diverted into harmless channels. In any organization such malfunctioning and changes are inevitable.

The correction most obviously takes the form of firing, but more subtle means are frequently used, such as open or concealed demotion and arrest of further promotion, which common parlance refers to as "kicking a man upstairs," "shunting him to another department," and "banishment to the sticks." Indeed, unless an organization is willing openly to remove personnel from important positions by outright firing or demotion, it must resort to less blunt tactics.[9] These techniques are well worth studying, for they are related to organizational functioning in determinable and important ways. Why a man is demoted or blocked, how, when, and what are his responses, may be fateful, or at least significant, both for the person and for the organization.

Unless the incompetent individual is fired, he frequently is not told bluntly or directly that he is being removed from a position because of failure in meeting company requirements. The typical procedure is simply that the man receives his orders from an appropriate superior, usually without much choice of alternative, and must shift to the new position within a matter of days. He may know or guess that he has failed, but there are hedges for his hurt ego in so far as he is shunted or promoted rather than openly fired or demoted.

Such removals from positions have been termed "cooling out" by one sociologist, Erving Goffman,[10] who has borrowed the term from the con man's vocabulary. There it refers to the psychological disturbance which arises when the "mark's" ego is hurt after he discovers that he has been "taken" by the con man; therefore, the latter usually provides a mechanism whereby the victim will be

[9]The recent *Fortune* magazine article on *"How To Fire an Executive"* (October, 1954), by Perrin Stryker, suggests that expulsion of top personnel is neither a simple matter nor necessarily the method of demotion most practiced.

[10]Erving Goffman, "On Cooling the Mark Out: Some Aspects of Adaptation & Failure," *Psychiatry,* XV (1952), 451-63.

cooled out; otherwise he will go to the police or create other embarrassing disturbances. Like the con man, any organization, Goffman suggests, must protect itself against the consequences of demoting its members by seeking to minimize humiliation and loss of self-esteem.

There are numerous organizational methods for cooling out, but any given organization cannot make casual selection among them. These methods flow both from the organizational structure and from accepted ways of behavior. If horizontal movement, for example, is used, then a flexible organizational structure must exist. Otherwise there would be no place to shunt these men. Assigning them to staff positions requires the practice of a staff philosophy of management. Movement per se, indeed, must be a part of the accepted ways of behavior.

Thus in one concern studied — an organization with a broad and flexible system of positions — horizontal shunting, either within branches or between branches, is combined with honorific or terminal promotions. Occasionally, and especially at the upper ranks, a relatively functionless post is created to slide a man into. Staff positions, therefore, frequently function as receptacles for incompetency. These methods of removing men are closely linked with the nature of the vertical and horizontal mobility routes in the company.

Among other methods for cooling out, we might mention the following: use of seniority to slow up promotions, destruction of mobility drives, forcing of resignation, open demotion, bribing the failure out of the organization, progressive down-grading by merging departments, continual and rapid transfer from one branch to another, and continued bypassing. In some instances an organization has occasion to cool out men temporarily, often with the tacit or overt understanding that the move is not permanent. Sometimes this happens when a man is promoted too rapidly to be competent at handling his post. He is then shunted to another department or division at the same rank. If he fails again, he is given a terminal promotion.

RESPONSES TO BEING COOLED OUT

There are both short- and long-range responses to the cooling-out process. The former are probably less important, both for the men themselves and for the company. Some men, as we have pointed out, temporarily withdraw, become hostile, apathetic, and morose. Overt hostility seems to be more characteristic of men at lower levels; higher up, there appears to be an attempt at covering up, carrying on, and putting a good public face on the matter. The long-range responses are more serious. We have already pointed out some of these in our illustrations of the effects of sponsors dropping proteges. At lower levels, supervisors may become antimanagement in orientation. They may strongly identify downward, turning, as it were, to face-to-face relationships with employees for their chief work satisfaction. At higher levels executives may become increasingly intractable and develop a tough, hard-boiled quality and an individualistic philosophy which makes them treasure autonomy. They may come to look upon their departments or divisions as private bailiwicks and develop possessive attitudes toward them. Along with this goes a rationale or myth of indispensability. Superiors find them unduly centered upon their own departments and complain that communication between themselves and these department heads is poor. They tend not to delegate authority properly, gathering control into their own hands. This means that they provide inadequate training for rising subordinates.

Such long-range effects of personal failure within the organization call forth answering responses from the organization. We might visualize this as a series of gestures taking place over a lengthy period of time. The company makes judgments upon men, cools out those who fail in specific ways, is met with answering responses from the men, and in turn must respond to their responses. The company has to set some of its internal policy, therefore, to take into account such untoward and unforeseen eventualities as the intractableness of executives who have been cooled out.

There are several approaches which companies use in responding to such situations. Training programs and seminars frequently are useful in broadening the perspectives of these men. Attempts are made to build up their self-esteem by broadening their responsibilities and giving them special assignments. In still other instances companies respond by formalizing channels or communication — by forcing such executives to make periodic reports. Frequent horizontal shifting tends to break down departmental thinking and possessiveness and to nip in the bud any potential colleagueship of these executives stemming from their similar predicaments. From the standpoint of organizational structure, it may even be necessary to create staff positions to house those who have been kicked upstairs.

Thus the organizational strategies for handling partial or complete failures of personnel are many and add up to a complex system of policy acts. Such a system for handling failure is integral to getting men allocated, jobs done, and administrative leaders, high and low, picked, trained, and developed.

A stable organization and a systematic meshing of methods of cooling out thus go hand in hand. A system of mutually supporting methods wherein those methods do not run excessively afoul of one another cannot exist when the organization is undergoing great policy changes or has just terminated a major power struggle. Major organizational changes eventuate not merely in the supplanting of old demotional procedures by new ones but in the piling-up of old. The picture is further complicated because in large organizations shifts of power go on continually with different degrees of speed and intensity in the several component divisions. These may be expected to affect, directly or indirectly, the cooling-out procedures of each.

IMPLICATIONS

It is believed that the ideas set forth in the preceding sections provide a substantially correct picture of certain significant aspects of the mobility structure found within industrial organizations. The main outline of these ideas should serve to provide a basis for further investigation into this highly relevant facet of industrial management.

We have pointed out several important elements of mobility structures and have emphasized the necessity to view this structure within the context of the over-all organization and its history. In venturing this interpretation, we have pointed to some of the significant problems which must be faced as a result of the malfunctioning of the mobility process.

Further research and ultimate refinement and expansion of these ideas are, of course, necessary. Different types of mobility patterns are certain to be found, for it may be predicted that varying types of companies will evolve differing sequences of movements through the management hierarchy. Comparative studies of occupational mobility in different industrial concerns, both simple and complex, are surely in order to add to our understanding both of organizations and of careers within them.

The systematic procedures for cooling out can also be viewed from the social-psychological or career perspective. To ask what happens to a man as he moves through these successive positions is equivalent to asking what effects his occupation has upon him both sequentially and in the long run. It is no easy matter to pin down the steps in the psychology of his change. Psychologists usually are content with characterizing the personalities of executives either without saying much about how the person got that way or speculating fairly generally about the social context within which personality is affected. The impact of occupational position upon personality can be studied more pointedly by tying the psychologist's kind of research into organizational and career investigation. It is just here that further studies of the effects of demotion and the arresting of promotion should prove most valuable. The fateful periods in a man's life are frequently associated with personal and public recognition of failure. In so far as the type of failure and the handling of it are not unique but are common and related to organizational structure, there is the possibility of determining and studying the crucial turning points in personality development within occupational worlds.

THE SHAPE OF MOBILITY*

Direction, distance, timing, rate, temporal commitment, and the articulation of concerns are all relevant to the form or "shape" of the careers of mobile persons (or of other units such as families and labor unions). In attempting to manage those careers, the implicated participants are concerned with exactly those features of mobility. Hence, a principal analytic issue is that of control, especially who is in control over various features of mobility, and how they manage to achieve or maintain control.

Among the major conditions which affect control are whether mobility occurs primarily as a solo effort (individualistically) or whether as either a collective effort or at least along highly institutionalized routes (medical schools, law firms). Who controls what, and how, will be related to whether mobility careers are routinized, or need to be newly generated or at least require the search and discovery of existing routes. All those considerations form the organizing framework for analyzing shape.

INDIVIDUAL MOBILITY

The standard American story of success or failure tends to overemphasize individual ability and responsibility; however, there is implicit in those stories the contribution of the family, at least, to the person's mobility. In sociological literature also, the emphasis is mainly on individual (or aggregate) mobility but social class, family, community, and organizational factors are given considerable representation in the mobility. Yet, one cannot help but be struck by the difference between the American emphasis on indi-

*Reprinted by permission from
THE CONTEXTS OF MOBILITY
Chicago, Aldine Pub. Co., 1971, pp. 228-51
Copyright © 1971, Anselm L. Strauss

vidual mobility (especially in the more standard literature)[1] as contrasted with the insistence on family mobility by an Austrian scholar like Joseph Schumpeter, who was raised in a less individualistically-oriented country.[2]

An ideal picture of individual mobility would show an individual in complete control of its every feature and phase. Furthermore, he would have neither help nor hinderance from any known agent (friend, kinsman, sponsor, enemy) or from any unknown agent. If fortunate or unfortunate accidents occur, he alone takes advantage of, or succumbs to, or copes with them. Of course, there can be no mobility career like that. Even as personally controlled a mobility step as the permanent passing of a Negro may depend on the occasional or continual silence of others who recognize his passing. Analytically, however, if one focuses on individual mobility as such, then the person can be regarded as the chief agent in his mobility while all other agents function in roles subsidiary to his. He may require teachers or coaches during certain phases of his mobility, and from time to time he may seek advice or assistance, but all other persons are subordinate to his mobility goals. Even submission of self during some undesirable phase — such as when an aspiring actress becomes mistress to a Broadway director — is only a means to climbing upward. Even to generate a new route, let alone follow or discover a routine one, a mobile individual needs to bend the energies of others to his purposes.

Inevitably these will engage him in contests for control over one feature or another of his mobility route. The older sociological literature of "culture conflict" between first and second generations portrayed vividly the anguish of both parties to the mobility con-

[1]See also Joseph Gusfield's criticism in his "Political Equality and Social Stratification in India and Japan: A Comparative Analysis," unpublished manuscript presented at the meeting of the American Sociology Association, 1967.

[2]Joseph Schumpeter, *Imperialism and Classes, 1951;* see the excerpts in R. Bendix and M. Lipset (eds.), *Class, Status and Power* (New York: The Free Press of Glencoe, 1953), p. 44: "Class barriers are always . . . surmountable and are, in fact, surmounted, by virtue of the same qualifications and modes of behavior that bring about shifts of family position within the class. . . . The ultimate function on which the class phenomenon rests consists of individual differences in aptitude . . . The differences . . . do not relate to the physical individual, but to the clan or family." Compare this with even such a non-individualistically focused sociologist as E. Digby Baltzel: "in this paper, the *elite* concept refers to those *individuals* who are the most successful and stand at the top of the *functional* (objective) class hierarchy. . . . On the other hand, in any comparatively stable social structure, over the years, certain elite members and their families will tend to associate with one another. . . . The *upper class* concept, then, refers to a group of families, descendants of successful individuals (elite member), one, two, three, or more generations ago. . . . " See his "Who's Who in America' and 'The Social Register,' " in Bendix and Lipset, *ibid.*, p. 267.

tests.[3] Parental attempts at control over mobility — direction, distance, and so on — begin early and they and later tactics scarcely need description here. One or two points only perhaps are worth special emphasis. When children discover routes that a parent does not understand — even when following them may exceed parental expectations or dreams — then the contest over control may be ferocious. If parents have already ceded control, generally after he approaches adulthood, then the contest may be attenuated or replaced by puzzled but ineffectual protest. (As Moss Hart reported after he sold his first play and had announced the great news in "ringing tones" to his parents, they "received the news with an air of amazed disbelief and infuriating calm." Even the check was regarded "with irritating detachment and a quite evident distrust. 'I suppose you know what you're doing, taking all that money,' said my mother warily, 'but I wouldn't touch it until after you've worked with this Mr. Kaufman for a while — in case he asks you to give it back.' " After the play began to appear in newspaper announcements, his mother still did not understand that her son would become famous and rich, "but simply . . . that my activities, always so mysterious and faintly spurious in the eyes of her friends, had taken on the aura of respectability.")[4] Parental control over the direction or distance of a child's mobility is threatened, of course, by "outside influences" of various kinds. When parents are not aware of those influences, then they can suffer such consequences as were met by immigrant parents who sent their children to school and college expecting them to become "successful" only to find them so successful that a growing gap between child and parents could not be bridged. Even when the unfortunate conditions are understood, as when Negro mothers understand all too well the untoward influences affecting their children, they may be unable to control their children's tendencies "to go bad."[5]

[3]Thus a father states:
We had no trouble with him in Europe. He was a fine child . . . I had great ambitions for him to become an educated man, maybe a doctor or a lawyer or a rabbi. But all my hopes have gone to pieces . . . My word counts for nothing with him and he is teaching the younger boy to be as bad as he is. . . . I can't even tell you what he does for a living. He always wears fancy clothes and jewelry and I am sure he doesn't get it in an honest way . . . This is America, where children are not children but wild animals.
William Carlson, *Americans In the Making* (New York: Appleton-Century Co., 1939), pp. 276-77.

[4]Moss Hart, *Act One* (New York: Random House, Inc., 1959), pp. 275-76 and 319.

[5]Cf. one intelligent mother whose boy had become a poor reader and a problem child at high school: "Melvin was having three study periods in a row . . . studying what? I went to see this study hall . . . there's very few lights, and there's children everywhere, male and female, and about the only thing they can do there is make love. Most . . . can't read anywhere, but if they could, they wouldn't be able to see." Studs Terkle, *Division Street: America* (New York: Pantheon, 1967), p. 17.

Although marriage is a "mutual mobility bet," to use the felicitous phrasing of Everett Hughes, wives can also complicate the picture of a mobility which ideally is without contest. There is protest bearing on "how far" and "how much": "I've let Bob know I would sooner have him in a lower job than knocking himself out as a v.p." "When Edgar's work gets so it's interfering with his health and happiness, it's not worth it. I keep telling him we're a lot better off than most — another car and things like that aren't necessary."[6] There is also contention over timing: " 'All right' he said, 'maybe I'm licked, and maybe I don't give a damn.' 'I suppose you're going to say I've always been pushing you because I want us to get on,' she said."[7] By such tactics, wives succeed in changing the shapes of their husbands' mobility careers, or lose both the contests and their husbands. Friends also may be a complicating feature in decisions about mobility, especially those taken about assisting agents and about timing. Thus the manuscript of Moss Hart's first successful play was sent to a famous producer through a friend. " 'Jed Harris would go for this play like a ton of bricks. . . . Don't wait to re-write it — just send it to him the way it is — tomorrow morning, if possible!' " Hart protested Harris wouldn't read the play for a long while, he was so busy, and then the play's timeliness "will just evaporate into a collection of old Hollywood jokes." So his friend pulled the strings of family connections to reach an agent, who arranged to get his play a quick reading.[8] When Harris did not then say either yes or no, the discussions among Hart's friends over the next two or three days on what to do next "were loud, violent and opposite." As Hart remarks in his account, "One of the grave dangers inherent in the various stages of any theatrical career — whether it be budding, quiescent or diminishing — is the advice of friends." As for the influences of those organizations (and their representatives) in which individuals elect or are forced to satisfy their mobility goals, those are of course many and varied.

AGGREGATE MOBILITY

Although an individual can be "on his own," he may be considered only one of a large aggregate by some agent or organization. While each individual may regard himself as a single person who will succeed or fail, depending on his own performance, analytically one

[6]Quotations are from the wives of corporation executives; see William H. Whyte, *Is Anybody Listening* (New York: Simon and Schuster, 1952), p. 169.

[7]John P. Marquand, *Point of No Return* (Boston: Little, Brown and Company, 1947), p. 540.

[8]Hart, *op. cit.*, pp. 243-44 and pp. 259-60.

must examine what happens to him as part of an aggregate processed through agential or organizational machinery. (Members of aggregates tend under certain conditions to form at least loose collectivities.)

First, let us examine the possible contests between single agents and the aggregate members who choose him in order to further their mobility designs. The major contingent issue derives from these facts: each mobile person usually considers himself in solo movement, and often voluntarily selects his agent while actually the latter is juggling an aggregate. For instance, unscrupulous dealers in automobiles or furniture contribute to blocked mobility by managing aggregates of lower class clients to cheat them out of considerable money, without most being either individually or collectively aware of his shrewd practice. And if a purchaser discovers that he has been cheated, he usually is quite powerless to institute retribution. In one instance, however, many purchasers began to complain about their individual cases to a Legal Aid Society newly established to help the poor; its lawyers eventually perceived a common pattern in the dealer's operations and filed suits against him in the name of one client.

More usually, agents are honest and more or less open in handling their aggregates. Ordinarily, also the individual understands perfectly well that his agent has many other clients. The agent's great problem is that he is juggling competing demands made by his clients and engages in appropriate tactics that allow him to juggle as successfully as possible. If a person clearly understands that he competes with others, or believes his own mobility important enough to warrant actively countering that competition, then he engages in counter-tactics — bribing, seducing or harassing his agent, or threatening to take his business elsewhere. He may also attempt to control aspects of his mobility route by indirectly taking competitors into advantageous account. Specialists, such as famed teachers of piano, are chosen because they have had valuable experience with "others like me." Precisely because of this past success, the individual may be quite willing to suffer the direct competition of others; and be willing to wait longer even to be accepted as a student, and then to put up with his teacher's idiosyncrasies, aggressiveness or unsatisfactory scheduling of some aspects of his own course of mobility. Agents gain extra control if they can establish awe or trust, or if they have few if any competitors. Yet there may be possibilities of bargaining with them, especially over matters of timing or rate of movement, under certain conditions — a competitive market among agents, sensitive assessment by the agent of necessity to compromise, too great an emotional involvement with the client by the agent, or even some dependence of the agent's

157

own mobility — that is, prestige or money — on the client's remaining with him. Contributions of an agent to mobility considered undesirable by members of an aggregate usually are not countered by collective action (as in the instance of the auto dealer noted above). Among the tactics are attempts literally to escape the agent's control (debtors leave town or go bankrupt, tenant farmers migrate North in the night), or to put on sufficient social pressure to get at least some slowing up of undesirable mobility.

When a complex organization is dealing with an aggregate of mobile individuals, the issue of control is likely to be somewhat more complicated. A convenient illustration of the processing of aggregates is how the movie industry used to, and probably still does, select and "build up" its future stars. An executive of Columbia Pictures tells about the discovery of Kim Novak:

> I sensed something. She had an unusual personality which we can spot in one of five hundred girls who are sent to us. I think it was those fantastic eyes that sold me—the eyes and the Slavic cheekbones. I told her to lose twenty pounds and come back to see me.[9]

As Orrin Klapp remarks, Miss Novak was then "taken over by the studio. A crew of dramatic coaches, photographers, dress designers, cosmeticians, and directors went to work on her. Each took credit for making her into a star, typically referring to her as a 'dumb blond,' who owed everything to him."[10] Minimum costs for producing stars at Columbia Pictures was in the neighborhood of $200,000.

Two contingent problems confront both the organization and its aggregate of mobile individuals. The organization (and its representatives) must, first, exert control over the shape of the total aggregate's mobility. Second, it is concerned with the shape of each individual's mobility, especially insofar as each may deviate from the norm for the total aggregate. Robert Merrill, the well-known opera star, has described how the director of the Metropolitan threatened to fire him when he insisted on giving too many individual recitals; Merrill came quickly to heel on whether to put his major time into recitals or into opera rehearsals and performances. Deviancies like his can cause organizational crises, but more important is that they challenge some measure of the organization's control over the total aggregate. (Mediocre or worn out boxers are

[9]Bill Davidson, "Kim Novak: A Woman Who Can't be Free," *Redbook* (March, 1959), p. 84. The title, of course, is expressive of many aggregate-organizational relations.

[10]O. Klapp, *Symbolic Leaders* (Chicago: Aldine Publishing Company, 1964), p. 28.

chosen by "the organization" as good enough to function, within its stable of men, as "set-ups" who will lose to promising boxers — or be fired if they don't act right.) The corresponding problem of the mobile individual is to secure some measure of control over his own mobility, using the advantage of or getting around the disadvantages of being part of an aggregate. Medical students who have decided beforehand to become missionary doctors have had to learn just as much medicine as they thought they should, but not necessarily to follow closely the ordinary types of student careers while in school; and graduate students in some disciplines have had to put together new combinations of courses and work out new career actions to create novel kinds of mobility routes.

In instituting and maintaining the proper shape of aggregate movement, the organization needs to pay careful attention to the quantity and quality of members of the aggregate when they are about to be accepted into the organization. (Miss Novak's recruitment and tutoring makes this point.) Quantity is important because too many or few recruits can create havoc with monetary or manpower resources. Recruiting the wrong individuals can also create grave problems; they might require too much effort to teach and control or might get discouraged and drop out, with consequent wasting of time, money, and effort. Other aspects of aggregate shape are debated within the organization; review of past organizational performance is transformed into changes of policies which pertain to the shape of aggregate passage. On the basis of "our current experience" should we drop more quickly those who fail or who move too slowly? Should we speed up some phases or omit some phases? Can we make the division of labor more efficient, with different personnel for varying phases, rather than each agent and his assistants taking responsibility of the totality of each individual's movement?

Organizational mechanisms for handling these and related problems vary according to diverse structural conditions. For instance, Morris Janowitz reports at the end of World War II,[11] "The Air Force was faced with the task of selecting fourteen thousand officers" so had recourse to a contract with a research institute which "produced an elaborate technique based on the so-called 'critical incident' device" supposed accurately to evaluate individual performance. But in the military, elaborate informal devices also operate to make such "cumbersome systems" as the efficiency report and the dossier workable at all. In large business firms, which have many hierarchially arranged positions and at least several

[11]Morris Janowitz, *The Professional Soldier* (New York: The Free Press of Glencoe, 1960), p. 146.

different workplaces, "Vertical and horizontal movement of personnel through the various positions making up the organization is executed so as to make certain that competent men get in the right places at the right time. . . . At the same time, the organization provides a number of channels through which mobile individuals can move to realize personal objectives."[12] In such organizations, to insure only a minimal contest with individuals over their demotions at various levels of the firm, a series of tactics are employed. These have been enumerated and discussed by Douglas More,[13] under the relatively self-explanatory headings of: lowered job status with continuation of the earlier compensation; lowered status with decreased compensation; retained status with decreased compensation; being bypassed in senority for promotion; change of job to a less desirable function; maintenance of status with decreased span of control; exclusion from a general salary raise; increasing the steps in the hierarchy above a given position; movement from line to staff authority but with the same compensation; retention of the same mobility level, with some job compensation, and carrying with it equal authority and responsibility, but transfer out of direct line of promotion; position elimination and reassignment. Thus the organizational tactics for handling partial or complete failures of their aggregate personnel are many and add up to a complex system of policy acts. The system is necessary for getting men allocated, jobs done, and both high and low administrative leaders picked, trained, and developed.

Under some conditions, organizational agents may be allowed relative autonomy in the management of their assigned segments of the aggregate. For instance, parole agents may be delegated considerable authority in their enterprises of restoring parolees back to society (onward and upward!) or returning them (downward) to the prison.[14] It is easy to see the kinds of conditions which mitigate against agent autonomy: when the organization is new and everyone is concerned with proper aggregate shape or when coordination of the whole enterprise itself is precarious (as with a new medical school); when agents are responsible only for certain phases of each individual performance so that articulation of phases is a necessity; when there are visibly untoward consequences to the organization of poor agential performance, including complaints or an emergency caused by agents' ineptness (as with parolees); when the entire organization is judged, or believes it is judged, by other orga-

[12]Norman Martin and Anselm Strauss, "Patterns of Mobility Within Industrial Organization," *Journal of Business,* vol. 29 (1956), p. 101.

[13]Douglas More, "Demotion," *Social Problems,* vol. 9 (1962), pp. 213-21.

[14]E. Studt's study of Parole, Center for the Study of Law & Society, University of California, Berkeley.

nizations in accordance with "the results," that is, with the performance of its products now or later (as with job corps trainees). A listing of such conditions suggests why and how organizations can run through cycles of tightening or loosening of the autonomy of its agents and, conversely, the relative freedom given to the individual members of its aggregate. Both the multiplicity of agents and the conditions which enable their relative autonomy also make possible a range of variations or latitude in individual phasing and timing and so affect the fates of those individuals. A parole officer may believe a parolee will stand a better chance at rehabilitation if he is allowed to live, "for stability," with a woman; or that this arrangement may save the agent extra work; it may even save him time so that he can moonlight on organizational time and so raise his own standard of living.[15]

An important property of aggregates is that under certain conditions they may become collectivities. This possibility is enhanced when the aggregate as a whole is handled by an agential group rather than by single agents, and by the necessity for the aggregate members often to appear at organizational locales. The probability of communication is increased if only because they are more likely to sit or stand near each other and spend time in each other's presence. In one business school, for instance, described in Blanche Geer, et al,.[16] the student body is essentially an aggregate, each student pursuing his own learning and relating directly to the instructor, with a minimum of interaction among these more or less ambitious students. In this setting, although the students have not much time to spend with each other, and all are at different stages in their learning, nevertheless a certain amount of communication occurs among them, mainly about how to handle the work and the instructor himself as well as about such vital specifics as the scheduling of one's time in relation to the lessons. At barber colleges, however, where the aggregate of students is much on its own, the students are constrained to learn mainly from one another, and so there is little contest for control between them and an instructor.[17] Compared with medical or law schools, however, only a minimum of student culture develops because the aggregate never evolves into much of a student body.

When aggregates evolve into active groups, they can cause organizational or agential havoc (as with the auto dealer and his aroused

[15]Ibid.

[16]Blanche Geer, et al., "Learning the Ropes" in Irwin Deutscher and Elizabeth Thompson (eds.), Among the People (New York: Basic Books, Inc., 1968), pp. 209-33.

[17]Ibid.

customers) and radically alter the normal shape of aggregate mobility. It is not unknown for inept or inexperienced organizational agents to take exactly the steps which turn an aggregate at least temporarily into an aroused group, even laying the basis for more persistent collectivities that have emergent conceptions of collective mobility. Recent events at city colleges — ordinarily these schools have minimal student cultures — are dramatic examples of student aggregates evolving, at least temporarily, into collectivities. Demands such as were made at the City University of New York (all minority students were to be accepted regardless of grades made in public school) if effected, will alter radically the very structure of the processing institution in addition to disturbing its handling of aggregate careers. However, such radical transformation insures the generation of novel careers, not merely the opening of existing ones to new types of individuals. It is no wonder that an aggregate turned collective would rather destroy an institution that it believes fails to serve its members—or does them disserve—than to permit continued operation as usual. Under such attack, organizations may knuckle under, compromise, go out of business, or call on higher authorities. In the history of labor-business relations, all those possibilities are exemplified.

COLLECTIVE MOBILITY

Mobility relations, of course, have other characteristics when collectivities deal with other collectivities. Contests for control then are raised above the level of individual efforts — though certainly these usually, or perhaps inevitably, exist — and collective mechanisms come into play, as in labor-management negotiation or in bargaining between Negroes (qua group) and whites. A set of major problems confronts any group which is in relative authority. First, it is concerned with instituting and maintaining a proper shape for the mobility of various other groups. Second, the superordinate group is concerned with managing individual mobilities which depart disturbingly from normal ones dictated by an expected shape of mobility. This set of problems is implicated in the efforts of all collectivities which attempt to control the mobility of other collectivities — whether it is one ethnic group controlling another,[18] or one racial group controlling another, or a medical school faculty controlling the movement of its student body (because students develop a "culture").[19] The subordinate groups face the following typical problems. First, they are concerned with achieving some measure

[18]T. Shibutani and K. Kwan, *Ethnic Stratification* (New York: The Macmillan Company, 1965); and E. C. Hughes, *Where People Meet* (Glencoe, Ill.: The Free Press, 1952).

[19]H. S. Becker, *et al., Boys In White* (Chicago: University of Chicago Press, 1962).

of control over the shape of their collective mobilities. Second, the members of those groups are concerned with gaining some control over their individual mobilities. Group interest and personal interests may support or run counter, depending on variable but determinable conditions, but the potential discrepancy between the types of interest is inherent in group membership.

A major variable in determining the character of all contests over control of mobility is whether the superordinate group is confronted by a cohort which shares collective features (as a faculty *versus* a student body, a prison administration *versus* a body of prisoners), or by another "true" collectivity (as one racial group *versus* another). Each type of confrontation deserves separate discussion.

Cohort mobility inevitably occurs on institutional or organizational terrains. To put a cohort through status passages or to arrange for its work within a division of labor (or just to hold it, as in a prison), there must be at least minimal organizational machinery. There always exists the possibility of disagreement among members of the controlling group about how that organizational machinery should operate and about details of cohort management — even about exact shape of cohort or individual mobilities. Internal dissension is minimized when the backgrounds of superordinate members are similar, and when there is minimal differentiation in their division of labor within the organization. Homogeneity of perspectives means maximum agreement about the desired shape of cohort mobility (say, in business corporations in regard either to personnel in general or to potential collectivities such as its Negro personnel). It also means that superordinates cannot easily be played off, one against another, by the subordinates. Also there is less likelihood that superordinate members will covertly maneuver against the intentions of the superordinate group at large. When organizations are rent with dissension, then the subordinate group may manage to play off one faction of superordinates against another, to what they believe is their own collective advantage (as may a student body, or some segment of it such as the "minority students"). Some of the strain of discrepant views among superordinates can be minimized when the pacing or timing of subordinate mobilities are less than rigorously prescribed and scheduled. Also when an organization is new or becoming revitalized (as some segment of military forces) and so can afford or even idealize its internal discrepancies of view, then there may be fair latitude in the management of cohort mobilities by superordinates.

Parallel to the institutional machinery is a greater or lesser degree of cohesiveness among the cohort members — so there is a potential

163

for collective action in its own perceived behalf. The longer the cohort members are in passage — also the more social structural bases, such as ethnicity or propinquity there are — the more likely are they to develop a consensus about what matters are of greatest moment for the cohort. Cohort culture arises, as studies like those by Howard Becker or Virginia Olesen and Elvie Whittaker make clear, primarily because the cohort members face common contingencies.[20] The more they realize these contingencies confront them all, the more they will share definitions about those contingencies, as well as ideas about how to cope with them. Also, the more collectively shared the contingencies are, the more probable is a collective perspective compounded in some part of a shared memory about past victories and defeats; for instance, an aggregate of workingmen develops a collective memory about relations with management.

It is safe to say that unless the life of the cohort is of very short duration and the members share a very homogenous background, there will be at least occasional strain among cohort members as they act on different ideas about how better to achieve their own mobility goals. Discrepant views can evolve over virtually all items discussed earlier: rate, timing, temporal commitment. Whenever such discrepancies evolve and an individual acts in accordance with his own viewpoint, he has to face the consequences of his action, if visible, as seen by other cohort members. His tactics may include, of course, keeping his action invisible to them, or at least to all except others with very similar views. At the other extreme, he may attempt to convert all others to his view of the aspect of mobility under question, either because he believes all will then benefit (as with local labor leaders) or more cynically because he at least will benefit.

Another implication of solo "within" cohort mobility, is that attempts to control aspects of personal passage lead to complex interactions among individuals in the cohort: Among the most consequential are competition and cooperation. When cohesion of the cohort is great, then virtually all may cooperate in keeping competition minimal, for instance, insuring that laggards in pace are coached — or their true pace concealed from superordinates — so as neither to be reprimanded nor flunked out (among students, for instance).

Inevitably moments arise when the superordinate members perceive actions by a cohort member which run counter to the proper shape of cohort mobility. Both to control that shape and to prevent a person who commits deviant acts from developing into a

[20]Becker, *ibid;* Olesen and Whittaker, *The Silent Dialogue* (San Francisco: Jossey-Bass, Inc., 1968).

thoroughly deviant individual, they will evolve appropriate tactics including the bringing of cohort pressure to bear on that individual. Deviant members may, however, also require superordinates' protection and aid. Under given structural conditions where dropouts from a professional school are believed undesirable, a faculty will work hard to bring the slow student up to snuff or stretch its concept of cohort shape and allow him to move through the school either at a slower rate or at a normal rate, although with inferior performance. Again the cooperation of other cohort members may be enlisted to insure success of these tactics.

One final point about the management of deviant acts and cohort members: insofar as the superordinate members are a diverse lot, either exemplifying their differences implicitly in their words and acts or openly disagreeing with one another, cohort members can model themselves after different superordinates. If the organization is so structured that the latter perform quite different organizational functions, then cohort members have increased opportunities to choose from different models somewhat different aspects to imitate or incorporate genuinely into their inner selves. Medical students may discover that they can become researchers rather than practitioners — and even learn to settle for less affluence and an academic life style. In such situations, of course, the judgments of cohort members are affected in no small measure by conversations among themselves, and differential choice of mobility careers and styles are viewed with relative tolerance by both the superordinate and cohort groups. Superordinates who cannot endure this amount of tolerance are likely to leave for more satisfying terrains.

Cohorts (and aggregates of individuals) are likely to act only sporadically as enduring units rather than to become more permanent collectivities. Perhaps the chief condition for relative permanence is the widely shared perception of "common fate," whether by ethnic groups, American blacks, unionized laborers, workingmen in a company town, prisoners, or families. Wherever such permanent collectivities evolve, they develop perspectives which probably include self-placement in some "social scale," and assumptions about whether the future augers better, worse, or the same for their placement. Future conditions may be changed through luck, the will of God, attention to proper virtues, or by hard work or cleverness. In their views of future conditions, they are very likely to take into account the presence of competing or conflicting groups, so that at least some future fortune is attributed to another group's evil or envious character, its increasing or decreasing power, and so forth.[21] These collectivities are concerned,

[21]Tomatsu Shibutani (ed.), "On the Personification of Adversaries," in *Human Nature and Collective Behavior* (Englewood Cliffs, N.J.: Prentice-Hall, Inc. 1970).

in some measure at least, with controlling their own destinies, even when fatalism looms large in their pictures of the world. Attempts at such control bring them into conflict — but also into coalition or cooperation — with other groups. There would seem little need to draw out discussion of those points, except perhaps to add that although social science literature is replete with descriptions and analyses of mobility conflict and cooperation between and among specific groups, it is not much concerned with developing a general theory about collective mobilities.[22]

A few theoretical propositions are worth noting about conditions, tactics, and consequences. For instance, when one group believes it is firmly in the superordinate position, then behavior from subordinates is tolerated that under more conflictful conditions would be regarded as "uppity," censurable, even downright threatening or punishable. Distinctions are made also between or among subordinates who are more or less uppity or threatening. (In 1949, John Dollard noted that Southern whites tolerated explicit criticism by Negro women that they would not have tolerated by Negro men. "Humility and lack of direct demands are elements of caste etiquette for Negroes . . . women are given more license than men.")[23]

When the positions of superordinate and subordinate groups are relatively, if not so firmly stabilized, then implicit understandings underpin the relationship, so that a few exceptions can be made without disturbing the basic positions of the groups. There can be occasional sharp contests over minor changes which will not represent real challenges to the existing order. In one New England factory, a "clearly definable system of ethnic sponsorship" for promotion existed, although "almost never explicitly declared." Both management and labor, including the union, recognized this system

[22]An excellent exception but on quite a macroscopic level is a comparison by Joseph Gusfield of two societies in his "Political Equality and Social Stratification in India and Japan: A Comparative Analysis" (unpublished manuscript.)

[23]He continues:

A middle-class Negro informant was asked to talk before a women's discussion group in one of the white churches on the topic, 'Our Manchurian Friends.' The chairman of the club introduced her as a *friend*. When she rose to speak, she said she was glad to be introduced as a friend and hoped she was one. She went on to take as the major issue of her discussion the fact that it was nice to be interested in Manchuria, but that the club might also be interested in its Negro friends in Southerntown. Right over on the other side of the tracks were plenty of problems nearer home than Manchuria. Probably no local Negro man would be asked to speak before a group of white men . . . but if a man were invited he would hardly dare to be as lacking in humility as this woman was.

John Dollard, *Caste and Class in a Southern Town* (New York: Doubleday Anchor, 3rd ed., 1957), p. 303.

of job expectations, and conflicts over promotions infrequently occurred. Nonadministrative levels customarily were filled by the
Irish. However, once when an Irish subforeman resigned the management replaced him with a well liked Yankee. A formal protest
plus informal pressure forced management to retreat, and Murphy
was promoted to the job. Conversely, Yankees customarily were
appointed to administrative jobs without any opposition from the
Irish. But once there was ambiguity about whether a new job was
administrative or merely supervisory, then a sharp conflict arose
between management and workingmen. Management finally agreed
to have candidates submit their names. All the "labor nominations
were, with one exception, both workingmen and Irish. Management
rejected all" and several days later appointed a Yankee. "The repercussions were violent, but the appointment 'stuck.' By changing
the title of the new job from 'foreman' to 'engineer,' management
had removed the job from *supervision* to administration. . . .
Labor's argument had lost its force."[24] Those episodes reveal some
conditions under which contests for control may be fought — new
jobs with unclear placement and vacancies in an old job which the
superordinate group is tempted to usurp. The episodes also suggest
some of the tactics used in these distinctly minor contests — customary mechanisms like formal protest and informal pressures
("bitching" or a slowdown of work), and outflanking (or face saving) maneuvers.

Relatively stabilized superordinate-subordinate positions are
sustained also by internalized convictions, so that subordinates
either do not much question their right to higher positions or keep
their doubts under strict behavioral control. When the older system
of relationships begins to break down then its advocates resort
more openly to the use of force, and so do its antagonists. The
latter also apply epithets to those still under its internal control
("white Negroes") or susceptible to external constraints and rewards ("Uncle Tom"). Those who are seen as beginning to sell out
to the superordinate group are enjoined and pressured to reestab-
lish allegiance (or silently "pass" among) or face the consequences
— which can be as dire even as assassination if the betrayals seem
to endanger members of the superordinate group. Members who
are believed to be agents of the superordinate group (Negro police,
scabs in labor strikes) also are subject to informal pressure and
threats or actual acts of violence.

As open conflict increases between superordinate and subordinate groups, some subordinates who are beginning "to make it"

[24]Orvis Collins, "Ethnic Behavior in Industry: Sponsorship and Rejection in a New England Factory," *American Journal of Sociology*,
vol. 51 (1946), pp. 293-98.

within the larger world (seemingly controlled by superordinates) are vulnerable to the accusations of pure selfishness because only collective action will raise the entire subordinate group — or keep it from dropping lower. Some succumb to those arguments and guiltily turn their backs on individual mobility. Others juggle their own ambitions and do something for "their people," perhaps compromising on both. Others use the threat of collective action actually to further only their personal interests. Still others generate new types of mobility careers in fighting for the upward mobility of their collectivity. These kinds of development are paralleled by reactions and behaviors among the members of the superordinate group, as a moment's reflection about the complex responses of whites to blacks today makes clear. Add then the responses of whites to blacks and blacks to whites, along with blacks to blacks and whites to whites, and that gives some inkling of the complexity and quick change of mobility perspectives when relationships among large collectivities are shifting rapidly. (A poignant example[25] is the bafflement of an elderly southern white liberal whose efforts in behalf of a potential "hunger campaign" to relieve the starvation of Negro children were rejected by a black minority on the grounds that this was palliative and would do nothing for the long-run improvement of Southern Negroes. They both hated to see children used as pawns in politics, but the gap between their respective priorities and ideas about timing was unbridgable.) Although these examples have used Negro-white relationships, one could just as well substitute (in other times and places) relationships between labor and management, nativist Protestants and immigrant Catholics, or populist farmers and town merchants and city capitalists.

Even so, the above discussion underplays complexity if only because it turns mainly on a contest between only two antagonists. Much collective mobility occurs under conditions where one group actively fights for what it believes is the welfare of another — for whatever reasons of its own — and indeed may owe its very existence to coalescence around this issue of mobility. A good instance is the pre-Civil War abolition movement which did so much to change public opinion in the North about the Negro and which so profoundly affected the management of white-black relations during the Reconstruction. The efforts of reformers, who have conspicuously, since the 1880's, fought to raise the poor or at least to build a floor against further degradation, are another obvious example of what might be termed mobility advocacy.

Less disinterested advocates who have not always the purest of motives can also enter the reform ring; for instance — and here I

[25]Brought to my attention by Helen Rowan.

168

quote from a recent communication written by the representative of a large corporation:

> [This] company is preparing a proposal to the Federal Executive Board . . . to upgrade 100 selected families presently on welfare to middle class status. The target income at the conclusion of the proposed effort would be $8,000 per year per family. Generally the program envisions making a survey of each family's present condition in the areas of language skills, educational levels, vocational aptitudes, adequacy of housing, and health and medical problems, including drug addiction. Following this a planned improvement program would be launched tailored to each family member to assist him or her to attain the norm in these various areas. To the heads of households, efforts would be directed to make him self-supporting initially, and to advance to the target income level subsequently.

Leaving aside the question of practicality (or naivete) of this proposal, it helps to focus attention on one essential condition for advocacy: namely, the advocate's history must properly intersect that of the group to be helped. In this instance, big corporations are beginning to cast about for alternative profitable ventures in anticipation of fewer defense contracts.

The above examples should suggest that an advocate does not operate within an uncontested context. The advocatee (to coin a word) may have its own ideas about its destiny, or indeed may be very divided among itself on this issue, and just as obviously there may be more than one advocate fighting over the prone or active body of the advocatee. (Sometimes the latter may not even know a battle is going on above itself — for instance, fights over how lower class children should be educated, and for what purpose, have long raged without the children or their parents necessarily being aware of the fights.) [26] Various of the service or professional occupations inevitably get involved, as Berenice Fisher has incisively discussed, [27] in competition over determining the fates of their "client groups" as each challenges the right or mandate of the other to serve the client group. This problem of "credibility" is compounded because the latter may also challenge an occupation's claim "to help." As Berenice Fisher remarks:

> the ideologies which the occupational groups carve out in the course of their rivalry are broad. They embody not

[26]For detailed documentation of many of these battles and their social placements see Berenice Fisher, *Industrial Education: American Ideals and Institutions* (Madison: University of Wisconsin Press, 1967).

[27]"Claims and Credibility: A Discussion of Occupational Identity and the Agent-Client Relationship," *Social Problems,* vol. 16 (1969), 423-33.

mere justifications of specific actions, or attacks on one another . . . but basic approaches to industrial and occupational life, and critiques of the premises on which the aspirations of their rivals rest. Hence, arguments concerning occupational life extend into arguments over the character of social mobility. Disagreement of the desirability of one or another type of mobility involves disagreement over the meaning of success and failure. Differences of this kind involve diverse judgments about the true character of helplessness and, therefore, about the kinds of helping occupations which should be developed. Such judgments, in turn, involve opinions on which of the nation's social groups should receive such help and how one or another kind of helping conforms best to the ideals of democratic life.[28]

Miss Fisher notes that when clients either reject or are unresponsive to an agential group's claims, the latter may move in several directions. It may attempt to alter its ideology and the nature of its claim to help, or try to alter its internal structure to better effect its claim or try to change the response of its clients or the composition of its clientele. Clearly, such strategies and tactics are not merely manipulative but may involve profound questions about identities — of oneself as well as those of others.

Not infrequently when contestants are fighting for control over their own mobilities, coalitions of temporary allies form to gain more purchase over respective fates. Alliances are rendered temporary not merely by opportunistic motives and shifting circumstance, but because actual and perceived situations so obviously change. For instance, by 1969 Chicago's previously notorious gangs of black youths were reported to have been "so successful at operating businesses in the city's west side ghetto that they are seeking professional education in management techniques just to keep up with their own progress." Progress in this instance meant ownership and management of various small business, and projects like street beautification drives or outings for children. Recently the men "started their malt shop partly on a grant from the Rockefeller Foundation and with matching funds from a local group, and they have received some other assistance" and are now "preparing to use another grant to bring some managerial experts into their projects to give advice." Presumably they got lots of advice from other allies, some of it requested, in their attempt within the ghetto to raise themselves by their bootstraps. But, the reporter remarks, "No matter who is involved with them — foundations, civil rights groups, businessmen — they are their own decision makers and spokesmen."

28*Ibid.,* p. 426.

Because none of the members of the organization "want to be a Horatio Alger character . . . it would not be considered polite to pat them on the back," meaning, presumably, that they want no benevolent paternalism from the boss but only helpful temporary (otherwise encumbering) alliances.

One striking aspect of coalition and advocacy is the question of the relative visibility of the collectivity "lower down." Periodic rediscoveries of the poor, for instance, always involve selective perception and selective choice. Not only do the poor exist before their recognition, but only certain of them are selected out as "the poor." Others remain invisible to their potential advocates and allies. Recognition may be furthered by the endeavors of outsiders who have access to the mass media such as journalists, or by members of the collectivity who are able to express themselves in ways outsiders can understand. Of course, recognition may be furthered also by unconventional and certainly by non-verbal means, such as rioting or striking or by the symbolic seizing of Alcatraz Island. It is worth adding that the recognition of collectivities can be curiously restricted to given localities. Watts was relatively invisible until after the great riot, but Detroit had later to explode before most of its white citizens linked their own Blacks with those of Los Angeles. This is why there is no guarantee that an increased visibility of any segment of population (say, the coal miners of West Virginia) to a sympathetic public will necessarily be extended to another segment in a similar plight (the miners of Montana). As for the poor themselves, some of the historical debate over their plight — whether by themselves or their advocates — bears on the proper choice of tactics for their achieving public recognition. The proponents themselves, however, may regard their tactics as bearing directly on desirable political and social change; but a necessary first step may be gaining more visibility. An aroused public may respond "positively," but because of what they conceive as stark necessity, not merely because of sympathy or conscience.

An exceedingly informative example of how attitudes are formed and transformed and coalitions formed only to end by disintegrating, is Barbara Solomon's account of the decades after the introduction of Irish immigrants into New England.[29] Each generation of natives and "foreigners" lived in a different social context than its predecessors, therefore were in a strikingly different situation *vis-a-vis* each other and their respective allies. This is the very stuff of which evolving movements — with their myths, leaderships, and organizational machinery — are made. In such movements —

[29]*Ancestors and Immigrants* (New York: John Wiley & Sons, Inc., 1956).

whether ethnically, regionally, or occupationally based — groups seek to exert control over collective mobilities not only through occasional force and threat of force, but through legislative and judicial action and through intermittent if not continual negotiation with enemies, allies, and important mediating agents.[30] This should lead the reader full circle to the real institutions and social movements (and the images relevant to them) characteristic of the nation's frontiers, countrysides, cities, immigrations, and its many varieties of industrialization.

Americans tend to forget, or never know that much of our mobility is collective rather than simply individual, aggregate, or cohort movement — and downward as well as upward. While many citizens have shrewdly hitched their individual stars to rising industries, towns, and regions, other Americans have been caught in the declines of entire regions, towns, and industries. Analytically, one ought not to regard those individual rises and falls as merely individual, because the respective units have acted collectively in behalf of their members.

Furthermore, one ought not to forget, however unpalatable the remembrance, that some collectivities have successfully kept others "in their places" and even attempted to prevent aggregates from becoming collectivities. Much of that maneuvering is relatively invisible to the potential advocates for underdogs. More widely known strategies can be forgotten with the passing of time and the changing of circumstance. Scarcely anybody could be aroused if told that legislation passed early in the century forbade Japanese and Japanese-Americans to own rural land in California (the law has since been rescinded) and that the legislation drove this ethnic group from its dry rice acreage after it had successfully developed this type of agriculture on previously sterile land.

That small case affords a convenient end to this book because the ethnic group then moved to urban areas in California, their migration (as well as the enforced one at the outset of World War II plus voluntary migration at the end of that war) reminding us once again of the major themes developed in earlier chapters. The combined sociological and historical perspectives thus lead to the conclusion that while individual mobility assuredly does occur, it needs to be studied in collective as well as aggregate contexts.

30In the United States, the executive arm of the federal government has sometimes acted as an ally of the weak, justifying its action as a needed balancing of unequal weights, for instance, in establishing the Freedmen's Bureau after the Civil War or in acting, however mildly and "belatedly" to redress balances for Negroes in the Army and in the South.

172

PART III

WORK AND ORGANIZATION

NEGOTIATED ORDER AND THE
CO-ORDINATION OF WORK[1]*

In this chapter, we shall pursue an inquiry that follows logically from those immediately preceding. It bears upon how persons with such diverse motives for working at PPI and such different psychiatric ideologies can manage to work together. It is not enough to answer that they share common goals. They have many and varied goals, personal as well as professional. Such goals as are shared must be developed and maintained through common actions. As we have seen, the one end that all do share — "getting patients somewhat better" — becomes fragmented in actual implementation. Neither can we ourselves accept the conventional answer that things are accomplished at such a hospital because of its organizational structure, for that answer avoids the question of what kind of structure can exist under the conditions we have sketched.

At such a hospital, the physicians are principally concerned with organizing treatments for patients, while nurses and aides are concerned both with achieving manageable wards and with significant involvement in therapeutic activities. The patients themselves seek to manage their sick selves and their institutionalized lives. Unlike the treatment services at Chicago State Hospital, where teamwork is relatively simple because team members are few, at PPI the teams are usually not even designated as teams. They are not only varied but immensely variable, forming and dissolving continually. The more formal, visible, and durable teams encompass the most import-

[1]The point of view expressed in this chapter has previously been formulated by the authors in their "The Hospital and Its Negotiated Order," E. Freidson, ed., *The Hospital in Modern Society* (New York: The Free Press of Glencoe, 1963), pp. 147-69.

*Reprinted by permission from
PSYCHIATRIC IDEOLOGIES AND INSTITUTIONS
(with L. Schatzman, R. Bucher, D. Ehrlich and M. Sabshin), N. Y.
The Free Press, pp. 292-315. Copyright © 1964

ant administrative relationships. The clinical teams formed around patients are among the most transient and ephemeral. In addition, a number of transitory arrangements, bargains, "deals," and other types of negotiation permit both administrative and clinical ends to be attained. All these considerations lead us in this chapter to emphasize the continual negotiative activity that, together with periodic reviews of activities, constitute processes vitally important to the structured life of this hospital. At the chapter's close, we shall ask what import such matters have for the sociologist's concepts of "structure" and "social order." While our commentary may surprise many readers, it simply makes explicit what has been implicit throughout this chapter.

THE ORGANIZATION OF TREATMENT

Like other medical specialists, who bring private patients into general hospitals, PPI's psychiatrists are principally engaged in organizing treatment for their patients. A major problem confronting each attending man is to achieve maximal control over the hospital's administrative apparatus, which is at his service but over which he has no official command. As a consequence, the degree of his control of relevant aspects of treatment is problematic: He must gain such control, and he must continually struggle to maintain it.

Certain special features of this specific hospital may also have to be reckoned with in attaining therapeutic ends. Among them are the rapid turnover of patients; the five-ward system; frequent transfer of patients from ward to ward; the system of private physicians in which each patient on a given ward has a different attending man; and the range of treatment philosophies found among these physicians. These various features constitute important resources in the total array open to any physician, provided he wishes to use them. They also can hinder treatment.

As we have already noted, the somaticists rely upon limited institutional resources to supplement their own brand of psychotherapy and regard nurses less as a clinical resource than as an administrative necessity. They are all the more willing to accept nurses' therapeutic maneuvers because most hospital conditions do not seem to them potentially antitherapeutic. The somaticists tend to distinguish sharply between administrative and therapeutic action, viewing the former as subordinate or unrelated to the latter. They are willing to cede most administrative jurisdiction to the house staff. In effect, they can comfortably tell the head nurse to "do the usual things" with their patients. We have adopted the term "blue plate special" to designate ready acceptance of the ward's usual fare. By contrast, most psychotherapeutically oriented men regard various features of

176

the hospital as potentially quite useful — or dangerous — to their patients' treatments. They do not sharply separate administrative and clinical jurisdictions and, as we shall see, cannot so easily assume that clinical ends will be served by administrative machinery.

OBSTACLES TO TREATMENT

Let us assume that a psychotherapist knows what he wishes the hospital to accomplish for his patient. Let us further assume that he is well liked by the personnel, is skillful at making them feel important to his therapeutic programs, and can therefore elicit excellent co-operation. Despite these ideal conditions, he may encounter hindrances to successful utilization of institutional resources. Before examining the problems facing any physician so unfortunate as to be thought unco-operative, we shall look at the situation of his "co-operative" colleague.

The latter's first obstacle may be that he cannot successfully place his patient upon a given ward for various reasons: because the ROD judges the patient initially inappropriate for that ward, because its beds are filled, or because the personnel refuse to receive the patient on the basis of his reputation. More important, the therapist may believe that he knows the qualities of a given ward and may place his patient there precisely because of those qualities. For instance, 2E is believed to offer relatively intimate contact, while 2W supposedly has more acting out patients. Sometimes, however, the wards depart from their "normal" shapes, and the qualities he relies on for his patient are actually absent. On 3N there may be a minimum of acting out this week, but the usual uproar may begin again tomorrow. On 2W, the ordinarily unruffled, depressed atmosphere may for the moment be supercharged. Wards are always changing shape, despite physicians' images. Generally speaking, the more time a physician can spend at the hospital, the more aware he can be of the wards' current qualities. (The youngest physicians tend to be most "up" on the hospital for this reason.)

Besides advantageous placement, physicians may attempt to gain therapeutic control by leaving orders and talking with the head nurse. Despite the best of intentions, however, such communications can be misunderstood or orders neglected. During their interviews, most psychotherapists insist upon the near impossibility of giving orders for establishment of proper therapeutic relationships. They must wait for such relationships to develop, encouraging them and hoping for their continuation. The nurses exert pressure for early directives ("be firm," "give contact"), however, as well as for detailed directives if the patient responds slowly. A physician may discover that the staff cannot comprehend his program, and the "most co-operative" spend much time attempting to convey some insights into patients'

177

conditions and problems. A common saying among psychotherapists at PPI is that the staff is able to be firm but unable to be permissive with patients. Types of regressive therapy therefore require enormous patience from the therapists. With stoic fortitude or with disgust, the physicians transfer patients around the ward chessboard, in search of personnel with whom patients can form useful relationships. Sometimes they abandon the search.

Certain problems also arise for the co-operative therapist if his patient seems to the personnel not to envince fairly steady improvement. They may grow impatient and wish to transfer his patient to a "more appropriate" ward, especially if he is very troublesome or aggravating a ward already badly out of shape. If he has markedly improved, on the other hand, the personnel may reason that now he belongs elsewhere. While they are accustomed to having troublesome patients transferred back, they occasionally refuse to receive a returning patient because his condition is unchanged or worse. Even if a patient seems to the physician to be making progress, the personnel may believe that he is growing worse, for their respective standards of judgment, as we have noted, can differ widely. But the co-operative physician may talk the staff around to his point of view or may at least elicit tolerant co-operation by careful explanation of what "is really going on with" his patient.

If the physician manages to overcome most of these obstacles, he can expect good feedback of information from the head nurse, who in turn can rely upon her staff's reports. Whether or not the physician knows it, he can also depend upon the staff to give more attention to his patient than it ordinarily would. Although staff members' attention to a patient depends also upon other variables — how well the patient is liked and the effectiveness of his own demands for attention, for example — nevertheless a co-operative physician commands an additional important resource. That resource is suggested by the comments of one head nurse:

> These doctors are really interested in their patients . . .
> oriented to hospital work too, they like hospital work . . .
> they have a good idea of how the hospital functions; they
> either write it or they speak to us. . . . They make us feel
> as if the work we're doing really contributes to what they're
> doing. . . . If we get the feeling from the doctor that it doesn't
> make any difference whether we understand or not, we'll
> muddle through all right and be angry. . . . [The others]
> are telling us what they expect right away; that makes it
> simple for us to perform, to carry through what they expect.
> . . . We can depend on their coming around and telling us
> what is happening and what they expect us to do further.

... Yes, they do give us more information about what happened during their sessions with the patients; so that we have something to go on again. We know a little bit what is happening and what kind of reactions we can expect from the patient [Can you expect him to talk to the patient about things that are on *your* mind about the patient?] Yeah, they'll be much more supportive of the nursing staff in general.

Before spelling out this nursing personnel's perspectives upon how physicians organize treatment, let us consider the obstacles facing an "unco-operative" physician who wishes to utilize hospital resources beyond EST. Once his unfavorable reputation has developed, the staff tends to withhold information or at least to keep communication to a minimum and to transfer his patients readily. Staff members ordinarily do not overextend themselves with his patients. Occasionally they will have his orders countermanded. More quickly than he believes warranted, they isolate his patients — or, as a concession for keeping those patients, they wring from him certain orders for drugs and restricted privileges. If relationships grow tense, the staff may call up certain administrative pressures, which the offending physician is tempted to regard as measures to thwart his own good therapeutic intentions. Commenting about one of these men, another head nurse said:

I think he is very little concerned about the unit as a whole and about other patients on the unit. His patient is the prime consideration, and everything good for his patient should go. He very easily changes his mind about what is therapeutic. . . . At times, he leaves the nursing staff in the cold, when he says one thing this minute and another thing the next. . . . We're never clear about our role with patients. . . . How do we handle such a patient as that? We either try to bring in the administrator or get an administrative stand, or we throw up our hands in disgust. When a patient of his is transferred off the unit, we try not to get her back.

The first head nurse also remarked that:

Dr. Syth is notorious for telling patients what the nurses have been saying on the charts. "The nurses have been complaining about this sort of behavior, now what have you got to say about it?" It may not be that he means to get the nurses in trouble, but he uses the information in this way. Good God, this thing has horrible repercussions! Sometimes we get so mad that we could just shoot him, but he does it all the time, and we are just a little bit wary of what we're going to put down. . . . There have been some patients of his,

179

particularly Joan, who I see in retrospect should have been transferred but we didn't because I didn't know him well enough to know that some of the stuff he was handing me was crap. I really believed him when he said that this unit was the only one who could do it: "Let's not send her away. You've got to love her, you've got to understand," and all that. . . . I was new here so that I thought — oh boy, if I couldn't play a hero's role I could certainly try. I wouldn't do it again because I learned. But a patient of Dr. John's, of Smith's, of Jay's — any of the younger ones who will stand with us while a patient does a lot of acting out, will probably . . . get consistent treatment and care, and we will see the patient through the rough spots. . . . The doctors who don't pay very much attention to what the nurses need, and want by way of support from them, find their patients shunted around a little bit more.

Both nurses are touching upon their principal means of reprisal against the offending physician. Other measures — confining patients to their rooms ("seclusion") or sending them overnight as punishment to the closed ward ("guesting") — are addressed more directly at patients. From the therapist's point of view, all such measures are obstacles to effective treatment.

THE STAFF'S MULTIPLE RESPONSIBILITY

The head nurses' remarks suggest how the views of the staff, including those of aides and administrative residents, are tinted by eagerness to co-operate in the therapeutic enterprise and with concern for controlling the condition under which it works. These desirable goals must be attained under three important, but not always compatible, sets of responsibilities. First, personnel are responsible to the central administrators, who expect the staff members to maintain relatively orderly wards. Second, they are responsible to the attending men, each of whom expects to protect his patients' interests from the damaging behavior of other patients and from the unanticipated effects of another physician's requests for *his* patients. While each doctor can participate in only a few clinical teams, the staff, with many patients simultaneously, participates in many clinical teams. Finally, personnel are responsible to the patients. In fact, under certain conditions in which a patient seems not to be receiving adequate therapy, the staff will develop its own therapeutic program. The staff quite often finds itself caught in the crossfires of these different responsibilities. We turn now to some of the consequences.

The Staff's Organization of Treatment

We have caught occasional glimpses of personnel developing modes of treatment behind the backs of attending physicians. The conditions under which they do so are worth noting because they reveal something about work co-ordination in this kind of hospital. We already know that somaticists give permission for supplementary handling of their patients when the staff believes such efforts can help. An irate staff may take its case against a somaticist to central administration when a youthful patient is receiving EST without visible salutary results. But the staff may also embark, under certain conditions, upon its own therapeutic program without the explicit knowledge or consent even of a co-operative psychotherapist. The staff may grow restless because a patient "is not improving," is not showing any progress, and indeed seems to be retrogressing. Sometimes the physician, disagreeing with the staff's analysis, persists doggedly in his own program, so that the staff feels it must institute a supplementary program. When a physician ruffles the feelings of the staff by not letting members in on his program, and if his program — whatever it may be — seems not to be producing results, then conditions are almost perfect for supplementary programming. Furthermore, if the physician seems genuinely confused, seems not to have "doped out" his patient, or has confessed bafflement, then the staff members may reach consensus about a reasonable line of action and may pursue it even if he rejects their advice. Immensely troublesome patients are likely to be regarded as "manipulating" their physicians, "just as they do to us." Having lost faith in the "manipulated" physician's efforts to control his patient, the staff is inclined to develop its own program. In all such instances, consensus may be imperfect, but it involves at least several people, including the head nurse. Among parties to the agreement may be the ward resident, the ward co-ordinator, and even members of the central administration. Consensus is reached not only through informal chats at the station but in actual formal conclave. Weekly conferences also tend occasionally to draw paternal unit co-ordinators into the therapeutic act, providing that they cannot dissuade the staff from giving the offending physicians a few more days of grace.

Among the conditions that propel the staff into its own programming is one characterized by much fanfare: when patients become so enmeshed in mutual problems that the staff feels individual programs are no longer either manageable or therapeutically realistic. During our stay at PPI, there occurred a famous incident known as "the adolescent scarification." To the staff's mounting dismay, a number of adolescents continued for days to slash their own hands and wrists, and no action seemed able to stop this distressing fad. The staffs of the wards involved never achieved genuine consensus, so that the continued "scarification" spawned a number of individualistic and group programs. The attending physician regarded staff action variously, according to their respective philosophies. Some openly accused staff members of throwing therapy out the window in favor of control, but there is little reason to believe that these personnel were actually concerned only with safety and management. Not only was the principle of fair play at stake (Mary should be transferred; keeping her here is not fair to Joan, who imitates her), but direct therapeutic responsibility to patients was also involved. In reply to accusations that they were simply overanxious, frightened, and concerned for ward orderliness, the personnel charged that the psychiatrists were ineffective with their patients — and that something must be done. Harsh judgment was made of various psychiatrists precisely on the grounds that they refused to act as a therapeutic body when the situation called for collaboration rather than individualistic programs.

THE SHAPES OF WARDS

The personnel on each ward share certain general notions about their ward: its qualities, what kinds of patient "fit," what kinds of behavior "are appropriate" or "inappropriate," and its place in the hospital's scheme of things. All these notions taken together are commonly referred to as the ward's "shape."

The concept of shape arises from the staff's efforts to keep relative order in the face of continual change, albeit order consonant with therapeutic conscience. In the nature of institutional conditions, each ward is subject to changes in patients, physicians, and personnel. Understandably, the various personnel wish to manage the ward successfully — for their own comfort and pride, as well as to satisfy their various responsibilities — yet they also want their wards to be maximally therapeutic.

Central administration gives a certain impetus to prevailing notions of shape, both by its general conception of how each ward relates to the others (what has earlier been termed the hospital's "map") and by its publication of a few rules for each ward. Yet these notions of shape and the term itself arise from the daily "wear and tear" of ward activity. From time to time, these wards change sufficiently to change the personnel's notions about them too. Ward 2E gradually became recognized as the ward for adolescents, and its nurses developed conceptions of themselves as overseers and therapists for adolescents. Such conceptions are sustained both by physicians' expectations and by central administrators' implicit and explicit affirmations.

From time to time, the staff recognizes clearly that its ward is "way out of shape." With resignation, the 3N personnel note that they have far more medical patients than usual, with all the extra physical labor that entails. Personnel on 2E complain that their ward's sex ratio is askew. In general, the situation is more endurable when not all dimensions of shape are awry simultaneously. Unusual ward shapes are regarded as occasionally inevitable, rectifiable only by time: More women will eventually arrive on 2E, and the medical patients will someday disappear from 3N. In essence, the staff assumes that the ward swings from equilibrium to disequilibrium and back again.

The staff is not always so fatalistic, not always so patient about waiting for the disequilibrium to right itself. If the ward seems dangerously out of shape, then something should be done about it now! We have already seen what tactics can be used: seclusion, restriction of privileges, sedation, and eventually transfer if necessary. One unit resident whose ward had "too many adolescents" made certain when he was made ROD that the next new adolescent was assigned elsewhere. The staff can thus at least prevent shape from becoming further distorted. Such tactics lessen the probability that the ward will get too far out of control or become untherapeutic or antitherapeutic in atmosphere. The staff has ample rhetoric to accompany its tactics: for instance, "the unit isn't set up for too many of those patients," or "it isn't fair to other patients," or "he's not appropriate for this unit, he'd do better upstairs."

But quite as important as the relationship of ward shape to both therapy and management is its influence on the staff's self-conceptions. When a ward is too far out of shape, the staff tends to feel useless, even violated. Of what use are we under conditions like these? What do the physicians think we are anyhow? This unit is set up to take care of mental patients, not physical ones! This ward is set up to take care of sick patients, not adolescent brats! When appropriate tactics restore a unit to near its usual shape, then the staff also begins to feel itself psychologically to rights again.

Because the definition of each ward's shape arises from daily activity rather than solely from administrative fiat, the definition is characterized by flexibility and ambiguity. Observers like ourselves are amazed at first to find personnel grumbling that a ward is out of shape when, to our untutored eyes, it is not very noticeably out of shape; conversely, what seems to laymen to be a badly misshapen ward is scarcely remarked upon by its personnel, who may readily agree that there is a bit more acting out than usual or a somewhat unbalanced sex ratio but who will add that things are generally quite in order.

Unquestionably this apparent inconsistency is related to subjective perspectives. When genuinely fond of a patient or interested enough in his fate, the staff endures behavior far beyond the confines of ordinary "fit." One woman patient who required constant physical care was kept on 3EW because its staff so emphasized with "how far she had come" from the regressed state in which she had entered the hospital: She was so deteriorated physically that other patients had been induced to help with her care. Similarly, when a co-operative physician arouses sufficient faith in his efforts, the staff tends to be more lenient in its definitions of shape.

Quite as relevant is how a patient happens to fit in with what is occurring on the ward. It is common to see the personnel transferring patients whose behavior under less tense conditions would fall well within their tolerance limits. A patient may be reluctantly transferred because he cannot be adequately "worked with" under present conditions, that is, he is currently outside the limits. An outsider cannot entirely predict which patients will be regarded as "stretching" shape unless he also knows something of the ward's immediately preceding history. Accident and chance also enter into the decision: If 3N's guesting bed is taken, then 2E may decide not to keep its troublesome patient another day but transfer her to 2W; if two or three patients begin to "provoke each other," then the staff may break up the combination by a transfer or two, although the same number of acting out patients who ignore one another can be endured.

An occasional immensely troublesome patient challenges not only each ward, as he is transferred successively to each, but also the very shape of the hospital itself. No ward is able to hold him for very long within its usual scheme of things: Tactics fail, strategies break down, consensus dissolves. The most closed ward is the last refuge; if it fails, the patient probably will be discharged from the hospital. As this process will be illustrated in detail in the next chapter, only one case will be noted here. 3N is set up to handle relatively violent patients. The evening nursing supervisor, among whose important functions is the quieting of potentially excitable patients, was at his wits' end because he could not control an exceptionally violent patient. This patient was not unusually violent but violent in an unusual way: He hit out at everyone, indiscriminately, suddenly, and apparently without knowing what he was doing. Every tactic to quiet him and to anticipate his violence failed.

Yet the principal danger to each ward is not the inappropriate patient; it is the recalcitrant doctor. The patient can always be disciplined or transferred or eventually expelled from the hospital. The doctor may be susceptible to discipline and pressure, and he may be open to negotiation, but the personnel possess no power to evict him from the hospital. If they must work with his patients, then they must work with him. But the doctor tends to see ward shape somewhat differently from the way in which the staff sees it, for he focuses on single patients rather than on groups of patients and perceives the ward's characteristics mainly in relation to his patient's therapy. He has what may be termed a conception of therapeutic shape or therapeutic potential, rather than the staff's more complex conception of shape, which stems from its own multitude and often conflicting responsibilities. The physician's idea of therapeutic shape may even run counter to the personnel's notions — including their therapeutic notions. For instance, what they define as drastically out of shape may be precisely what the doctor thinks best for his patient. When crossed by the personnel, a physician sometimes utilizes his psychiatric vocabulary to accuse them, calling them "rigid," "overanxious," "compulsive," and so forth.

Neither he nor they are entirely correct, of course, for behind their potential conflict of perspective and interest lie the considerations we have already touched upon. There is also a certain inevitability about disagreement in their respective interpretations of some patients. In an earlier chapter, we noted that nurses or aides are likely to focus upon a patient's daily behavior, of which the psychiatrist sees little, and to interpret it differently. Furthermore, as the hospital houses many emergency patients, even the doctor may be uncertain about his patient's "real" character. To potential disagreement over ambiguous and changeable shape must be added potential disagreement over the patient's sickness.

All this disagreement necessitates a tremendous amount of talk, a phenomenon noted by various investigators and commented upon wonderingly by many who work in such hospitals. This talk is composed of various elements: wonder at events and how they are handled; argument over proper interpretation of events and patients' behavior; efforts to persuade oneself and others, including physicians and patients to particular points of view. At various places in preceding chapters, the staff's attempts to influence physicians' actions and to elicit explanations from them have been mentioned. In addition, much communication directly involves negotiations between parties who must work together. In the following pages, we shall discuss negotiation in detail. Here we shall remark only that, except in relatively routine types of treatment (the "blue plate specials"), the staff and physicians must negotiate. They must strike bargains, make verbal agreements, or at the very least achieve implicit understandings. Such bargains, agreements, and understandings are not fixed for all time — nor do they necessarily cover everything. Some arrangements are less extensive in time and scope than are others, but all are necessary for what we call "negotiated consensus," which must be periodically reviewed and reconstituted.

CLINICAL AND ADMINISTRATIVE ARRANGEMENTS

To understand fully the establishment of negotiative consensus, it is further useful to distinguish, according to the intentions of the contracting parties, between clinical and administrative arrangements. A physician's arrangements with the head nurse for clinical purposes are clinical arrangements. By contrast, when she persuades her unit resident to stand firm against an attending physician who wishes to give a patient excessive privileges, that is an administrative arrangement.

The chief initiator of most clinical arrangements is the physician, the leader of the clinical team. He usually makes the major decisions about what will be done to and for the patient and by whom. At PPI most clinical arrangements are inherently unstable for several reasons. To begin with, the personnel the physician counts on may be on rotation or absent. Although the head nurse is a relatively stable feature of ward landscape, the remaining members of the specific clinical team assembled for his patient are not. Furthermore, with changes in the patient's state, either he or she may decide to add or subtract members from that team. Each time the patient is transferred, whether by his physician or by the house staff, the physician must make new clinical arrangements. All such unstable arrangements are partially supported by long-standing agreements like those between certain physicians and head nurses, and by a given patient's lengthy stay on any ward. It is unnecessary to dwell upon the similarly unstable character of clinical arrangements initiated by the personnel, since they are subject to identical conditions, in addition to the physician's frequent exclusion from their programing.

By contrast, administrative arrangements vary from quite stable to very unstable. The former include all the routine uses of the administrative apparatus for administrative purposes. One example is the institutionalized procedure by which the ROD examines and assigns new patients; another is the daily collection of information from head nurses by the nursing supervisor. Certain other routines are not matters of official ruling, nevertheless are quite reliable. The evening nursing supervisor can be telephoned by night nurses, who know from experience that he will support them if a patient becomes unruly. Many other administrative routines are inherently unstable because of changes in the personnel supposedly involved in the routines. Because the ROD rotates daily, night nurses cannot accurately predict what to expect in an emergency, unless they know exactly who the ROD is. Whenever a unit resident is appointed, a period of administrative uncertainty follows, until firm understandings develop between him and at least the head nurse. The same strictures apply whenever a new unit co-ordinator or head nurse is appointed.

To understand the phenomenon of negotiation, it is important to recognize that many administrative arrangements do not rest firmly upon either administrative rulings or relatively established procedures. Like clinical arrangements, some administrative arrangements must be continually renegotiated. They must also be initiated by someone. Just as the physician has a choice of whom he will ask to do certain things for his patient, so a nurse can choose with whom she will negotiate for specific administrative purposes. The nursing personnel have an array of potential allies: the unit residents, the unit co-ordinators, the RODs, the central administrators, and the nursing supervisors. For administrative purposes, nursing personnel can call upon one another, as well as other echelons in any combination. Who are chosen for partners in such enterprises depends, as we shall see, not only upon established procedures but upon the past history of relationships among personnel and the severity of the administrative problem.

Under optimum conditions, the administrative and clinical arrangements mesh neatly. Whenever physicians accuse the staff of too much concern with management or whenever the staff believes physicians insensitive to hospital requirements, it can safely be assumed that administrative and clinical purposes are not entirely harmonious — and that special arrangements will have to be negotiated if indeed they are not already operative. Such arrangements do not always proceed according to Hoyle. The nurse may draw the physician into an administrative arrangement, persuading him to use the therapeutic sessions to calm down his patient. A physician may secretly draw the unit resident into a clinical arrangement, persuading the resident to "work on" the nurses to keep an unruly patient and to take responsibility for blocking potential transfer. Sometimes, however, nurses have so much invested in a patient that they are unwilling to give up on him and will persuade the resident and even the attending physician to "give us two more days." More than once we observed the nurses' requests eventually, if reluctantly, overruled by a unit co-ordinator or other higher administrator.

All the more understandable is the nurses' eagerness for action that might reconcile clinical and administrative ends. If the physician will not offer such a program, they seek to force it upon him, but if he will not negotiate, then they will either pursue their own program or decide reluctantly in favor of administrative ends. During the most uproarious battles, even central administrators may offer suggestions for clinical programs that seem eminently reasonable to the staff precisely because they are balanced nicely between clinical and administrative ends. When such suggestions are opposed by a staff member, it is usually because of an imbalance between those ends.

In all instances where administrative or clinical intentions are in conflict, special arrangements are required. Understandably, the contracting partners are not always happy about being drawn into an arrangement. The unit resident is especially vulnerable because he is exposed to requests both from attending physicians and nursing personnel. The latter, however, especially the head nurse bear the brunt of misalignment between clinical and administrative ends. Since the nursing personnel are torn between desires for involvement in the therapeutic enterprise and for manageable wards and since they have multiple responsibilities to central administration, the physicians, and the patients, they stand at the very center of institutional conflict. They have much to gain from harmonizing administrative and clinical arrangements.

THE WEB OF NEGOTIATIONS

Prescribed and Unprescribed Behavior

What have been designated as relatively stable administrative procedures are in effect procedures governed by hospital rules. The rules governing action at PPI are far from extensive and are not clearly stated or clearly binding. As in most sizable establishments, hardly anybody knows all the rules, much less in exactly what situations they apply and to whom. This confusion reigns, if for no other reason, because of considerable turnover of the nursing staff. Also noticeable to us as observers was that rules, once promulgated, would fall into disuse and would periodically undergo administrative resurrection after the staff had either ignored or forgotten them. As one head nurse, smilingly said, "I wish they would write them all down somewhere." The plain fact is that staff members forget not only the rules from above but those that they themselves have agreed upon "for this ward." Periodically, informal rules are agreed upon, enforced for a short time, and then forgotten until another ward crisis elicits their revival.

At the very top of PPI's administrative structure, there is a tolerant attitude toward rules. The point can be illustrated by a conversation with the chief administrator, who recounted with amusement how some members of his original staff wished to have all the rules set down in a house rule book, a movement that he had staved off. This administrative attitude is also influenced by a profound belief that care of patients calls for a minimum of rules and a maximum of creativity and improvisation. In addition, in this hospital, the multiplicity of medical purpose and theory, as well as of personal investment, is openly recognized. Too rigid a set of rules would only cause turmoil and affect the hospital's over-all efficiency.

Furthermore, the hospital must recognize the realities of the attending physicians' negotiations with patients and their families, negotiations carried out beyond the physical confines of the hospital itself. Too many or too rigid rules would restrict the medical "entrepreneurs'" negotiations. Any hospital with attending men must allow this kind of leeway.

The area of action covered by clearly enunciated rules is therefore really very small. As observers, we began to become aware of this point in our first few days, when we discovered that only a few general rules guided placement of new patients within the hospital. Any rules that are clearly enunciated and generally followed can be regarded as long-standing shared understandings among the personnel. Except for a few legal rules stemming from states and professional prescriptions and some rulings pertaining to all of Michael Reese Hospital, almost all house rules are more like general understandings than commands. In general, punishments are not spelled out, and most rules can be stretched, negotiated, argued, ignored, or applied at convenient moments. Frequently they are less explicit than tacit, probably honored as much in the breach (and the stretch) as in application. In addition, no rule is a universal prescription; each requires judgment of its applicability to a specific case. Does it apply here? To whom? In what degree? For how long? With what sanctions? The personnel can only point to analogous instances in the past or give "for instance" answers when queried about a rule's future application.

Nevertheless, such rules can be used to organize certain actions by one status occupant (head nurse) toward another (unit co-ordinator). As in other establishments, personnel call upon certain rules to obtain desired ends. All categories of personnel are also adept at breaking rules when certain exigencies arise. Stretching the rules is only a further variant of that tactic, itself less attributable to human nature than to an honest desire to accomplish things properly. In all such instances, the respective parties must negotiate; they cannot simply declare rules applicable or inapplicable. Conventional behavior, governed by long-standing understandings among personnel, is also subject to qualification and review, requiring negotiation.

Patterns of Negotiation: The Unit Resident

These negotiations do not happen merely by chance: They are patterned. They occur in discernible proportions among the occupants of the various hospital statuses. While such statuses do not rigidly determine how a person will act, they do determine whom he has to take into account and therefore which situations are likely to recur. To illustrate these probabilities and to probe further the characteristics of PPI's web of negotiations, we shall discuss certain negotiations carried on by the unit residents. These negotiations do not exhaust the universe of their agreements but are typical enough to afford excellent illustration.

First- and second-year residents are assigned to each unit on a rotational basis. Their assignment is justified administratively in terms of education, which is the *raison d'etre* of residency. Both administration and residents rank learning through supervision and classroom as primary. Experience gained as an administrator is regarded as distinctly secondary. Yet the residents are caught up and often absorbed in the daily events on their wards. A resident cannot help himself, for he is exposed to various personnel who involve him in perennial knotty problems. Making demands upon him and seeking to strike agreements with him are head nurse and other ward personnel, the unit co-ordinator, other unit residents, the attending physicians, the ROD, and on occasion the central administrators. Most demands, except those made by physicians, are of an administrative rather than a clinical nature, although occasionally the resident's clinical advice, judgments, or services are requested. But his administrative capacities are more in demand, for he is useful in effecting or blocking transfers and in mediating between nursing personnel and physicians. The topics on which he will be asked to negotiate and those persons by whom he will be asked, and when, are scarcely accidental.

The unit resident's principal coworkers are the co-ordinator and the head nurse: These three must establish new agreements whenever a new resident is rotated to the unit. Exactly what arrangements will result depends upon such variables as the respective experience of nurse and resident and how much responsibility is ceded to the resident by the co-ordinator. If the latter finds that his resident can be safely trusted, he will delegate virtually complete command over the unit. As one co-ordinator said, "I have . . . followed pretty much what . . . [my co-ordinator] did with me, now that I am co-ordinator. When I was unit resident, after a while, he told me 'you can make administrative decisions' which were actually his role." Asked about his current agreements and understandings with his unit resident, he replied:

> I have an agreement with him that we aren't going to have regular meetings, except for once a week meetings with the whole staff. If anything comes up he should let me know, and we will talk it over, anything that he feels he can't handle. . . . What happened was that originally . . . I told

him that I wanted to wait and see how things were running. After a month maybe I told him, why don't you take this over. . . . So that is the kind of agreement we have had, and things have run smoothly on the unit. . . . I felt that he ought to try to run the personnel meetings as much as possible and I would comment whenever I thought it necessary and helpful.

When the co-ordinator does not trust his resident (and especially if he himself is a resident, spending more time at the hospital than those co-ordinators who are residents), then he is less likely to make such special arrangements.

I didn't feel as free in delegating the power of the unit and his making administrative decisions. For a while he did and got things all fouled up and I thought that I ought to take it over, and did. . . . Yes, I probably had more direct dealings with the head nurse then. . . . Yes, she tended to shortcut this resident and come to me. I tried to get her to go to him sometimes; one time she called me about transfers and I said it was his job. She acted as if he wasn't capable of doing it.

Usually a nurse prefers to deal with her unit resident, once he has won his spurs after a short trial period, since he is much more available than her co-ordinator. That period may not be entirely free of jockeying, for the residents sometimes grow restive waiting for more responsibility.

Beside general agreement ("for the most part, he has let me run everything"), a few other contingencies may necessitate specific agreements between the two men. For instance, they may feel that personnel are rejecting certain patients and decide that "we were going to try to tolerate more severely disturbed patients. We have done this, and the unit has gotten back to where it should be." Faced by an identical problem, one co-ordinator even went so far in backing up his resident as virtually to give therapy to the head nurse: "We worked through some of this and she became less apprehensive and began to accept more freely these patients, and these transfer problems lessened." With particularly difficult attending men, the co-ordinator may be asked by resident and nurse to intercede.

But most of the resident's specific understandings and special arrangements involve his relationship with his head nurse. Not only does he mediate between her and the physician, while she in turn mediates between the physicians and her staff, but some ambiguity exists in their respective administrative powers. The more experienced the nurse, the less disposed she is to cede authority to her resident, especially during the early months of his residency. Yet residents, as everyone recognizes, are soon eager to take responsibility and sensitive at being denied it.

Under these conditions, what arrangements are likely to be worked out between resident and nurse? To begin with, the resident who has a trustworthy nurse may delegate certain administrative powers to her, much as the co-ordinator has delegated to him, in order to save himself time and trouble. For instance, he may sign sedation orders and allow the nurse to write them out each evening.

> Transfers are another thing that are kind of a delegation of responsibility. Sometimes this gets out of hand and one has to know the nurses to be able to know which patient she can transfer without my OK. Officially, I have to OK each transfer, especially when to a more open unit. [Then] . . . they like to have my OK and the OK of the resident of that unit. . . . I have found that to talk about every transfer is really again a waste of time.

If there is mutual trust, the resident need not fear that patients will be transferred behind his back. Incidents like this one happen when such trust does not exist:

> I had very definite orders and a very definite understanding that this patient should stay unless something particular comes up. One morning . . . Miss Jay said "we just transferred him [through the ROD] and that is all. You can't do anything." . . . I was very angry and thought this was very poor judgment. I was even angrier at her smile, which seemed to be a sign that if you don't go along with me, you will just have to suffer: Your principles mean nothing to me.

Through proper negotiation, the head nurse can induce the resident to be very helpful. If her personnel are in an uproar about the possibility of another adolescent or another "psychotic" being transferred to their ward when it already has several, she can ask her resident to block the transfer. This request forces him to negotiate with either the ROD or the other unit resident or both. ("Miss Jacks was very hesitant about accepting this man. I felt I had to go along with her. . . . I felt that I had to sort of stand behind her.") Frequently they strike quick agreements to persuade an attending man to increase drug dosage, to reduce privileges, to communicate more information, to attend the staff's weekly meeting and talk about his patient, and even to ask for the patient's transfer. Any resident sensitive to staff claims upon him is quick to take up "his responsibilities" for the transfer of patients, despite the wishes of the therapist. In speaking of the therapist who wanted to house his patients only on 2E, one resident remarked:

> He is famous for bringing in bizarre patients to an open unit . . . in my experience it doesn't work out. As a unit resident, I already have the feeling that it is not going to work out, so I'm looking to transfer his patient, Janet. . . . They so totally exhaust the nurse that she can't give time to the other patients.

But sometimes the personnel want to work with a patient despite extreme difficulties in managing him. They may enlist the resident's support in eliciting further co-operation and information from the therapist. ("We were not 'hot' to transfer the patient off, but we wanted to know how we could keep him there without it being harmful to the patient.") The resident "carries the ball" in such negotiation.

The resident, in his turn, becomes absorbed in effecting certain actions — all the more important to him because, as a learner, he wishes to try out his own ideas — and may therefore initiate understandings with his personnel. One resident was exceedingly eager to have adolescent self-mutilators worked with for as long as possible.

> We had two "cutters" and we agreed that we would try to do everything to keep them and help them progress. . . . I had an agreement with the staff which I think was almost universal there, that self-mutilation is not a reason for transfer. We would try to handle all these things ourselves, unless it comes to the point where we can't.

Conversely, the personnel may be against receiving certain patients. ("The nurses were against it. I kind of pushed them into giving it a try.") Or the resident may attempt to talk the nurses into transfer — the nurses sometimes "develop such attachments to patients that you can't get the patients off. I suggested that we may have to transfer this patient, and the nurse began to cry." The resident tends to be most active in initiating negotiations when he has definite ideas about what philosophy should prevail upon his unit, that is, on how the unit should function in the total hospital.

Less crucial for the resident's peace of mind than his relations with the head nurse are his relations with attending physicians. Yet the physicians can initiate negotiations that upset this equilibrium or flatter him, especially as some are supervisors and others are actually residents treating service patients. Caught between nurses and a physician, the resident may succumb to the latter's persuasion and agree that a patient should not be transferred.

Then he gives you the story that it is traumatic to the patient and plays upon the guilt of the resident, which works in the beginning. . . . Then I have to admit that I was inclined to give his patient a little extra, to allow a little more acting out than some of the others, but after I saw that he was taking advantage of it, I just told him, well I'm sorry. I have to check with my co-ordinator, usually, but he gives me a pretty free hand.

Frequently, a therapist will ask the resident to intercede with the nursing personnel to ensure that a patient remains longer on the unit.

None of her behavior, of course, is ordinarily tolerated on this unit, but this was a special case. It was finally resolved with my talking with the nurse . . . if this patient is upsetting her, then I too would be in agreement to postpone it another week. By these delaying tactics, which was a test agreement between myself and him, we tried it for three days. . . . We tried getting her to calm her fears . . . and little by little she became aligned again with this therapeutic effort, and after three days this patient had completely calmed down. . . . I had told him that I agreed with him about the handling of this patient, that as the resident I would do everything possible to allow him to align thinking along this direction. . . . [At one point] a meeting was held . . . he appeared. The co-ordinator, too . . . [who] sided with the fact that the nurses were getting anxious and it was time to transfer the patient.

The resident's footwork in maintaining balance is revealed in these remarks about that meeting:

I remember one little incident that I purposely sort of brought to bear: I asked him whether or not this patient was raking him over the coals like we were doing. Everybody laughed. This made the condition a little more handleable all the way around.

Occasionally, because the resident also is a physician, his professional services are called upon by attending men. A child analyst, who rarely hospitalized patients, asked one resident — who felt he was asked because the analyst had not much time to spend at the hospital — to "take the case over and . . . to write all the orders and see him once in a while . . . the patient is an interesting fellow. So I did that. I felt I was somewhat pressed into it, but also that I could learn something from it." Another therapist about to go on vacation had a patient who "had a tremendous difficulty in building up new relationships and I had known her for some time and she had a fairly good relationship with me. So he asked me to take over that patient [for] . . . five days." Occasionally residents are asked to oversee drug prescriptions by physicians who believe their own knowledge is deficient: "He has been an analyst for many years and has been away from drugs. This was an interesting case for me and I put her on a new kind of thorazine compound." The analyst more than upheld his end of the bargain by making himself accessible by phone and coming twice to ward meetings. "So there was a real active agreement: He gave more than he usually would to the unit by coming to our meeting and talking to me about the patient; I have more to do than usual because I followed the patient from a medical point of view." Such symbiosis may, however, easily turn into or seem to turn into exploitation. One physician:

> Had the habit of bringing patients to the hospital and giving them to residents so that they will see them an hour a day and he will kind of do some therapy . . . but the resident would really take the bulk of the patients, the management and the therapy, while he got the money. . . . Early in my residency he had one patient acting up and two residents treating this patient. Each saw that patient for three full hours a day, and then he saw the patient for about a half hour intermittently. He had another; I had worked him up, I think. He came and said: Smith likes you as a therapist, you are a good therapist and I think you would be good for her. Would you please do me the favor, or would you be interested in seeing her every day for some time? I said I was sorry, I had my own time and I would like to see my own patients. I would be glad to see her once in a while for five or ten minutes. He said: that is not what I mean. . . . He went around to every resident and finally he found one who would do it, for about a month. . . . There is nothing wrong with it, if he gets something out of it, that is fine . . . [but] it is kind of taking advantage. . . . I resent this and I know that the other residents resented this too. . . . Yes, some do have him as a supervisor.

Occasionally, from lack of a clear understanding, an attending physician may believe that a resident is stepping beyond administrative bounds to interfere with clinical proceedings. There was "a case in which I was interested. She was used to talking with me, when Dr. Fleet was not around. I went to see her twice. After . . . Dr. Fleet came up to me — he was very angry — and asked me what I was doing seeing his patient. 'When I have a patient I want all of the material resolved with me, I want all of it, I want it concentrated.' "

But a unit resident is likely to have even more delicate negotiations with other residents, whether or not they themselves are treating service patients upon his unit, are acting as ROD's, or are unit residents themselves. "He wanted me to be the administrator for his patient, and write the administrative orders. I told him I didn't think it was indicated and he agreed; now if Johnnie [with whom he was more friendly] had asked, I probably would have done it as a personal favor." When he himself was treating a patient upon Johnnie's unit, "it was an unsaid statement that my patient wouldn't be transferred off until I said that she was ready." Because resident therapists can spend more time with their patients than can the attending physicians, greater administrative demands can be made upon resident therapists by the unit residents. One resident therapist, who had a great investment in keeping a particular patient upon the open ward, said that the unit resident "has the feeling that anyone who is able to be on 2N doesn't need an administrator, so I took over fully the administrative duties. The only understanding I had was if she makes one wrong move, she goes." Asked whether or not other residents come to him, in their turn, when he is unit resident, he answered, "Yeah, like Joe comes to me about his patient, and we meet from time to time in an attempt to keep her in line well enough that we can keep her on the unit. He wanted very much to keep her on the unit." Occasionally negotiation involves as many as three residents. Here, for instance, is a resident whose patient is on 3N striking a bargain with two other unit residents whose consent he needed. "What he wanted to do was to take my patient to 2N. Mel is the resident on 2N, and Jim is the resident on 3N. So we have all that we need. . . . We have to have the agreement of the [head] nurses too, so we would be sure to get this for a day [at least], until the evening nursing supervisor comes on."

Whether acting as administrators or therapists, the residents are easily able to negotiate with the RODs because all are colleagues. A typical situation is that of a unit resident who requests that a newly admitted patient not be placed upon his ward. The ROD may not accede, but he is likely to say, "Well, Mike, if you any trouble within the next hour, I will transfer him, or any time you want." Sometimes the ROD, feeling dubious, will check on the unit before long. Asked whether or not this sort of activity leads to disagreements, one resident remarked, "You see in most cases if there isn't a disagreement, there doesn't have to be an agreement. When your philosophies aren't alike all of the time, one guy will often say, 'well gee, I will go along with you.'" Nevertheless as residents do have different ideas about managing wards and treating patients and, in addition, may dislike one another, their differences may affect their respective negotiations. Refusal to negotiate or an attempt to drive a hard bargain ordinarily heightens bad feelings. Despite ideological differences, the men may co-operate, either because the issue is unimportant or because it is not important enough to warrant a firm stand.

This web of negotiation in which residents are involved is only one segment of the total web of negotiations spun throughout the hospital. It is possible to trace systematically the typical negotiations linking each hospital status — from the point of view of the principal actors — but those of the unit residents underscore several important points. First, once having been placed in status positions, personnel are confronted with the necessity for acting toward certain other occupants. While some rules and conventions do exist, usually they merely serve as general guides. Furthermore, various contingencies arise outside their jurisdictions. In that large area beyond, negotiations are affected by such matters as relative hierarchical positions and ideological commitments, as well as by periodic staff rotations and ward tensions. The form and direction of negotiation are also, as we have seen, affected by personal relations. While the general pattern of negotiation is recurrent and can be observed and analyzed, many precise outcomes are relatively unpredictable. In this regard, it is well to keep in mind Herbert Blumer's sage remark:

> Social organization enters into action only to the extent
> . . . it shapes situations in which people act, and to the extent . . . it supplies fixed sets of symbols which people use
> in interpreting their situations. . . . [The] most important
> element confronting an acting unit in situations is the actions of other acting units. . . . [With] increasing criss-crossing lines of action, it is common for situations to arise in
> which . . . actions . . . are not previously regularized and
> standardized."[1]

One striking phenomenon at PPI — and probably at other mental hospitals — is the recurrence of identical situations, which personnel then argue out almost as if they had never before faced them. This recurrence is not entirely attributable to staff turnover and rotation. Sometimes personnel recognize that "we have been through all this before" and ask piteously whether or not there is an end to going around in circles, but more often they seem not to recognize that they are treading similar if not identical ground. The structure of the hospital causes the problems, but specific solutions are not determined strictly by structure.

[1]Herbert Blumer, "Society as Symbolic Interaction," in Arnold Rose, ed., *Human Behavior and Social Process* (Boston: Houghton Mifflin Company, 1961), p. 190.

The Temporal Dimension of Negotiation

Negotiation has many dimensions. It can be overt or covert, periodic or extraordinary, standardized or novel, general or specific in scope. But the dimension that we wish most to emphasize is the temporal one. Whether negotiations result in "agreement," "understanding," "contract," "compact," "pact," or some other form, it is for a limited period, whether or not the period is specifically defined by the contracting parties. As one listens while agreements are being made or understandings established, he often becomes aware that a specific termination period has been written into the arrangement. A physician, after being accosted by the head nurse, may agree to transfer his patient after she has agreed to "try for two more days." What he has done is to issue to her a promissory note: "If things don't work out satisfactorily, then I shall move the patient." Sometimes the staff breaks the contract, as we have seen, by transferring behind his back, especially if the patient is especially obstreperous, the ward out of shape, or staff tempers running high. If the patient improves or shape springs back, however, the staff's demands may subside. Interestingly, it often happens that both sides will negotiate further, seeking some compromise. On less tender and less specific grounds, physicians and head nurse may reach nodding agreement that a new patient should be handled in certain ways "until we see how he responds." There is clearly a continuum ranging from specific to quite unspecific terminal dates. But even those explicit and long-term permissions that physicians give to nurses in all hospitals are subject to review, withdrawal, and qualifications.

The very terms "agreements," "understandings," and "arrangements" — all used by hospital personnel — suggest that some negotiations are made explicitly, while others are established with scarcely any conversation. The more explicit or tacit kinds of contract are called "understandings." The difference is high-lighted by the following contrasting situations: When a resident suggests to a nurse that an established house rule be temporarily ignored for the good of a given patient, it may be implicit in their arrangement that the resident must take the responsibility if administrators discover the infraction. But the nurse may make this clause more explicit by demanding that he promise to assume any possible public guilt before she will assent. It follows that some agreements are simultaneously explicit and specific about termination, while others are explicit but nonspecific. What may be called "tacit understandings" are those that are neither very specific nor explicit. When a physician is not trusted, the staff is likely to push him for explicit directives that have specific terminal clauses.

NEGOTIATION, APPRAISAL, AND
ORGANIZATIONAL CHANGE

This discussion raises knotty problems about the relationships between any negotiated order and genuine organizational change. Since agreements are patterned and temporary, the sum total of today's agreements may very well be different tomorrow — and surely quite different next week. Agreements are continually being terminated or forgotten in the hospital, but they are also continually being established, renewed, received, revoked, revised. Those in effect are considerably different from those that have been or will be in effect.

A skeptic, thinking in terms of relatively permanent or slowly changing structure, might remark that the hospital remains the same from week to week, that only the working arrangements change. This argument, however, raises the further question, already touched upon, of the relationships between today's working agreements and the more stable institutional structure of rules and statuses. Practically, we maintain, no one knows what the hospital "is" on any given day unless he has a comprehensive grasp of the combination of rules, policies, agreements, understandings, pacts, contracts, and other working arrangements that currently obtain. In a pragmatic sense, that combination "is" the hospital at the moment, its social order. Any changes that impinge upon this order — whether ordinary changes, like introduction of a new staff member or a betrayed contract or unusual changes, like the introduction of new technology or new theory — will necessitate renegotiation or reappraisal, with consequent changes in the organizational order. There will be a new order, not merely the re-establishment of an old order or reinstitution of a previous equilibrium. It is necessary continually to reconstitute the bases of concerted action, of social order.

Such reconstitution, we would hazard, can be usefully conceived as a complex relationship between the daily negotiative process and a periodic appraisal process. The negotiative process not only allows the daily work to get done; it also reacts upon more formal permanent rules and policies. An illustration taken from our field notes should be helpful. For some time, the hospital had been admitting increasing numbers of nonpaying adolescent patients, principally because they made good supervisory subjects for the residents. As a consequence, the hospital began to develop the reputation for being more interested in adolescents than previously. Some attending physicians were encouraged to bring adolescents for treatment to the hospital. The presence of many youngsters on the wards raised many new problems and led to feverish negotiation among the various actors implicated in the daily drama. Finally, after some months of high adolescent census, a middle-level administrative committee formally recognized the change. The committee was forced to such recognition primarily because a mass of adolescents was much harder to handle than its adult equivalent. Yet the situation had its compensatory aspects, for adolescents remained longer and therefore could be given more interesting types of therapy. After some debate, the committee ruled that no more adolescents be admitted after a stated number had been reached. The decision constituted a formal proclamation, with the proviso that, if the situation continued, the policy should be reviewed at high administrative levels in light of "where the institution was going." The decision was never enforced, for shortly thereafter the adolescent census dropped and never again rose to such heights. The decision has long since been forgotten, and, if the census were again to rise sharply, a new discussion would doubtless take place.

Yet it is precisely this process by which novel policies and new rules are absorbed into what is conventionally called "hospital structure." In their turn, of course, such policies and rules serve to set limits, and some directions of negotiations. We suggest that future studies of complex relationships between the more stable elements of organizational order and the more fleeting working arrangements may profit from examination of the former as a background against which the latter evolve — and sometimes as the reverse. What is needed is both a focus upon this kind of metaphor and development of a terminology adequate to handle it. But whether this metaphor or another is adopted, the question of how negotiation and appraisal influence each other and rules of policies remains central.

THE NEGOTIATED CHARACTER OF RULES[2]

So far in this chapter rules have been discussed as if they were relatively exempt from negotiation, as if negotiation occurred almost exclusively beyond the jurisdiction of rules in a realm where rules were either inapplicable or debatable. The realm of rules could then be usefully pictured as a tiny island of structured stability around which swirled and beat a vast ocean of negotiation. But we would push the metaphor further and assert what is already implicit in our discussion: that there is *only* vast ocean. The rules themselves are negotiable.

This statement is much more radical than a statement that rules, like other agreements, are temporally limited and stretchable, breakable, or selectively applicable. We noted in passing that "most rules can be stretched, negotiated, argued, ignored, or applied at con-

[2]We owe to Harold Garfinkel the full recognition that rules are also negotiable, that organizational life is not, in his words, "a series of flights (negotiations) and perchings (structure)."

venient moments." In fact, if the formulation, change, and application of rules are examined closely, the conclusion must be that there is a "negotiated order" within which rules fall. The remainder of this chapter [and the next paper] should clarify that statement.

Rules are not disembodied standards. Like other negotiable products, they are human arrangements. In large-scale organizations, they tend to be written down, codified, and specifically sanctioned. Probably the tendency to emphasize rules as part of structure is derived both from the rise of bureaucratic phenomena and from an inherited language of law and politics. But the assumption that rules (or values) stand outside a negotiable realm assumes a consistency of conduct that surely exists only in the eye of the beholding theorist.

When one asks actors why they have acted as they have or what rules obtained, neat answers are sometimes forthcoming. Whether one asks them directly or simply adduces their answers — from observation or oblique interviews — one is seeking their grounds for action. Those grounds are sometimes stated as rules ("I acted this way in accordance with the rule that . . ."); but one man's grounds may not be the grounds of another. It is only when all agree that the grounds for action are "this rule" that consensus obtains. Not only may rules be broken consciously or stretched or avoided with supporting rationales, they must be implicitly negotiated to be applicable in specific situations. ("Implicit negotiation" is based on a history of explicit negotiation about similar rule applications.) Once the parties disagree, negotiation becomes explicit, sometimes ending in actual formal revision of a rule.

Clearly the sociologist must examine rules within a rhetorical framework, regarding them as historical pronouncements, usable in future situations. Rules enter into current and future conduct in that actors define rules as relevant to situations, which means that they must define situations as related or unrelated to specific governing rules. Consequently, in our hospital and elsewhere, people expect rules to control their own and others' behavior. They also counter other's claims to be rule-appliers with claims of their own. [In the chapter on nurses such maneuvers will be illustrated.] Here we wish only to reiterate that rules do operate within a negotiable arena. To restate a previous metaphor in which rules were to be viewed alternately as background and foreground for more fleeting working arrangements, rules may be regarded as background in current consensus and foreground in current argument. When action runs into censure or counterstrategies, then the actor is exposed to the full glare of rhetorical activity. This exposure highlights not only actor and act but also past history (the rules), possibly showing that he acted "outside history," unless he can make his particular rationale convincing. In the ensuing debate, the actor himself may be persuaded otherwise.

If rules are regarded as within the negotiated order, then we need no longer raise questions of where negotiation takes place in the hospital or on what issues. We are concerned instead with discovering among whom it takes place and its forms, content, timing, directions, and outcomes. (The usefulness of such questions ought to be readily apparent for the study of organizations like hospitals, where new concepts and practices — the hallmarks of medicine — have a way of making a shambles of current order. Such order can be imagined as temporarily frozen history.) In sum, the orderly character of hospital activity can be discovered by answering those questions.

THE NURSES AT PPI*

INTRODUCTION

The parallel growth and intimate association of psychiatry and psychiatric nursing are often proclaimed, since both are developing quickly and especially since psychiatric nursing depends upon psychiatric theory for much of its orientation. We believe, however, that the full import of the links between the two specialties has been insufficiently appreciated even by those who best visualize them.

The most informed opinion tends to underemphasize two points. The first is that what psychiatric nursing will become necessarily must depend upon what psychiatric ideology and practice — especially in hospitals and clinics — eventually become. In schools of nursing virtually everywhere, the major emphasis is upon the therapeutic relationships that psychiatric nurses ought to build with patients.[1] As a corrective, we wish in this chapter to shift emphasis to the nurse's problems with the psychiatrist himself, noting how he affects both her work and her image of herself as a professional.

The second aspect of psychiatric nursing that is usually overlooked, although pragmatically appreciated by nurses themselves, is the tremendous impact of hospital settings upon psychiatric nursing practice. This point has far greater implications than that one hospital encourages high-quality nursing while another does not. The *specific* practices that develop — whether "good" or "poor" — develop within hospitals and are molded by much that happens there. What nursing will become is inevitably linked with what happens at influential psychiatric hospitals.

[1]Marion Kalkman, *Introduction to Psychiatric Nursing* (New York: McGraw-Hill Book Co., Inc., 1958); Morris Schwartz and Emmy Shockley, *The Nurse and the Mental Patient* (New York: Russell Sage Foundation, 1956); and Hildegard Peplau, *Interpersonal Relations in Nursing* (New York: G. P. Putnam's Sons, 1952).

*Reprinted by permission from
PSYCHIATRIC IDEOLOGIES AND INSTITUTIONS
(with L. Schatzman, R. Bucher, D. Ehrlich and M. Sabshin), N. Y.
The Free Press, pp. 206-227. Copyright © 1964, The Free Press

We shall focus in this chapter upon two perplexing problems that beset PPI's nurses. Each problem inevitably involves both the institutional setting and its psychiatrists, often simultaneously.

1. The nurse must work out relationships between her managerial — or purely administrative — tasks and her therapeutic ones.

2. She must answer one question at the heart of her professional identity: What does therapeutic action toward patients actually involve for a psychiatric nurse?

To introduce the first problem, we need note only that managerial duties (charting or giving medication) are not necessarily identical with therapeutic actions ("giving contact" or "confronting patients with reality"). As for the second problem, the nurse at PPI does not engage in formal therapeutic sessions, as do psychiatrists; neither does she merely "help" patients (as do aides in state hospitals). What is she supposed to do? What kinds of psychiatric care can she actually give to patients?

At PPI the nursing students, who work on these wards during three-month training periods, need not confront these two problems. The student does not have to reconcile her therapeutic and administrative tasks because they are relatively separate: Either she works with patients on the floor, or she does routine chores at the nursing station. She need not face up to the disturbing problem of defining nurses' therapeutic action, partly because the psychotherapeutically oriented ideology she has been taught keeps her focus upon the relationship between the patient and herself and partly because she has almost no contact with physicians. After graduation, if she joins the PPI staff, she confronts the same major problems as her colleagues.

If PPI nurses were recruited differently, perhaps some of their problems — and certainly the solutions that they devise — might be different. PPI has rarely, if ever, recruited a nurse trained at a nursing center that might be considered more "advanced" than is PPI. Frequently nurses are recruited from institutions that PPI's personnel tend to consider less advanced. Yet in the Chicago metropolitan area — indeed in the Midwest generally — psychiatric nursing is relatively backward, ideologically speaking, unlike psychiatry itself. It is interesting to speculate what nursing practice, and psychiatric practice too, might be at PPI if the nurses had been trained in a more unified ideological style. We suspect, however, that the basic problems would remain the same: Only the answers would be somewhat different. The reasons for our belief will be given at the chapter's close.

We shall in the next pages be interested in how nurses cope with a set of primary problems and especially with the conditions that block formation of a stable and entirely satisfying therapeutic ideology. The data bearing on these problems were gathered in two years of fieldwork on PPI's wards, which included countless informal interviews with nurses, supplemented by formal interviews with former student nurses and with head nurses. At PPI, during the day, each ward is administered by a head nurse, assisted by a variable number of nurses. The division of labor between nurses and aides overlaps, but generally nurses do much more paper work, give medications, and are more self-conscious about their therapeutic maneuvers. As in other hospitals, the evening and night staffs have less contact both with attending physicians and with central administration. PPI's nurses number approximately twenty-eight. They are recruited from Michael Reese's school of nursing and from other hospitals, including nonpsychiatric ones. The teacher then responsible for the nursing school's psychiatric program was psychotherapeutically oriented and in good communication with PPI's head nurses and nursing director.

KEEPING ORDER ON THE WARDS

The nurse's managerial, administrative, and nursing-care (nonpsychiatric) tasks are less problematical than the therapeutic aspects of her work life. She has been trained for the former at nursing school and possibly on nonpsychiatric wards. Nevertheless, certain problems concerning those particular tasks arise repeatedly in the psychiatric hospital. These problems are similar to problems that confront nonpsychiatric nurses, but some features are probably unique to psychiatric nursing.

Two of the repetitive administration problems arise from the ambiguity surrounding the nurses' administrative and managerial authority and the potential of psychiatric wards for eruption into sudden "emergencies." We caution the reader against concluding that these problems are central for nurses. We shall attempt later to demonstrate that they become so *only* in combination with the therapeutic side of nurses' work, for, as we have already mentioned, one immense nursing problem is how to put together "management" and "therapy." Before discussing that problem, we turn first to the relatively minor ones concerning authority and emergencies, conveniently isolated, for analytic purposes, from therapeutic issues.

AMBIGUITIES OF AUTHORITY

Psychiatric hospitals everywhere share a common administrative feature. The institutional structure is headed by psychiatrists who are responsible for major administrative decisions; but below these high ranking officers are the nursing personnel, who are responsible for daily operational decisions with or without the assistance of ward psychiatrists. This arrangement places at least one medical functionary, sometimes without extensive adminstrative experience, in charge of the hospital. At the same time, it gives the nursing personnel a central role in administration, for they must quite literally keep the hospital in good running order. The nurse is even more important in the hospital's universe if attending physicians treat private patients at her hospital. The nursing staff finds itself thrown into special relationships with these physicians, who are much less concerned with administration than with the treatment of individual patients.

PPI also has unique features. Its administrative chain of command links each head nurse to the chief of the hospital and his two assistants, who are all psychiatrists; the director of nursing, who is directly responsible to the chief of the hospital; and the day and evening nursing supervisors, who are responsible to the director of nursing. In addition, there is a "unit administrator" for each ward, who is a first- or second-year resident. As his stay on the unit is only three months, the nurses periodically find themselves working with different residents. Also attached to each ward is a "unit co-ordinator," who is either a relatively recently graduated resident or a third-year resident. The duties of the co-ordinator and the unit administrator are not clearly defined. The various attending physicians who treat private patients at PPI have no administrative rights or functions except through negotiation with or counseling of the nurses and administrators.

During PPI's early years, the general adminstrative picture was different because the chief and his assistant were more involved in the administration of wards. Nurses had much less authority and consequently found themselves acting as buffers between irate attending physicians and the central administration. Nowadays, the nurses have considerably more autonomy over the daily operations of their wards. None of the psychiatrists at the administrative apex ordinarily enters authoritatively into the daily adminstration of the wards; for each is more deeply interested in research, writing, and residency training than in hospital administration *per se*. Each enters into ward operations from time to time, as we shall see. The chief enters mainly during great emergencies, while his two assistants keep daily and weekly tabs upon the hospital and its wards. But the nursing personnel regard their administrative psychiatrists as relatively distant, although accessible and occasionally "interfering." (Some regard the evening nursing supervisor as the chief's administrative right arm, although this view is probably more widespread among residents.) Relationships with unit administrators and co-ordinators

206

are variables since the amount of collaboration, counsel, and control asked by nurses or imposed by these functionaries must be worked out. Between the head nurses and nursing administrators, communication flows freely.

This formal picture of the organization of adminstrative action is, as always, considerably modified in the *actual* organization. We shall not discuss the difference in detail; it suffices to point to only one important fact. The nurses repeatedly find themselves in ambiguous situations, for the locus of major administrative decisions on each ward is indeterminately variable. That locus cannot always be predicted: Its indeterminacy hovers over nurses whenever anything approaching the dimensions of an emergency occurs.

Normally, each head nurse and her assistants will be inclined to make the decisions necessary to the ward's daily management. But one or another adminstrative officer above the head nurse may choose to step into the managerial process. He may be her unit resident, who has ideas about the running of wards or the handling of particular patients; he may be her co-ordinator who has been persuaded to act either by the unit resident or by an offended attending physician, whose patient may be threatened by an undesirable transfer; it may be the nursing supervisor, whose intervention, like the ROD's, can easily take place, especially during evening hours; it may be central administration, which is laying down emergency measures, perhaps because of the excited state of the hospital at a given time; it may be the chief himself who suddenly rules from above because, for instance, relationships with the general hospital across campus are involved; it may also be one or more committees, like the committee in charge of the adolescent population, which challenges the head nurse's decision or lays down policy counter to her convictions. All those administrative agents may enter in, and they frequently do in combination or in alliance. When the hospital is at its most tense, then the cross fire of authority is probably at its maximum and head· nurses feel most buffeted and frustrated in discharge of their duties. In a later chapter we shall discuss certain subtle maneuvers among the nursing personnel during this game of shifting authority; here it is only necessary to emphasize how unsteady the ground is under the personnel.

Yet nurses, and especially head nurses, have been given a mandate to maintain order upon the wards. One of their primary jobs is to prevent wards from getting unduly out of hand. Like any cadre of workers, also, nurses seek to gain maximum control over their conditions of work. The more authority in ward management they possess, the more they can control conditions. If other administrators intervene in the managerial process, they may improve conditions of work, but they are more likely to achieve the opposite. Nurses therefore develop a vocabulary of blame and accusation to explain why things go wrong on the wards, frequently blaming the administrators and meanwhile feeling frustrated and angry. Lest this picture appear too black, we hasten to add that the nurse's regulatory functions are often unimpeded and that administrators are not only frequently helpful but can become allies in whatever battles for control nurses may be waging. It is not accurate to assume either that all nurses actually want complete control over their wards. The important point is not how much or little control nurses have; it is the ambiguous nature of that control. The highlights of that ambiguity have barely been touched upon; we leave until later the discussion of how nurses seek to cope with such ambiguity.

EMERGENCIES AND THEIR CONTROL

Certain specific features of PPI heighten the possibilities of emergency, although this hospital does not admit or keeps to a minimum admission of certain kinds of patient who may cause undue disturbance. The greatest proportion of patients are new admissions and are also new to the physicians who have hospitalized them. The patients are mostly in acute phases of their illnesses especially when they arrive. There is a high turnover of patients, so that new faces are constantly appearing on each ward. There is much activity and stimulation in the hospital — and little disposition among physicians to quiet patients with drugs or unduly to restrict their movements. All these conditions ensure a fair amount of tension — and potential flare-ups on the wards.

The administration has certain policies to lessen the possibility of ward emergencies. The five wards are graded roughly by the amount of "acting out" that they can contain and by their restrictions of patients' activities. Upon entry to PPI, each patient is assigned by the ROD to whatever ward he seems most "appropriate to." On the wards where most acting out occurs, male aides are assigned to back up nurses in their handling of potential disturbances. Central administration also puts into the head nurse's hands certain procedures by which she may handle actual and potential crises. She may call upon the physician or the ROD for permission to administer sedatives and tranquilizers. She may also seclude the patient in his room if she deems it necessary to keep order on the ward. She may arrange for the patient's transfer to a ward where he may more easily and properly be controlled. She may even send the patient overnight to the most closed ward, in order to have him out of the way or to emphasize that he must henceforth control himself. She may also request additional temporary personnel.

In addition, nurses have at their command a great many tactics similar to a combination of fire drills for preventing panic and methods for preventing fires. We may term this "the organization of routines" for the prevention of emergencies. Shrewd nurses keep close watch of potential trouble-making patients. They establish a division of labor that minimizes the possibility that certain patients will get out of hand. Head nurses arrange for the strongest members of their nursing teams, usually men, to be positioned close to the troublesome patients. They keep a canny eye on rising tension and attempt by one device or another "to nip it in the bud" — to use a phrase that we have occasionally heard. They use many other common-sense methods like breaking up combinations of patients or scolding or reasoning with them. Giving "contact" to patients may also be used to keep the ward orderly and not merely for therapeutic purposes.

The nurses can and the head nurse usually will call upon patients' physicians to help in keeping order. Of course, the handling of a patient may be couched in the language of therapy rather than in terms of management. Nevertheless, the nurses seek sufficient information about patients to enable reasonable precautions for emergency behavior. A potentially suicidal patient, for example, should be reported by the attending physician — also how can the nurses be prepared for that possibility? Often nurses request and even pressure a physician to use the therapeutic session to encourage his patient to "put controls" on himself. It is not unusual for the physician to report back to the head nurse that he has done as requested and indeed to report further information so that she can better guard against the possibility of further eruptions. (Naturally physicians play a game of reassuring the nurses, too.) Nurses also want physicians to "co-operate" in matters of restricted privileges and transfer. If a patient does not properly "fit" the ward, then they believe the physician should arrange for a transfer.

Although nurses want physicians to co-operate, they do not have the absolute right to demand co-operation. Physicians may withhold their co-operation in varying degrees. More will be said about these matters shortly; here we wish only to emphasize the necessity for nurses' negotiations. With other hospital functionaries, negotiations are also necessary. The more skilled the head nurse or her assistants, the more resources they can bring to staving off potential emergencies. They make appeals to and bargain with physicians, administrators, resident administrators, supervisors — in an effort to have more drugs prescribed, more privileges withheld from certain patients, more transfers effected, and more troublemakers kept off the wards. Nurses must be alert to the possibility of selecting the right authority, the right ally, and the right action in order to minimize emergencies or handle them effectively.

Those who do not choose to co-operate with her or who do not sympathize with her specific efforts accuse the nurse of rigidity, anxiety, compulsiveness, rule-craziness, and overemphasis on management to the detriment of therapy. This assessment may be accurate in regard to particular tactics used by nurses. In general, though, it ignores the point that nurses seek to control important facets of their work. They attempt to do what every occupational group, including physicians, does — to gain maximum control over important conditions of work — because of concern both with their own ends and with helping patients. In this battle for control, they understandably utilize various weapons sanctioned by central administration, calling frequently upon hospital rules to justify action taken. It would be a mistake to believe, however, that nurses can depend only on those rules.

Finally, it is important to understand that the nurses' problems in foreseeing, preventing, and handling emergencies are compounded by the very ambiguity that surrounds their claims to ward authority. As we have seen, those claims can be challenged so successfully as to jeopardize what nurses believe is the integrity of the wards. Any patient or behavior that "does not fit the ward" is a potential danger. Because nurses' authority is subject to sudden challenge and can be overruled, the danger is more difficult to combat: Nurses believe so, and there is little reason to question that belief.

Nurses' ideas on how wards should be managed and patients handled are transmitted to residents, administrators, and even to attending physicians through a delicate and often unconscious process. Nurses are adept at obliquely expressing their own perspectives to authorities. Their conversations with physicians are replete with indirect requests and preferences. An immense amount of communication in the hospital serves the same end, however, without the nurses' actually having to maneuver conversations. On each ward, one hears a tremendous amount of talk about various patients. Nurses and aides, after carrying out their duties, return to the closed stations and talk about patients or incidents. They reminisce too about former patients and memorable events. Frequently residents and co-ordinators join in this talk or are drawn into it. Some of this conversation consists of gripes, complaints, and criticisms of those in each echelon. Staff meetings also stimulate such conversation. An unintended consequence of all this talk is the education of all personnel in the dominant concepts of ward shape and proper handling of patients. These concepts cover a major portion of the do's and don'ts of ward life, rules that are partly implicit, partly explicit. This education of personnel other than nurses is especially important at PPI, for the nurses must work closely with young residents. Each autumn new residents are educated by the nurses, who think of themselves as teachers of the young and are supported in this perception by the central administration. They initiate the resident into the atmosphere of negotiation that permeates each ward. The prevention and proper management of emergencies loom large in this negotiation.

THE NURSE AND THERAPY

The nurses would not consider themselves psychiatric nurses unless their work also included therapeutic action. At PPI, there is no public statement of the position that nurses play no part whatever in the therapeutic drama. The hospital's main business is to make patients well enough to function again in the outside world, and everyone in the hospital who works with patients is supposed to be contributing to the institution's goal. A sense of genuine colleagueship in a common enterprise is shared by all echelons, even the lowest.

The sense of common enterprise, however, shatters upon the shoals of certain critical events. Then the various personnel discover how far apart are their respective judgments of who is contributing what and how much to the therapeutic enterprises. Nurses are in a peculiarly perilous position: They take their therapeutic duties and prerogatives very seriously, but intermittently they cannot ignore the at least partial rejection of their specific claims by the psychiatrists. Furthermore, nurses have vested interests in therapeutic action sanctioned by a universal professional ideology, which teaches that they are psychiatrists' right-hand men, their auxiliary agents. When they fail to serve this function, it is supposedly their own failure and casts no doubt upon the tenet that nurses should be useful participants in the therapeutic process. Unfortunately for the nurses' peace of mind, this ideological teaching overlooks certain operational questions. Exactly *how* is the nurse an auxiliary agent? In what ways ought she to supplement or complement the doctor's efforts? What specific therapeutic roles should a good psychiatric nurse play? How can a nurse know when she is successful in helping the patient to improve? How does she determine the kind of credit she deserves for success in this co-operative venture with the physician? Across the nation itself, nurses do not agree upon the answers to these questions and reflect profound disagreement among psychiatrists themselves upon the same issues.

THE WORTH OF THE NURSE AND HER WARD

Both the nurse's professional ideology and the hospital's general philosophy support her professional self-regard. In addition, psychiatrists often remark that her efforts have supplemented their own in helping patients, indeed may have been more important than their own therapy. Since many patients come directly to PPI without previous treatment by their physicians, the latter are freer to compliment the nurses. From time to time, psychiatrists encourage specific nurses to continue working with specific patients because they believe the nurses have been successful. Even when they do not single out special actions or personnel as helpful, they may indicate that the ward's environment has been beneficial. The patients themselves, either during their stays at the hospitals or when they leave, may acknowledge that the staff has been very helpful, and of course the staff is not inclined to dismiss this kind of evidence.

But the nurses can also see for themselves how well they have functioned therapeutically. They may disagree with a physician's therapeutic program and note the beneficial effects of their own actions upon his patient. They may take action when a psychiatrist does not seem to know what to do or will not state his program, again noting how well their own program works. They may observe that a doctor is not "getting through" to his patient, although one or another of the nursing personnel is. Indeed, it is common knowledge that some patients cannot or will not talk to their doctors but talk freely to at least one member of the staff. Nurses tend to believe that they know the patients best, especially the patients of psychiatrists whom they little respect, for they see more of the patients and in more natural situations.

In addition, certain general procedures and conventions characteristic of PPI lend support to nurses' sense of therapeutic worth. A patient placed upon or transferred to an "inappropriate" ward becomes highly visible when it is clear that he does not "fit" and thus grows worse. To nurses, this change signifies that the ward cannot be therapeutic for that particular patient. Conversely, it implies that the ward is therapeutic for "appropriate" patients. Whenever a psychiatrist disregards the nurses' advice to order a transfer from a ward that is not benefiting his patient, then further retrogression of condition is likely to be heralded as confirmation of the disregarded advice. Conversely, nurses may obtain a psychiatrist's permission to work longer with a patient whose progress on this specific ward seems dubious; then if the patient shows improvement, the staff feels that its therapeutic efforts have been vindicated. Most patients do improve, and this success is underlined for the staff by the propensity of most therapists to transfer improved patients to more open wards.

All this improvement leads nurses to believe that their efforts are useful, sometimes very useful. They do not always clearly distinguish between therapeutic improvements due to their own individual or

212

collective efforts and those due to the general atmosphere and physical structure of the ward itself. Sometimes, however, that distincttion is clearly made — as when a patient "pulls himself together" with astonishing rapidity on the most closed ward after "falling apart" on a relatively open one. The closed ward itself is then regarded as having been beneficial. In other instances, the credit is given to specific nursing actions or programs. Distinctions cannot always easily be drawn. In addition, nurses believe that the quality of ward life rests not merely upon the physical attributes of wards but also upon how the personnel govern them.

THE NURSES' VULNERABILITY

Nurses are accountable both for ward management and for therapeutic behavior. The second is the price that nurses must pay for recognition as important agents in the therapeutic process. Nurses are exposed to criticism from the administration and from colleagues for actions that should have been therapeutic but were not. They may be reproached by attending physicians for becoming "over-involved" with patients and thus producing untoward effects on them. In fact, nurses are open to criticism and accusation by physicians — and by one another — on many grounds, quite aside from imputed laziness or simple error. These grounds are expressed in psychiatric terms: The nurse is compulsive or anxious or interjects herself so that her interaction with patients is ineffective or actually harmful.

It is important to understand that nurses stand exposed to this sort of attack, whether justified or not, from a whole host of critics: by her colleagues, by the aides, by her head nurse, by the nursing administration, by various psychiatric administrators, and by each and every attending physician with whose patients she comes in contact. The ward meetings themselves are sometimes seized upon by administrators as occasions for directing criticism at the nursing personnel, although usually at the personnel in general rather than at individual culprits. In addition, every nurse is open to criticism by patients, who may shrewdly find chinks in her protective armor or genuine deficiencies in her therapeutic performance.

The nurse as a single individual often accuses herself, blaming and scolding herself and feeling guilty, ashamed, or in other ways self-derogatory. This self-criticism is not couched in terms of mere error but in the same stinging psychiatric jargon that others use against her. She sees herself as culpable because she has "acted out" or been "compulsive" and so on.

She is especially vulnerable to accusations, her own and others,' for at least two sets of reasons. In becoming a nurse, she has absorbed enough of the psychotherapeutic orientation to act and think in its terms. This terminology is a double-barreled gun: It can, and indeed should, be used on oneself, as well as on the patients. (Stanton and Schwartz note that this generalized use of psychotherapy as a weapon throughout the hospital is an extension of the psychotherapeutic hour.) [2] Nurses are generally much more vulnerable than the aides, because they are much more likely to assimilate psychotherapeutic concepts. By participating in the wider psychiatric community, they become what may be termed "minimal psychiatrists." Psychiatrists appear to be considerably less vulnerable to this kind of therapeutic criticism, both from others and probably also from themselves, because they are institutionally protected against it. In the hospital, they stand in superordinate relationships to most personnel, which affords some protection. They spend far less time at the hospital than do the nurses; they are principally assailable only by their own patients; and they are less easily reminded of criticism by having to remain all day long at the locale. The nurses have only the stations to which they may flee from patients, and it is difficult to forget the remarks of critical colleagues and administrators while at the hospital.

Perhaps nurses are also more vulnerable than psychiatrists (although this point is far more speculative) because they operate with a minimum of psychiatric knowledge. Having far less systematic and extensive psychiatric education, they have less conceptual equipment with which to defend themselves against criticism. They are more open to accusation about their motives, because they are less practiced in thinking about themselves in theoretical terminology and at a psychological distance. This observation by no means implies that nurses are always vulnerable to higher psychiatric authority or that they have no answering rhetoric — far from it! — but only that, having learned a little psychiatry, they are then in the position of all beginners in that trade: somewhat shaky, if somewhat knowledgeable, about their own "true motives."

COMMUNICATIVE DESPAIR

If not shaky about motives, they are certainly often unsure of what therapeutic actions they should take toward specific patients. They are very aware that they may do little good for some patients and may actually harm others. If we put together nurses' doubts about certain of their actions and their vulnerability to potential criticism from psychiatric authorities, then we need not be astonished at nurses' intense preoccupation with wresting two things from at-

[2] A. Stanton and M. Schwartz, *The Mental Hospital* (New York: Basic Books, Inc., 1954), pp. 146-50, 200-6.

214

tending physicians — adequate information about patients' illnesses and advice (or commands) on how best to act toward the patient.

The most common grievance against attending men is that they fail to communicate sufficiently. Nurses are always complaining that physicians do not bother to write down information about patients and proper — if any — orders, that they skip in and out of the ward, not stopping to transmit information. One of the nurses' major criteria for judging psychiatrists is ability to communicate well; that is, whether or not they let nurses in on therapeutic programs. Quite aside from the programs' relevance to ward management, nurses wish to know about them because of their hopes for patients; they wish to know because they consider themselves legitimate participants in the treatment process.

Nurses consider themselves much more instrumental in recovery when psychotherapy is being practiced than when the psychiatrists merely treats his patient with shock and with little or no psychotherapy. In the latter instance, there is not very much for nurses to do therapeutically: Time and shock and perhaps the patient's isolation from his family are the main therapeutic agents. The psychotherapist who communicates well, who invites them into the treatment program, who "co-operates," is not only liked; he is also able to foster genuine *elan* among the staff — providing that co-operative efforts result in improvement. Since the nurses' ideas about hospital practice are closest to those of the ex-PPI residents, it is among the latter that "the most co-operative physicians" are usually found.

The least co-operative — those who drive nurses to despair with their refusal to communicate — are to be found among the individualistic group described in the preceding pages. These individualists are less likely to tell nurses precisely what they are doing, partly out of deliberate choice and partly out of tendency to use the hospital unconventionally. What is more, their attempts at communication are all the more easily misread as being no communication at all. Even with the best behaved of attending men, there are days or weeks when a wide communicative gap exists. The men also differ in the clarity of their expression; in the amount of time available for talking to nurses; in their estimate of the value of talking with nurses about certain types of patient or the stages of therapy they have reached, and whether or not they care to transmit their own sometimes slight knowledge.

It is not too extreme a statement to assert that despair over the communicative gap is ever-present among the nursing personnel. Aides share in this despair but can more easily shrug off the psychiatrists' silence, since the latter are much more distant from their world. Within the nurses' world, however, the psychiatrist looms large. It is to their charge that his patient is given over. Nurses are also much more dependent than aides upon the approval of psychiatrists. When the men show their appreciation of nurses' efforts, the women glow with pleasure and even with a kind of subordinate professional colleagueship. When the men seem to indicate that nursing effort is really of no importance for the therapeutic project, then the women find it difficult not to react strongly. They do not feel ashamed, as they might if they had committed therapeutic errors; they feel deprived of participation in the community of effort. They feel ignored, even denigrated or worthless. When angry at attending physicians for disrupting ward order or blocking ward management, they feel merely frustrated or indignant; when upset over rejection by therapists, they feel a blow has been struck at their professional identities. Communicative despair is only one step removed from the reactions that nurses experience when a psychotherapist lets a nurse know how little her therapeutic actions really mean in the sum total of his patients' improvement. Only rarely do the somaticists appear to evoke such responses, since the nurses do not regard themselves as especially important to somatic treatment.

Where Does Nursing Fit Into Therapy?

This discussion leads to two related questions, whose answers are vitally important to nurses. How is what nurses do for patients different from what physicians do? Exactly how does the work of each group of professionals contribute to the patient's improvement? We turn now to the nurses' answers to such questions — and why their answers take certain forms. Actually, we shall discuss nurses' conceptions of the proper division of labor that should exist between themselves and psychiatrists — as well as how nurses judge the success and failure of current collaborative efforts.

The nurses realize that certain attending men utilize their services unequally and somewhat differently. The somaticists ("EST men") are a class apart, for they are recognized as uninterested in nurses' therapeutic efforts or permissive with nurses who wish to behave "therapeutically" toward patients. The remaining physicians have reputations—a process we shall describe in a later chapter—according to how much and how wisely they utilize nursing personnel. The men are judged by their expectations that nurses will give support, give contact, be firm, point out reality to the patient, be maternal, and so forth. Nurses refer to their own actions in such terms, which is understandable, since that is how attending men write orders or verbally transmit their desires for nursing care. Such terms are common coinage that passes among the staff, as well as between staff and attending physicians.

This language does not, however, serve very well to distinguish between what the physician does and what the nurses do for a patient. Nurses at PPI understand that psychiatrists attempt psychotherapy with patients while their own therapeutic activity is either not psychotherapeutic or of considerably less depth and duration. But not all nurses have very clear notions of what psychotherapy is and how it differs from what they themselves do with patients. They understand that the psychiatrists' insights into and talks with patients may go deeper than their own; but this understanding is counterbalanced by a firm belief that nurses frequently know and handle patients better. When we asked point-blank whether the hospital could get along less well with psychiatrists or with nurses (therapeutically, not managerially), the nurses faced a difficult choice. While aides would unhesitatingly answer "us," nurses gave more scattered and sometimes more anguished answers.

What is unquestionably involved is the nurses' feelings that they cannot do without the psychiatrists, despite the absence of a clear conception of how their respective collaborative efforts actually combine in the total therapeutic enterprise. Nurses are pleased when invited into the drama of treatment, when the psychiatrist regards them as genuine participants, but they are scarcely more articulate about their respective therapeutic functions than at any other time. When nurses talk about a specific patient, they are frequently quite capable of formulating their presumed contribution to his improvement, sometimes using fairly sophisticated psychiatric terminology. To talk about their contribution to a specific patient's improvement is much easier than to talk about therapeutic functions in general.

Their lack of clarity in defining a "true" or desirable therapeutic division of labor is doubtless connected with disagreements among psychiatrists on this very question. Part of the nurses' difficulty surely is traceable, however, to genuine differences between the two sets of professional over what actually constitutes and may contribute to psychic improvement and deterioration. Naturally enough, nurses turn to attending physicians for judgments of whether or not patients are "moving," but they have their own eyes and their own standards for judging progress and retrogression. The obvious discrepancies between nurses' and physicians' perceptions and evaluations result in further muddying of waters.

Nurses are preoccupied with whether or not patients improve, for the daily life of each ward revolves around helping patients get sufficiently well to move along either to the outside world or to another ward. A visitor is struck by the nursing staff's constant reference to patients' "moving" or "not moving," to their "getting worse" or "looking better today." When recalcitrant sickness yields before devoted nursing, the staff may evince relief and even jubilation at the smallest signs of improvement. Patients who remain on plateau for weeks tend to depress the staff or to receive scant attention because the staff no longer feels that the effort is worth the candle and turns to more promising or newer candidates. Improvement in patients is a vital matter for the nursing personnel. Such improvement — whether recognized by them or the physicians — allows them to measure, to a considerable degree, their own success and failure at psychiatric nursing. (Their only alternative measures would have to be along lines of administration, management, and medical care.) Even when the standard is how much they are "learning," is associated with discerning improvement and retrogression in various patients.

How do the nursing personnel discern such improvement and retrogression? Both in common sense and in quasi-psychiatric ways. By "common sense," we mean judgment that is essentially the same as judgment by a lay person. The nurses perceive similar kinds of signs and interpret them in lay terms: It is clear that the patient is improving, for his speech becomes more coherent, intelligible, and sensible; the formerly regressed patient, who could not control his bowel movements or feed himself, is again able to manage those bodily functions; the noisy, violent patient has calmed down and acts more decorously; the ritualistic patient no longer goes through his routine motions. Or patients may grow more confused, more incoherent, more regressed, more uncontrollable. The great preponderance of nurses' perceptions and evaluations of patients' psychiatric conditions are akin to those of laymen, but some judgments do rest upon more sophisticated psychiatric knowledge. Nurses do develop the ability to observe keenly patients' behavior and symptoms. Their interpretations of patients' actions can often pass muster with persons who have been more extensively trained in psychiatry.

Whether most of the nurses' judgments are minimally psychiatric or closer to common sense is much less important than that they disagree, with considerable frequency, from judgments made by the attending physicians. We shall attempt to explain why. The physicians whom we interviewed are characteristically skeptical about the possibility that hospitalization will bring any profound changes to patients, except for infrequent special cases. They settle for the minimal improvement that will permit a patient once again to function passably, at least for a time, outside the hospital. Because psychiatrists, especially the psychotherapeutically oriented, think in psychodynamic terms, they do not believe that daily or weekly changes during hospitalization necessarily represent genuine improvement or retrogression: At best these changes are only preparations for further treatment at the office. When a patient begins to improve in the limited sense that these physicians conceive of improvement, the special signs that they read may be overlooked by nurses, let alone by laymen, and may even be read by nurses as deterioration. (As one nurse commented, "The doctor says she's making progress. I don't know how these doctors sometimes can tell what's getting better anyhow.")

To understand the nurses' perceptions of patient "movement," one must consider the implications of their daily contacts with patients, since nurses' ward work, when combined with their less than systematic psychiatric orientation and education, often causes their views of movement to differ from physicians' views. On each ward patients come and go as they get better or worse than is deemed appropriate for the given ward. Sometimes there is a rash of arrivals and departures; at other times, movement is reduced to a trickle. Sometimes almost all the patients seem to be getting better at once; at other times, everybody seems to be on a plateau, with no apparent movement. Sometimes patients get better swiftly, sometimes slowly. Sometimes patients improve, only to reverse themselves and become worse. Sometimes they get worse before they get better. Some patients pass through cycles, swinging from one extreme condition to another. Some patients enter the ward at very low points, while some enter almost well enough to qualify for a more "advanced" ward. Sometimes patients enter the ward when all its patients are relatively well and sometimes when all are relatively deteriorated. At any rate, nurses perceive a given patient's improvement against a backdrop of other patients' movements. Any patient's progression is perceived also in terms of the nurses' related conceptions of a current and ideal "shape" of their ward. If they believe their ward is ordinarily successful with patients and if their ward is at the moment terribly "out of shape" — as, for instance, when it contains too many patients who require medical care or too many adolescents who require long hospitalization — then their morale can be low because work achieves little success. How the ward's shape and its complement of patients relate to judgments of success with patients is easily pictured in another way. One need only imagine that each new patient becomes better in a day or two, so that the ward has an almost daily turnover of patients: The nurses' sense of accomplishment can then easily be imagined.

At PPI nurses are accustomed to patients entering in various conditions of illness, to divergent rates of improvement, and to various kinds of forward and backward movement. The nurses are prepared for almost anything, so long as it does not too radically disturb their wards' shapes. Nurses definitely prefer not having too many deteriorated patients enter simultaneously, too long a period of time without progress among patients, too many patients whose movements swing unpredictably from better to worse and back again, and even too many patients who are improving — if improvement brings troublesome behavior. Under such conditions, nurses feel neither successful with their therapeutic work nor capable of doing their best work.

Of similar importance for their judgments of patients' improvement is a phenomenon that can conveniently be called "patients reputations." Patients rather quickly, within perhaps two to four days, begin to gain reputations among the staff. The personnel talk among themselves about each new patient, describing his behavior, recounting interesting events that he has precipitated, and making judgments about his condition, his illness, and his behavior. The day-time personnel make log-book notations about each patient; this information is passed along to the evening and night staffs, abetted by the head nurse's report to the evening staff, which she often supplements with anecdotes. Each patient's reputation is composed partly of therapeutic judgment — whether he is getting better or worse and by how much — and partly of managerial judgment of how troublesome he is, for example.

Much of each ward's daily communication consists of phrases and stories passed among the staff about each patient, especially about those patients who are interesting, colorful, troublesome, or "moving." Each patient, unless he is remarkably unnewsworthy, is the subject of a continuing story: "He's the same today" or "You should have been here when he acted out again." Each day features episodes in the continuing stories of the more troublesome, loved, or colorful cast of characters. (We may term these episodes "focal events.") Each day is likely to have its single salient event, although of course many days may be devoid of truly memorable incident. Some of the stories are success stories — "You should have been here when she first began to eat!" — and some are stories of failure. On some days, indeed for days on end, the staff may focus principally upon its struggle for success with a single patient. (We may term this phenomenon "focal attentiveness," and we may call the patient the "focal patient.") The staff becomes engrossed in the continuing story of the focal patient. The jubilation or gloom that may pervade the atmosphere at the nursing station need bear no relationship to any objective statistical assessment of the progress of patients as a whole. One or more focal patients can have more impact upon the staff's sense of therapeutic worth than would seem warranted by considerations of mere arithmetic.

We leave to a later chapter discussion of how the nurses maneuver to affect the patient's continuing story; here we are concerned only with how and why their views of patients' movements are unlike doctors' views. The doctors, at least those who are psychodynamically oriented, not only think more systematically about patients, but they scarcely can view patients within such a rich context of ward life. Even the ex-residents do not: They may understand the staff's perspective, having once operated within it themselves, but one has only to listen to the ward co-ordinators advising nursing personnel to recognize that memories are short and that a practitioner's view is very different from a nurse's.

One qualification must be made, however: The judgments of nurses and physicians are not always so disparate as we have described. Occasionally patients worsen enough to be sent to a state hospital; much more often they improve sufficiently to leave for home. Concurrence of physician and nursing personnel does not mean that the two agree exactly, but at least there is agreement on the direction of change.

Yet even then, there may be no agreement on the causes of change. This point again raises the question of how nurses weigh the respective contributions of themselves and physicians. It is not always an easy question for nurses to answer confidently. When physicians have "co-operated" and everyone has "worked together closely," then the question is unlikely even to arise, whether the patient has improved or deteriorated. At the other extreme, when the nurses have carried out their own therapeutic program for a given patient, because his psychiatrist either seemed to have none or was unwilling to communicate it, then the nursing personnel can easily believe that their claims to success or imputations of blame have been justified. These divisions of labor — with quite co-operative and quite unco-operative physicians — together undoubtedly involve a majority of patients, exclusive of those given EST. Success and failure are relatively easily judged for the latter: Either shock succeeds, or it fails. But if nurses step in, believing shock inappropriate or unsuccessful, then they credit their own programs with any apparent success. In the remaining cases there may be some question about who has been the more effective (or destructive) therapeutic agent.

We are not concerned with detailing how that question is answered but with two issues. The first is that nurses may not find it easy to assign credit and blame. The causes of change in a patient's condition are difficult to ascertain, and nurses are aware of the difficulty, except when the credit or blame is exceptionally great. In addition, nurses face the knotty problem of vindicating their claims to success and their assignments of blame.

Actually, with most patients, this problem need not arise since open contests between physicians and nurses are unlikely. If there happens to be strong feeling among the nurses that a considerable share of the credit is theirs, they take it quietly through a variety of almost automatic tactics. They support one another as they talk about the patient and how he improved. They make assumptions about how the ward and their own action helped the patient. Most often they do not make a clear distinction between credit due themselves, credit due the ward itself, and credit due the psychiatrist's action and orders: All merge into an undifferentiated "helped the patient." As for the psychiatrist, he usually does not announce that credit is due to anyone, unless a particular nurse or aide has been particularly useful.

When a patient deteriorates, however, or is so troublesome that his treatment is called into question, then both physician and nurses are vulnerable to charges of error and blame. Then the central administration is most likely to enter the situation, sometimes acting as an interested mediator and sometimes as an interested participant. Other audiences also may enter or be pulled into the fray for at least two reasons. The patient's reputation may have traveled to far corners of the hospital, stories about him circulating among all levels of personnel. He and his treatment may have become something of a *cause celebre*. Various persons will have expressed different opinions and taken sides in judging him and his physician. Outsiders may also enter into the affairs of a ward when its nurses pull them in. Nurses may illegitimately bombard other attending physicians with questions that bear upon the vindication of their own position. Some attending men must invoke their professional code to remain neutral. Some do not remain neutral but get caught up in the issues; or become involved because of their own opinions of the colleague whose treatment is being challenged by the nurses; or attempt to placate the nurses. In their search for vindication, the embattled nurses will speak to almost anybody who enters the station — including sociologists! We may call this general process the "scanning of potential vindicators."

For the nurse, it is a very important process precisely because she is a minor partner in the collaborative therapeutic enterprise. She is in a weaker position than the psychiatrist, weaker because her formal status allows less claim to psychiatric knowledge and judgment and because she has less confidence. She must find people who will listen to her, to whom she can appeal, who will help her make her own claims and accusations "stick." If she can find such allies among the central administrators or among the colleagues of the offending psychiatrist, so much the better. When the nurses themselves are divided, the same processes occur — except that the atmosphere becomes more like that of a civil war. The entire search for vindication is of momentuous consequence for nurses, for it pertains to perhaps the central question that they face: Where does therapeutic nursing fit into the total treatment of a patient? To this abiding question neither the central administration nor the attending men offer clear answers. The nursing profession has no single ideological position that will give her a clear answer either; although, as we have said earlier, if PPI's nurses were more firmly trained in one ideology, they might have less difficulty in coping with this crucial problem. We believe the problem would still exist, however, as long as the attending men themselves either possessed no clear answers or were willing to reveal their private beliefs only to colleagues or researchers.

ALIGNING MANAGERIAL AND THERAPEUTIC FUNCTIONS

At the outset of this chapter, we named two major problems confronting psychiatric nurses, especially those who work with psychotherapeutically oriented psychiatrists. One problem has been discussed: How does therapeutic nursing fit into the total treatment process? A second problem arises from the necessity for nurses to align their managerial and therapeutic functions. To this second problem there is no easy answer, but answer it each nurse must. Even a firm answer has potentially hazardous consequences for her, since it may work better on certain wards in certain hospitals.

Around each psychiatric nurse at hospitals like PPI, there is a field of institutional forces, which pull her sometimes in the direction of her managerial duties and sometimes toward her therapeutic obligations. She is not allowed to forget that she is a *psychiatric* nurse and that her major function is therapeutic. This philosophy is explicitly enunciated almost daily and is implicitly expressed in continual interaction with colleagues. Her head nurse, the nursing administration, and the central administration all expect appropriate therapeutic action from her, as do some attending men. Even the patients may have such expectations. There are also other expectations, however, pertaining to the nurse's managerial, administrative, and custodial duties. The very same people who expect her to engage in competent therapeutic action also expect her to be a good ward manager. Even the attending psychiatrists may emphasize now one aspect of her work and now another, with respect to their patients' welfare, although differing in the weight placed on each aspect. All these expectations or requirements have the effect of catching each nurse in harrowing cross fire. They also intensify whatever internal struggles she herself may have over the proportional weights that ought to be given to therapy and management respec-

223

tively. Her safest answer is to make a commitment that harmonizes the two kinds of demand. Yet even this answer is constantly brought into question.

There is, however, a supporting structure for combining managerial and therapeutic functions. We have suggested that the dominant philosophy of this hospital emphasizes that those functions naturally work together. The very division of the institution into five separate wards gives symbolic and actual support to nurses, in the sense that, when an improved patient is transferred, the personnel on his original ward can believe that they and their ward have helped him. Furthermore, those physicians whom nurses consider among the best and with whom they work most comfortably take pains not to disrupt unduly the ward's orderliness. In working with these co-operative men, a nurse is able to combine the frequently warring aspects of her dual job. This collaboration between physician and nurse allows the latter considerable freedom to help the nurses to organize appropriate action toward and around the patient — action that can be *both* therapeutic and managerial. This action leads to results that the psychiatrist in turn can perceive and interpret. He then reports back to the personnel. Similarly, the nursing personnel can make observations about a patient that can be utilized by his physician. The physician's actual therapeutic sessions can also serve both managerial and therapeutic ends — when the physician is co-operative. Management and therapy can ideally be fused by the nurses provided they can act as the physician's delegated managers, performing certain acts that he himself cannot perform either because he is not there or is not trained to do them.

Another institutional support enables nurses to combine management and therapy. It consists of an effective terminology used throughout the hospital by every echelon. The terminology is sufficiently ambiguous to allow at least three possibilities: It can refer to therapeutic action, managerial action, or both. For instance, "giving contact" to a patient may be used to mean therapeutic action or that such action should be taken merely to prevent further troublesome behavior — or both meanings may be indicated. Virtually all the terminology used by and to nurses, except for certain strictly psychiatric terms like "hallucination," has dual meanings. A physician's orders to give contact, for instance, may be read in two ways by different personnel. His very diagnosis can be converted from therapeutic to managerial connotation, since certain diagnostic terms suggest how patients can be expected to behave. The physicians themselves play into this ubiquitous lingual system, because they use these very terms as a shorthand for giving both orders and managerial suggestions.

By accident or design, a nurse can find other supports within the hospital setting for softening the potentially sharp conflict between therapy and management. Especially if she is shrewd or creative, she can find opportunities for maximizing therapeutic at the expense of the managerial effort or *vice versa*. We shall cite a few examples. On 3EW, the head nurse is assisted by two younger women, each of whom has her own *forte*. One is good at and enjoys working with patients; the other is adept at the administrative work, which is principally performed at an enclosed station. Each nurse tends to function in accordance with her particular ability. Since 3EW is a large ward, its head nurse consciously tends to play along with her assistants' desires in the daily assignment of work. She herself is exceedingly busy with ward administration and finds it useful to have both an administrative assistant and one who can supervise "work with patients." On PPI's most open ward, there are relatively minor problems connected with keeping order and less paper work than on other wards; the nursing personnel can spend much time working with patients. Indeed the head nurse runs into much less trouble with physicians over managerial problems than she does with the nursing administration, since the latter is more managerially minded than she. During the evening hours, on any ward, a floor nurse can better escape surveillance and feel freer to work with patients if she wishes, especially since she is less burdened with paper work and other administrative duties. A nurse who puts therapeutic action relatively low in her scale of values, however — a few PPI nurses do — may discover on the night shift a relative freedom *not* to work with patients. Here are two final examples: One nurse reluctantly allowed herself to be made a head nurse and then, caught in conflict of management and therapy, attempted repeatedly to be demoted in order to escape the extra stress engendered by her administrative position. One nursing supervisor grew restive with her wholly adminstrative duties and stepped down to replace a head nurse who had quit her job. In short, the hospital as constituted offers potentialities for working out various kinds of nursing commitment, whether they lean toward management or therapy or fall between the two.

The hospital also erects barriers to the implementation of nursing commitments. Besides those already discussed or suggested, others can be listed. The perennial transfer of nurses from one ward to another and from one shift to another allows some nurses to discover genuine satisfactions in working at the hospital; but this transfer system can also be immensely disrupting to nurses who have nicely managed their environments. Transfer not merely shatters routine and necessitates the learning of new routines, but it also means that new alliances must be made, new channels of negotiation found, new conditions of work be handled. To some degree at least, a new environment must be managed. Yet transfer and rotation of nurses are frequent in most hospitals, which are perennially "understaffed" according to administrative criteria.

It does not require much observation to see that some nurses fail to learn how to bend the hospital setting to their desires. Some quit the hospital. Some battle it out, looking for or stumbling into conditions that will allow them to do what they wish. Fortunately, too, some are abetted in their search by their superiors. Other nurses swing back and forth between the managerial and therapeutic poles, leaving themselves exceedingly vulnerable to attack and clearly restive about their unresolved positions. Lest we give the impression that all nurses are trapped, we hasten to repeat that many nurses find or create conditions that give them relative freedom for what they wish to do at the hospital.

Nevertheless, the implementation of any nurse's commitments is directly affected by her conditions of work. She needs relative control over those conditions, or she cannot carry out the dictates of her convictions. This control is hard to achieve in a hospital administered by physicians and used by a multitude of attending men. Even when nurses obtain relative control over their conditions of work, it must constantly be guarded and reconstituted when undermined. Some situations that lessen control are perennial and are therefore partly predictable. They can be prepared for to some degree. Other disruptions are difficult to foresee for many reasons: For instance, the hospital itself may be undergoing rapid changes; new physicians and new kinds of patient may be appearing; new kinds of therapy are being tried; and, of course, the views of attending physicians about nursing functions are neither consistent nor entirely understood by the nurses themselves. All these elements are crucial to an understanding of the world and the work of psychiatric nurses.

TRAINED VERSUS UNTRAINED PSYCHIATRIC NURSES

One outstanding feature of the PPI nurse is that she is not a "trained psychiatric nurse." Because she lacks the specialized training given in programs of psychiatric nursing at collegiate schools of nursing, she lacks the ideological staunchness so typical of many graduates of those programs, who often share the ideological fervor exhibited by the social workers and psychologists at Chicago State Hospital. In a certain sense, the PPI nurse's lack of formal training is useful at the hospital. Since such nurses have no firm and articulate commitment to a clear ideological position, they can work with somaticists and psychotherapists, without undue violation of their beliefs. Generally they can even work well with the individualistic psychotherapists, which might be more difficult if the nurses were more self-consciously ideological.

At least one excellently trained psychiatric nurse has remarked, however, on hearing about this hospital and its nurses, that the situation would be quite different if PPI's nursing service were headed by a genuine specialist. There is some merit in this argument, for one might then imagine certain new consequences for the nurses' work. The nurses would be inducted by the nursing director — a militant professional — into some variant of psychotherapeutic ideology. They would receive solid personal support from her during moments of stress. She might also gain more purchase on the central administration in terms of therapy rather than merely management. The director might also leave her educational mark upon residents, if not upon attending men, conveying the truer work and functions of the psychiatric nurse.

Assuming that this hospital's central administration were to change its views about psychiatric nursing sufficiently to hire such a director, it would still be difficult for her to change the situation radically. The attending men are not easily converted or even influenced. The residents would surely be affected while administering the wards, but by the time they had become attending men three years later, the director's influence would unquestionably have been counterbalanced and probably far outweighed by the combined influence of supervisors and personal career aspirations. Furthermore, a core of nurses with staunch psychotherapeutic ideology would undoubtedly precipitate certain new problems. Somaticists would find it harder to deal with these nurses, whose contempt for somatic practices would be more explicit and certainly more pronounced. Perhaps more important, the greater claims of nurses to participation in therapy would surely make more explicit the currently masked opinions of most attending men about the minor contributions of nurses to the therapeutic process. As we have noted, even the most cooperative attending men rates the general contribution rather low. Unless this opinion were altered, it is not difficult to imagine the reactions of nurses. Meanwhile, central administration would bear an increased burden of mediation between the attending men and the nurses. That is, the director would be teaching her girls that management and therapy support each other and are not separable (or perhaps that management is subordinate to therapy), but the older attending men would hardly accept her views of therapy either in general or concerning specific patients. (She would sometimes be unable to convince all her nurses.) As long as the hospital's work is organized around the private patients of attending physicians, the director of nursing service would face, as sociologists are wont to say, a most difficult "structural" problem.

It is important to understand that another of the current basic problems among the nurses would be difficult to solve: The proper assessment of the relative contributions of physicians and nurses to a specific patient's progress. This problem, it will be remembered, rests partly on the differential reading of signs: Nurses read more behaviorally, more like laymen. The introduction of trained psychiatric nurses would change this situation of course, for then nurses would read signs much more professionally. We would anticipate that this change would only make the content of their therapeutic claims more explicit. While both echelons might now more frequently agree, their fewer disagreements would be far less masked and covert.

In painting so skeptical a picture of the value of introducing specialized nurses into a setting like PPI, our intent has not been to argue that it should not be done. Our purpose has been primarily to underline briefly what problems confront the various nurses and psychiatrists at PPI as they work together. Secondarily, our purpose has been to suggest *some* of the possible consequences of introducing strongly psychotherapeutically oriented nurses into hospital settings comparable to PPI. As the trends toward both psychiatric sections in general hospitals and specialized psychiatric nursing continue, we can expect that the kinds of problems outlined here will figure prominently — because for many years the nurses who man our psychiatric hospitals will not be formally trained in psychiatric nursing.

THE INTENSIVE CARE UNIT:
ITS CHARACTERISTICS AND
SOCIAL RELATIONSHIPS*

A country with as many different kinds of hospitals as ours cannot possibly develop a new type of medical facility such as the intensive care unit without also developing variants of it. Once adopted, the original idea is adapted in accordance with contingencies of space, available finances, and institutional politics. Innovative experiment also plays a part in implementing the original idea. Nevertheless, the variation in ICU's is not so great that features general to most of them are not discernible.

THE ROLE OF THE ICU IN THE HOSPITAL

Perhaps the best place to start is with two diametrically opposed views of these services. Paradoxically, they are sometimes viewed as much different from other services (for instance, more patients die there; specialized nursing takes place there), but sometimes nurses believe that ICU nursing is very much like nursing anywhere in the hospital. Both views are wrong, although each possesses an element of truth. How is the ICU like the rest of the hospital, and how is it different?

If one views any hospital as composed of a set of spaces, he will see that "critically ill" patients are always placed in some special place or places—even when the hospital consists of only one ward. The ICU's have developed as special locales for certain types of very critically ill patients: for those who have high potential for dying, or for suffering retrogression unless cared for closely and carefully—but only if they are worth saving or can be prevented from worsening. Moderately ill patients usually are not sent to the intensive care unit; neither are patients who are too far gone for anyone to wish to save them.

*Reprinted by permission from
NURSING CLINICS OF NORTH AMERICA
Vol. 3, March, 1968, pp. 7-15
Copyright © 1968, W. B. Saunders Co.

Functionally then, in any particular hospital, the ICU's are spaces where the most critically ill (as defined above) are sent. Occasional fights occur, of course, around who belongs there and who does not. The personnel of some ICU's complain that other services try to dump hopelessly dying patients on them; while the latter services complain either that they cannot get patients received on the ICU or that very ill patients are discharged from there much too soon. Also, nursing administrators and physicians at various hospitals may squabble over who should control admissions to the ICU.

Typically the ICU's have been carved (literally carpentered) out of existing space in the hospital. As these specialized services prove their worth, and as the ICU movement grows nationally, spaces occupied by ICU's become brand new spaces rather than reconstructed old ones. Most still occupy the older spaces.

One consequence of old space is that it is not as efficient as it might be if planned de novo, but in any case there is rarely enough space in the ICU. Maximizing space around each patient (including the visual and auditory barriers between patients) may mean that fewer patients can be serviced there. Even purposeful bed placement so that the staff can see everywhere on the unit means that they in turn can be seen by every sentient patient. When the placement of beds is not carefully worked out, private conversations — between patient and nurses or kinsmen — are rendered impossible, and, especially in emergencies, effective functioning of staff is reduced. All these consequences mean, in turn, that sentient patients are visually close, hence involved willynilly in some of the dramatic emergency scenes, and open to disturbance by the frequently accompanying commotion and staff traffic. On the unit and afterward, patients frequently complain about the noise, and the fright of hearing and seeing what is going on around them. Rather obviously this must affect the quality of their medical and nursing care, as well as their willingness to return for necessary stays on the intensive care unit.

Another feature of ICU's is the extensive resources that they have or can command, because of the kind of medical and nursing care given there. Sophisticated medical technology is characteristic. Machinery abounds. Staff is in high ratio to patient load: nurses work virtually in one to one (or one to two) ratio to patients. Nurses are backed up by more medical personnel — and more quickly on request — than in virtually any other place in the hospital.

Besides saving lives, there are other important consequences of these considerable resources. For instance, nursing administration "upstairs" may not agree with the ICU nurses, or their supervisor, that such a high ratio of nurses is necessary. Why do they need so many people or such skilled people? And especially if the census fluctuates, why must there always be the same high ratio of staff? The head nurse or supervisor bears the brunt of this disagreement.

THE NURSE IN THE INTENSIVE CARE UNIT

The presence of complicated machinery is one of the chief stresses for new recruits of the ICU. Most have not worked on these units before, and probably they require two or more weeks to feel comfortable with the equipment. Quite possibly some nurses remain anxious for a longer time. Unless properly taught, they may use some equipment inefficiently or ineffectively (for instance, when suctioning patients). The presence of machinery also gives the nurse a major task: she may need to explain to the frightened patient, and to his family, that the machinery is for the patient's good and certainly will not harm him.

A characteristic feature of intensive nursing care is that the nurse's focus is very intensive and narrow. She works with one or two patients. Virtually minute by minute she watches vital signs. During survival crises, her work is even more focused and intense. She has immense responsibility for her patient's welfare. And because this is such a medically and procedurally oriented service, she tends to concentrate far more on the medical aspects of her patient than on the "patient as a whole." Furthermore, this is one of those rare places in the modern hospital where she works in rather close — sometimes literally shoulder to shoulder — relationships with physicians. From this complex of features, various consequences flow.

Nursing morale tends to be high (but see the qualifications below) because the nurse feels she is saving lives. She can literally and quickly see her patient improve. This is, as some say, "what nursing really is — or should be." Working with medically interesting cases keeps interest high — so high, indeed, that the nurses tend to think of themselves as among the elite of the hospital staff. Learning the medical aspects of the case is relatively easy here, because the physicians also are interested in the cases; often they are enthusiastic about their handiwork or medical management, willing to talk about it spontaneously or when prompted by the nurses' questioning.

Because the nursing is or seems so medical, and because it is also frontier nursing, prompted by new technology, new operations, and new procedures, the physicians take a hand in educating or helping the nurses with their nursing problems. On brand new units, the physicians are often self-conscious teachers of their nurses, believing that only they know enough to teach the nurses — a belief fortified by medical responsibility for their critically ill patients. This teaching may make for high morale and close ties between the respective staffs.

It may also lead to considerable strain between nursing administration (including the ICU supervisor) and the ICU nurses, as well as between nursing administration and the ICU physicians. The staff in the unit feel that nursing administration knows little about the actual care that goes on, or should go on, at the locale. Administration may believe (or know) that procedural and even legislative rules are being violated by the nurses. They are upset by nurses becoming "junior doctors." The ICU nurses may believe the hospital rules are unrealistic or outmoded. There may even be strain between a "progressive" nursing director and her "old-fashioned" assistants — or, stated otherwise, between more and less cautious or conservative nurses.

The close ties between ICU physicians and nurses lead to a tendency to equate good nursing care with technical competence. Many of the nurses adopt this attitude. Since many nursing administrators and nursing educators recognize that high-level nursing care involves much more than technical competence, there is another basis for a clash with the physician and sometimes with the ICU nursing staff. At university hospitals where nursing educators wish to send their advanced graduate students into the ICU, the latter may find themselves appreciated only by relieving the work load and for whatever technical competence they possess, rather than for anything more "sophisticated" which they can add to the unit's knowledge — unless, of course, they feed it directly into the routines or into persistent problems encountered by the staff.

As a consequence of the intense procedural and medical focus of the ICU nurse, she tends to pay less attention to the psychology of her patient. Most of her formal and informal training for ICU nursing is not concerned with psychological and social relationships. Luckily for both her and the patient, he is very likely to be wholly or semi-comatose much of his time on the unit. When he is not, then he tends to receive poor quality "psychological and social" nursing. Indeed, I recollect one nurse telling me about a patient who lingered on her unit several days before his transfer to a surgical service: she found herself, as did her colleagues, quite embarrassed not to have "anything new to say to him" day after day. As for conscious patients who die on ICU's, or shortly after transfer from there, it can only be concluded that they get short shrift in their desires to talk about their dying with the staff. The same can be said of patients in considerable pain, since a need of these patients may be to talk about pain and what it means, as well as about the relief of their pain.

The nurse's protection against all these implicit, and occasionally explicit, demands is to turn to the details of her work. Since those details are so many and the work so intense, she is likely to get as effective a protection as her colleagues on other services who can more easily retreat to the distant nursing station. On the ICU, with all that machinery and all those vital signs to watch, the nurse is aided in escaping the full brunt of the patient's demands or entreaties, although obviously she cannot always minimize that stress.

THE PATIENT IN THE INTENSIVE CARE UNIT

A characteristic feature of these units, already alluded to, is the nature of their patients. The patients are not only very ill, and often comatose; they are either getting better or worse. Not all are saved, and so the death rate tends to be relatively high. It is high on other types of service also, but here it follows special patterns. Dying tends to be rapid; typically the patients die within a few days of their arrival. Hence the nurses do not know the patients very well as persons. Often the patient has been nontalkative or comatose most of the time on the unit. The nurses do not know the family very well either.

In consequence, though the death rate is high, the nurses may not be very depressed or upset when a patient dies. They did their best, and that was that. Just a few days later, even the nurse who was chiefly responsible for his care may hardly remember him. And though the death rate is high for the entire unit, she may not have had any patient die "on her" very recently. Nevertheless, ICU nurses observe that when their patients die in bunches, the morale of the service is affected adversely, much as on other services where multiple deaths occur.

Paradoxically, staff morale may also suffer because so many patients are comatose. One supervisor remarked to me that when there is a run of nonsentient patients, all of whom have to be suctioned and worked with in repetitive ways, her staff gets restive and blue. Therefore she regularly schedules long weekends. In contrast, medically interesting cases, though they require close attention and hard work, are a welcome relief from the run-of-the-mill cases.

On the other hand, the constant potentiality (if not actuality) of crises makes for considerable strain in the nurse's life. Although there is great challenge in averting or conquering a crisis, there is also great danger when it cannot be averted and great output of energy when it occurs. Also, while there is extraordinary risk that the nurse, or others, may feel that she has been negligent if errors have been committed during crises, the "backup" system is so dense, and other people within such ready call, that negligence accusation is perhaps less a danger than on services where nurses are more isolated or are working more on their own. Nevertheless, when there has been little formal training for the staff on an ICU, they may in a pinch feel very uncertain: "Do I know enough?" Probably this anxiety is added to when new or unfamiliar types of patients are housed on the unit.

THE PATIENT'S FAMILY

Another feature of the ICU is its relative inaccessibility to the kinsmen of the patient. Generally the nurses there have little training in how to handle families' psychological and social problems, although some nurses are superbly knowledgeable by experience, by nature, or through the good fortune of excellent training. The ICU nurses are relatively protected against the family's invasion of their work space, because of the physical separation of the unit from the outside world. Typically the kinsmen are allowed to visit for only a few minutes at a time, and at stated intervals. And typically the family members are at first very concerned, alarmed, or even hysterical at the sight of their critically ill relative. Only on successive visits, if the patient seems to be improving, are they more relaxed when in the ICU.

In consequence, the nurses function as reassurers (the machinery is for the patient's good; he is really getting better all the time). Also they coach the family members as to how to behave in such restricted, specialized space and before other very ill patients. Nurses also act as time keepers announcing the end of a visiting period and sometimes even ordering the relatives out of the unit. In extremis, they may pressure the physician to forbid the visit of certain kinsmen. Each trip outside the door of the ICU, the nurse may find family members awaiting her appearance so that they can ask how the patient is "doing," holding her transfixed with beseeching looks and long-winded colloquies. Nurses learn or devise various tactics for handling all these contingencies so as to minimize inconvenience to themselves and interference with their work.

On the whole, it has been my observation that families do not get much good nursing care as a result of those tactics. How one judges this matter depends of course on whether or not family management is regarded as "nursing care." An especially skillful competent head nurse may act as a support to her nurses in dealing with families and simultaneously be very supportive to anxious, even terrified, family members. On exceptional, but not rare occasions, such a kinsman if not properly managed may greatly disturb the other patients by his behavior and even throw the entire unit into an uproar, as with one husband who had an hysterical fit in the ICU when his wife finally died.

EFFECTS OF THE ISOLATION OF THE ICU

A final characteristic of the ICU is its relative isolation from other services. The ICU tends to be tucked away in the hospital — in the basement or at the ends of corridors, cut off by the doors as well as sealed off by its style and by posted warnings against outsiders' intrusions. Quite probably also, its nurses tend to eat together and spend coffee time together in the dining room. Patients are discharged from other services into the ICU and then perhaps are returned to those or still other services, with little communication between the respective services.

One consequence of the ICU's isolation, combined with its relatively high death rate, is that nurses elsewhere tend to think about the ICU in terms of a death image. As noted earlier, the ICU staff therefore may have to fight to prevent the "dumping" of dying patients onto the ICU. And, in turn, the other services may complain that they cannot get their dying patients into the ICU, or that they are sent patients who are not yet sufficiently recovered and belong rightfully inside the ICU.

A more fortunate consequence of isolation is that the ICU staff, working closely and frequently under crisis conditions, tends to attain a fair degree of intimacy. This may help to minimize the turnover of personnel. However, when someone must or does resign, the isolation from other units, combined with the lack of specialized skill in most potential recruits, means that the ICU cannot readily draw from other services for quick replacement. One supervisor is so bothered by this that she plans to train a nurse from each of several other services, giving them the usual two weeks of ICU training that each new recruit receives. This will make for quick replacement when an ICU nurse resigns, and allow for additional manpower when the ICU census is unusually high; in addition, it will help to improve the care of ex-ICU patients when they are moved to other services.

Her last goal suggests another important consequence of the ICU's relative isolation. The ICU has been thought of as a specialized service, and nurses have had to be specially trained to work there, but little thought has been given to the patient's total career while he is in the hospital. It has been assumed that when in the ICU he will get a certain kind of highly skilled care, and when he becomes less critically ill he will get another kind of care — equally skilled but of a different order. Unfortunately, for several days after being transferred from the ICU, many patients need nursing care that is not essentially different from before, but the nurses on other services have not been trained to give that kind of care. Indeed, the gap between the intensive care unit and other services is so great that there tends often to be relatively little transmission of nursing knowledge about specific patients from ICU nurses to those nurses who will next give care to these patients. So the defect is compounded: the latter nurses have neither the necessary specific knowledge about the patient nor the requisite special training to give him the best care.

OBSERVATIONS AND PREDICTIONS

Now, let us make an observation or two about the meaning — in the largest sense — of these units for contemporary nursing itself. The ICU's represent places within the hospital where some of the most sophisticated medical technology and medical knowledge are brought to bear on the patient. On some patients, at least in some hospitals, frontier medicine is being practiced. As always, nursing as well as medical care follows behind the technological and scientific aspects of medicine. This means, as noted earlier, that there is a strong and probably inevitable tendency for physicians to participate, at least in initial phases, in the evolution of nursing care for these special patients. What finally evolves is, of course, not merely a set of techniques developed by the physicians alone: the nurses contribute much to the process, and probably in increasing proportions during later phases of the evolution.

Because this type of nursing care is new in some of its important details, there is inevitably a gap between what an ICU nurse must know and what she was or is taught at nursing schools. Indeed, unless an instructor has worked intensively on such a unit, she is likely to feel uncertain about teaching for such a unit, and certainly her students feel uncertain when first they enter the unit either as students or as staff nurses. Nevertheless, the kinds of knowledge imparted in schools of nursing are relevant to what transpires on these services, as should be obvious from the "consequences" traced in this paper. Presumably what is needed next is to wed academic training with clinical experience — to teach more than procedures and techniques to ICU nurses, and in schools to begin to train people for their future jobs on the ICU.

This suggestion links up with another observation. Above all, what the ICU means to nurses who work there is more challenge and excitement than they can find elsewhere in the hospital. This *is* nursing. One works against onrushing death. One has great responsibility. Nevertheless, one works in close conjunction with *the* doctor — which is "as it should be." Although there are plenty of other places in the hospital where skill is needed and excitement runs high, it is well known that nurses with the greatest amount of formal education tend to abjure or quickly leave the hospital for other kinds of nursing, finding, among other reasons, that the hospital is too restrictive and relationships are too authoritarian. The ICU is one place where this accusation makes no realistic sense. But the same highly educated nurses who find hospitals uninteresting or restrictive would tend to characterize nursing on the ICU as "too technical." Their training has tended also to emphasize the interpersonal aspects of patient care. Hence some of the best trained and/or highly educated nurses are not being recruited to the ICU.

Yet, if they become public health nurses, they will see some of these same patients at home. For the modern hospital has virtually become transformed into a site where chronic illness is managed during its most acute phases. The ICU is only one of many spaces where chronically ill patients are cared for during their periods of maximum danger or tribulation. Like the rest of the hospital staff — but a little more so — the ICU nurses are predominantly focused on the knife-edge present: They are little concerned about what happened to their patient before he came or what will happen to him afterward.

I predict that only when physicians and nurses recognize that chronic illness is the nation's major medical problem, and when a system of health care is developed that can cope adequately with that problem, will specialized services like the ICU become what they could maximally become — a place for giving more than mere survival care, important as that is.

ACKNOWLEDGEMENT

The points made in this paper are based on many observations and interviews but at only a few hospitals (during a study of terminal care), on a reading of the literature, and on data gathered by Mrs. H. Mildred McIntyre from a number of other intensive care units. Over the years, Mrs. McIntyre and I have had many conversations about ICU's. I owe her additional thanks for her careful reading of this paper and for several suggestions that certainly improved it.

DYING TRAJECTORIES AND THE
ORGANIZATION OF WORK*

Any study of dying — not merely of death, the end of dying —
must take into consideration the fact that dying takes time. In hospitals where death is a common occurrence, the staff's work is organized in accordance with expectation that dying will take a longer
or shorter time. Sometimes the organization of hospital work fits
an individual patient's course of dying — his "dying trajectory" —
but at other times the work pattern is, at least in some respects, out
of step with the dying process. Here we will discuss the most general
features of this interplay between the organization of work and the
temporality of dying.

TEMPORAL FEATURES OF TERMINAL CARE

When not entirely medical or technical, most writings about
terminal care focus on the psychological or ethical aspects of behavior toward dying persons.[1] Those emphases flow from the psychological, and often ethical, difficulties that accompany death and
dying. However, much of the behavior of people toward the dying
may be just as legitimately viewed as *work*. This is as true when a
person dies at home as when he dies in the hospital. Usually during
the course of his dying he is unable to fulfill all his physiological
and psychological needs by himself. He may need to be fed, bathed,
taken to the toilet, given drugs, brought desired objects when too
feeble to get them himself, and, near the end of his life, even be "cared
for" totally. Whether persons in attendance on him enjoy or suffer
these tasks, they are undeniably work. Wealthier families sometimes

[1] *Cf.* Bibliography in Robert Fulton (ed.), *Death and Identity* (New
York: John Wiley, 1965), pp. 397-415.

*Reprinted by permission from
TIME FOR DYING
(with Barney G. Glaser), Chicago, Aldine Pub. Co., 1968,
pp. 1-7, 237-242, 148-178.

hire private nurses to do all or some of this work. In the hospital, there is no question that terminal care, whether regarded as distasteful or as satisfying, is viewed as work.

This work has important temporal features. For instance, there are prescribed schedules governing when the patient must be fed, bathed, turned in bed, given drugs. There are times when tests must be administered. There are crucial periods when the patient must be closely observed or when crucial treatments must be given or actions taken to prevent immediate deterioration — even immediate death. Since there is a division of labor, it must be organized in terms of time. For instance, the nurse must have the patient awake in time for the laboratory technician to administer tests, and the physician's visit must not coincide with the patient's bath or with the visiting hours of relatives. When the patient's illness grows worse, the pace and tempo of the staff's work shifts accordingly: meals may be skipped and tests may be less frequent, but the administration of drugs and the reading of vital signs may be more frequent. During all this work, calculated organizational timing must consider turnover among staff members or their absence on vacations or because of illness.

With rare exceptions, medical services always include both recovering and dying patients. Even on intensive care units or on cancer services, not all patients are expected to, or do, die. On any given service, the temporal organization of work with dying patients is greatly influenced by the relative numbers of recovering and dying patients and by the types of recovering patients. For instance, on services for premature babies, babies who die usually do so within 48 hours after birth; after that, most are relatively safe. The "good preemie" does not stay very long on the service, but moves along to the normal babies' service. Hence the pace and the kind of work in the case of a premature baby vary in accordance with the number of days since birth, and when a baby begins to "turn bad" a few days after birth — usually unexpectedly — the pace and the kind of work are greatly affected.

The temporal ordering of work on each service is also related to the predominant types of death in relation to the normal types of recovery. As an example, we may look at intensive care units: some patients there are expected to die quickly, if they are to die at all; others need close attention for several days because death is a touch-and-go matter; while others are not likely to die but do need temporary round-the-clock nursing. Most who die here are either so heavily drugged as to be temporarily comatose or are actually past consciousness. Consequently, nurses or physicians do not need to converse with these patients. When a patient nears

240

death he may sometimes unwittingly compete with other patients for nurses' or physicians' attention, several of whom may give care to the critically ill patient. When the emergency is over, or the patient dies, then the nurses, for instance, return to less immediately critical patients, reading their vital signs, managing treatments, and carrying out other important tasks.

Each type of service tends to have a characteristic incidence of death, which also affects the staff's organization of work. Closely allied with these incidences are the tempos of dying that are characteristic of each ward. On emergency services, for example, patients tend to die quickly (they are accident cases, victims of violence, or people stricken suddenly and acutely). The staff on emergency services, therefore, is geared to perform urgent, critical functions. Many emergency services, especially in large city hospitals, are also organized for frequent deaths, especially on weekends. At such times, recovering (or non-sick) patients sometimes tend to receive scant attention, unless the service is organized flexibly to handle both types of patients.

The already complex organization of professional activity for terminal care is made even more so by several other matters involving temporality. For one, what may be conveniently termed the "experiential careers" of patients, families, and staff members are highly relevant to the action around dying patients. Some patients are familiar with their diseases, but others are encountering their symptoms for the first time. The patient's knowledge of the course of his disease, based on his previous experience with it, has an important bearing on what happens as he lies dying in the hospital. Similarly, some personnel are well acquainted with the predominant disease patterns found on their particular wards; but some, although possibly familiar with other illnesses, may be newcomers to these diseases. They may be unprepared for sudden changes of symptoms and vital signs; taken by surprise at crucial junctures, they may make bad errors in timing their actions. More experienced personnel are more likely to be able to take immediate appropriate action at any turn in the illness.

Experiential careers also include the differing experiences that people have had with hospitals. Some patients return repeatedly to the same hospital ward. When a familiar face appears, the staff may be shocked at the patient's deterioration, thinking *"Now* he is going to die," and may therefore react differently than they would to someone new to the ward. Likewise, the extent of the patient's familiarity with the ways of hospitals or of a particular hospital influence his reactions during the course of dying. In short, both the illness careers and the hospital careers of all parties in the dying situation may be of considerable importance, affecting both the interaction around the dying patient and the organization of his terminal care.

One other type of experience is highly relevant: the differing "personal careers" of the interactants in the dying situation — the more personal aspects of the interaction. We shall later discuss instances where the reactions of young nurses and physicians indicated "involvement" in the deaths of young terminal patients — much more so, generally, than in the deaths of elderly patients. Similarly, if an older woman patient reminds a young nurse of her own deceased mother, the nurse's actions toward her may be affected.

Another aspect of the effect of personal career on the dying situation is in the conception of time. Recognizing his approaching death, an elderly patient who has had a long and satisfying life may welcome it. He may also wish to review that life publicly. His wife or nurse, however, may refuse to listen, telling him that he should not give up hope of living, or even cautioning him against being "so morbid." On the other hand, other patients may throw the staff into turmoil because they will not accept their dying. Nonacceptance sometimes signifies a patient's protest against destiny for making him leave "unfinished work." These various time conceptions of different patients in the dying situation may run counter not only to each other, but also to the staff's work time concepts; as, for instance, when a patient's personal conception prevents the nurse from completing scheduled actions.

One further class of events attending the course of dying is of crucial importance for the action around the dying patient. These events are the characteristic work required by medical and hospital organization which occurs at critical junctures of the dying process. That the person is actually dying must be recognized if he is to be treated like a dying person. At some point, everyone may recognize that there "is nothing more to do." As dying approaches its conclusion, a death watch usually takes place. When death has ended the process, there must be a formal pronouncement, and then an announcement to the family. At each point in time, the staff's interrelated actions must be properly organized.

Taken all together, then, the total organization of activity — which we call "work" — during the course of dying is profoundly affected by temporal considerations. Some are evident to almost everyone, some are not. The entire web of temporal interrelationships we shall refer to as the *temporal order*. It includes the continual readjustment and coordination of staff effort, which we term the *organization of work*.

242

DYING TRAJECTORIES

The dying trajectory of each patient has at least two outstanding properties. First, it takes place over time: it has *duration*. Specific trajectories can vary greatly in duration. Second, a trajectory has *shape*: it can be graphed. It plunges straight down; it moves slowly but steadily downward; it vacillates slowly, moving slightly up and down before diving downward radically; it moves slowly down at first, then hits a long plateau, then plunges abruptly to death.

Neither duration nor shape is a purely objective physiological property. They are both perceived properties; their dimensions depend on when the perceiver initially *defines* someone as dying and on his *expectations* of how that dying will proceed. Dying trajectories themselves, then, are perceived courses of dying rather than the actual courses. This distinction is readily evident in the type of trajectory that involves a short reprieve from death. This reprieve represents an unexpected deferment of death. On the other hand, in a lingering death bystanders may expect faster dying than actually occurs.

Since dying patients enter hospitals at varying distances from death, and are defined in terms of when and how they will die, various types of trajectories are commonly recognized by the hospital personnel. For instance, there is the abrupt, surprise trajectory: a patient who is expected to recover suddenly dies. A trajectory frequently found on emergency wards is the expected swift death: many patients are brought in because of fatal accidents, and nothing can be done to prevent their deaths. Expected lingering while dying is another type of trajectory; it is characteristic, for example, of cancer. Besides the short-term reprieve, there may also be the suspended-sentence trajectory: the patient is actually sent home and may live for several years thereafter. Another commonly recognized pattern is entry-reentry: the patient, slowly going downhill, returns home several times between stays at the hospital. All these generalized types of trajectories rest upon the perceivers' expectations of duration and shape.

Regardless of the particular attributes of a specific patient's trajectory, ordinarily there are certain events — we shall term them "critical junctures" — that appear along the dying trajectory and are directly handled by the temporal organization of hospital work. These occur in either full or truncated form (in the next chapter we shall discuss the latter): (1) The patient is defined as dying. (2) Staff and family then make preparations for his death, as he may do himself if he knows he is dying. (3) At some point, there seems to be "nothing more to do" to prevent death. (4) The final descent may take weeks, or days, or merely hours, ending in (5) the "last hours," (6) the death watch, and (7) the death itself. Somewhere along the course of dying, there may be announcements that the patient is dying, or that he is entering or leaving a phase. After death, death itself must be legally pronounced and then publicly announced.

When these critical junctures occur as expected, on schedule, then all participants — sometimes including the patient — are prepared for them. The work involved is provided for and integrated by the temporal order of the hospital. For instance, the nurses are ready for a death watch if they can anticipate approximately when the patient will be very near death. When, however, critical junctures occur unexpectedly or off schedule, staff members and family alike are at least somewhat unprepared. This book will offer many examples of both anticipated and unanticipated junctures. The point we wish to emphasize here is that expectations are crucial to the way junctures are handled by all involved.

TIME, STRUCTURAL PROCESS, AND
STATUS PASSAGE

In our opening pages, we remarked that the temporal features of work are of the utmost importance for understanding how organizations function. On virtually every page of this book, readers have found materials pertinent to the temporal features of work organizations and trajectories. Now those features will be discussed within the more general context of the sociology of time.

It is useful to begin by thinking of the hospital career provided for a dying trajectory as a succession of "transitional statuses" in the status passage between life and death,[1] as it takes place in the hospital. In contrast to Wilbert Moore's concepts[2] of sequence, rate, synchronization, rhythm, routines and recurrence, which simply denote time unrelated to social structure, transitional status is a concept denoting *social structural* time. How does a social system keep a person in passage between two statuses for a period of time? He is put into a transitional status, or a sequence of them, that denotes a period of time during which he will be in a status passage (*e.g.,* he is put on the ICU, thereby denoting a quick passage). As a concept for ordering social structural time, transitional status has great advantages over Moore's concepts. His concepts help us talk of the social ordering of behavior; but they are not automatically linked with social structure; they are only applied to it, if the analyst is so inclined. In contrast, reference to the transitional statuses of a status-passage, on the other hand, automatically require locating the discussion within a social structure.

In general, sociological writing about groups, organizations and institutions tends to leave their temporal features unanalyzed.[3] When

[1]Glaser and Strauss, "Temporal Aspects of Dying as a Non-Scheduled Status Passage," *American Journal Socoiology,* Vol. 71 (1965), pp. 48-59.

[2]See *Man, Time and Society* (New York: John Wiley, 1963), Chapter 1.

[3]The following paragraph is adapted from the introduction to *George Herbert Mead on Social Psychology* ed. by Anselm Strauss, (Chicago: University of Chicago Press, 1964 edition), pp. xiii-xiv.

they are handled explicitly, the focus is on such matters as deadlines, scheduling, rates, pacing, turnover, and concepts of time which may vary by organizational, institutional or group position. The principal weakness of such analyses stems from an unexamined assumption that the temporal properties worth studying involve only the work of organizations and their members. For instance, the work time of personnel must be properly articulated — hence deadlines and schedules. Breakdowns in this temporal articulation occur not only through accident and poor planning, but also through differential valuation of time by various echelons, personnel and clientele. But from our analysis the temporal order of the organization appears to require a much wider range of temporal dimensions. We have assumed in this book that, for instance, people bring to an organization their own temporal concerns and that their actions there are profoundly affected by those concerns.[4] Thus, woven into our analysis were experiential careers (hospital, illness, and personal), as well as the patient's and the families' concepts of time. In our analysis, we have attempted to show how temporal order in the hospital refers to a total, delicate, continuously changing articulation of these various temporal considerations. Such articulation, of course, includes easily recognizable organizational mechanisms but also less visible ones, including "arrangements" negotiated by various relevant persons.

The kind of analysis required when studying temporal order brings our discussion to the other topics of this chapter — structural process and status passage. Such a conception of how to study temporal order emphasizes the continual interplay of structure and process. Critics who incline toward a processual view of society have frequently criticized — and in our judgment effectively — the over determinism of structuralists. But that critique need not necessitate an abandonment of the tremendously useful mode of thinking which is called "structural." That analytic mode need only be combined systematically with an allied concern with process. The study of dying trajectories within hospital organizations happens to have led easily to *thinking generally* about "structural process" and "status passage." Let us consider each in turn.

STRUCTURAL PROCESS

One of the central issues in sociological theory is the relationship of structure to process. What implication does this book have for this issue? We have, in previous chapters, discussed explicitly the structural adaptations of hospitals to various phases of dying tra-

---

[4]This kind of view is implicit in the writings of G. H. Mead. Herbert Blumer has attempted to make the view more explicit in his writing about Mead and in various papers about symbolic interactionism. *Cf.,* his "Society as Symbolic Interaction," in A. Rose (Ed.), *Human Behavior and Social Processes* (Boston: Houghton Mifflin, 1962), pp. 197-92.

jectories. If one considers dying as a process extending over time, then the hospital's structure can be seen as continually changing to handle different phases in that process. Its structure, then, is in process; which phenomenon we call "structural process." We have seen how a person may be brought into one section of the hospital and then moved to another, as his trajectory is redefined or as he reaches certain critical junctures in an anticipated or defined trajectory. Even when a dying patient remains on one ward, he can be moved around within that ward so that different aspects of its "structure" can be brought into play. If he is never moved, the ward's or hospital's varying resources of manpower, skill, drugs or machinery may be brought into play as his trajectory proceeds. What is true for the staff's relationships with a patient is also true for its relationships with his family.

Sociological analysis ordinarily does not join structure and process so tightly as our notion of "structural process" does. Structure tends to be treated as relatively fixed — because it is what it is, then certain processes can occur. Or inversely, because the major goals involve certain processes, as in a factory or in a governmental agency, the structure is made as nearly consonant with the processes as possible. New processes are conceived as leading to new structural arrangement; while innovations in structure similarly lead to associated processual changes. A major implication of our book is that structure and process are related more complexly (and more interestingly) than is commonly conceived.

We have, for instance, remarked how during a given phase of a trajectory a ward may be quite a different place than before. For instance, when the sentimental order has been profoundly disrupted, the structural elements that can be called on are not quite the same as before; some elements no longer exist and may never again exist. If afterward an "equilibrium" is reached, it is a moving equilibrium with the ward calmed down but forever at least a somewhat different place.

So rather than seeing a relatively inflexible structure, with a limited and determinable list of structural properties, we have to conceive of a ward, hospital, or any other institution as a structure in process. It therefore has a potential range of properties far greater than the outsider (the sociologist) can possibly imagine unless he watches the insiders at work. He can be surprised at the ways in which staff, family or patients can call on diverse properties of the hospital or local community, for bringing in resources that he never dreamed existed but which became permanently or temporarily part of the structural processes of the ward.

In a previous work, one of the authors and his colleagues made a similar point, but neither gave it a name nor developed it as we are doing here.[5] It was remarked then that ordinarily state mental personnel, when observed closely, exhibit great variation not only in how they use the obvious resources of the hospital but also in how they draw upon outside resources. If we interpret that latter set of operations in terms of structural process, we would say that the innovating personnel are making use of the outside resources (say, a young psychiatrist who asks colleagues to give lectures, or asks his own analyst to advise him, however indirectly, on how to handle his subordinates). These resources are as much a part of the hospital "system" — at least for the time being — as anything found in the hospital itself. And they come into play during determinable times: they function neither independently of time nor of circumstance.

Perhaps we need especially to emphasize that the clients of an institution — patients or family members — are also structural features of it. Thus, a Japanese mother who cares for her dying son at a hospital becomes part of the hospital's structure. If the family gathers around during a patient's last days, then the hospital's structure is amplified. If familes are banished or voluntarily "pull out" during certain phases of dying, then they do not loom large as structural possibilities for the staff to call on or to handle.[6]

Structural process relates to the various participants' awareness. They will vary, of course, in their awareness of which structural properties are operating, or can be brought to operate, during various phases of the dying process. Misperceptions are involved as well as awareness; a doctor, for instance, may assume that he can call on some structural resource (e.g., an oxygen tank) when it no longer exists. He may discover its "disappearance" too late; or he may never discover his error, if it is not very consequential. Others, such as the nurses, may or may not be aware of the absence or presence of his knowledge. The relationships of these "awareness contexts" to structural processes are neither accidental nor unpredictable, as staff and patients sometimes believe.

Perhaps the point that most requires underlining, is that structural process has consequences which themselves enter into the emergence of a *new* structural process. For the sociologist, this fact implies

[5] Anselm Strauss *et al.*, *Psychiatric Ideologies and Institutions* (New York: Free Press of Glencoe, 1964).

[6] Herbert Simon makes the point that clients are as much part of an organization as its personnel, but he makes the point statically. See his *Administrative Behavior* (New York: Macmillan, 1948).

an important directive: part of his job is to trace those consequences that significantly affect the unrolling course of events called "structural process" — not for particular cases, but for *types* of cases. Sociologists, for instance, are not interested in *a* dying person, but in *types* of dying persons and the patterned events relevant to their dying. When focusing on the consequences of structure and process, it is all too easy to settle for lists of consequences for, say, various personnel or for the repetitive functioning of an organization or institution. But the explicit directive given by the concept of structural process is that the sociologist cannot rest until he has analytically related the interactional consequences to the next phases in interaction — or, in our terms, present structural processes to later structural processes.

LAST WEEKS AND DAYS

Unless a person dies abruptly, with virtually no warning, the dying trajectory includes a stage of "last days" and perhaps even "last weeks." The hospital staff responsible for his care usually finds itself engaged in a complex juggling of tasks, people, and relationships. Analysis of that juggling is the principal aim of this chapter. Because of its complexity, we cannot fully detail the myriad of variants that arise, but a schematic treatment should be sufficient to carry the dying trajectory forward to its next phase, the hours just prior to death, and then to the death scene itself.

JUGGLING

The staff's juggling consists, first, of organizing a number of potentially shifting treatment and care tasks. As a patient becomes visibly sicker and weaker, the staff typically stops certain activities and simultaneously initiates new ones. The comfort care activities may become very detailed and may now require considerable nursing skill; the medical care necessary to keep him alive may remain quite complex, although different from earlier medical care.

Meanwhile, the staff must also juggle people and relationships whose existence can cause great disruption to the ward's work and sentimental orders. If the patient is visible to other patients, their reactions to his last weeks and days must be taken into account, particularly insofar as they may see his dying as a rehearsal of their own. The problems of family management also are potentially great. Family members must be warned about the oncoming death, prepared for it, perhaps given occasional emotional support, and warned against bringing the patient into awareness if it is undesirable for him to know about his approaching death. The patient himself, unless he is virtually comatose, also represents a range of potential problems for the staff. He may not die acceptably, according to ward standards; may not come to terms with his dying; may ask uncomfortable questions, even if he is not aware of his oncoming death. Like the treatment and care tasks, the management of people and relationships shifts as the trajectory moves along. Whenever their handling of such work is inadequate, both the staff's work and the accompanying collective moods are profoundly affected. Things are, so to speak, out of order.

STRUCTURAL RELEVANCES

The range of potential problems a staff faces is measurably reduced by the systematic routing of dying patients into the appropriate wards of a hospital. Each ward, as we noted in Chapter III, tends to have its own limited range of probable dying trajectories, with personnel geared to coping with various phases of those trajectories. When unusual trajectories occur on a ward, the personnel are far less prepared to cope with either the medical treatment or the social-psychological aspects of the last days. They may not even anticipate various social-psychological problems that accompany those last days.

For the usual trajectories, however, the ward possesses considerable resources of skill, organization, and perhaps equipment, which can be brought into play when warranted. In short, the ward's structure is adaptable to specified phases of its typical trajectories. This structural adaptability is also found, as we shall suggest later, on the large, all-purpose, and therefore infinitely multitrajectoried wards characteristically found in countries outside Western Europe and North America. But although the structural resources of each ward are brought into play at appropriate moments, our familiar key variables (awareness, social loss, etc.) are also likely to affect whether and how this is done.

TEMPORAL ORDER AND CRITICAL JUNCTURES

Despite the institutional mechanisms for standardizing trajectories and the structural resources available for dealing with them, the organization of work is constantly in delicate balance. So much can go wrong: so much is unexpected. This would be true even if dying were "timeless" or took place only over a short period. But last days take time; hospital personnel must juggle tasks, people, and relationships that can and do change daily. And the three orders of change affect one another. This is why we earlier emphasized that the total organization of activity (which we call work) during the course of dying is profoundly affected by temporal considerations. We referred to the entire web of such relationships on a ward as its temporal order. This order includes the continual readjustment and coordination of staff effort.

Temporal order is threatened by a whole host of changes, which we shall detail below, and considerable staff activity during the patient's last days is likely to be directed at maintaining a workable temporal order. Since every ward has many patients, usually including some who are not dying, the entire matter is rendered all the more complicated than if the staff needed only to balance one patient, his "kin" and its own involvement.

One final point before we turn to detailed discussion of the last days: As we have seen, there is much variation in the duration and shapes of trajectories. Among trajectories that do include recognizable last weeks or days, three major classes are especially important. The first is when death is uncertain but, if it occurs, is quick. The second type is when death is certain but the time of death is relatively uncertain; the patient may linger with reprieves, plateaus, and even partial reversals. The third type is when both death and time of death are relatively certain. Each type tends to involve the staff in a somewhat different range of problems with patient, family, and neighboring patients. Each type also gives rise to somewhat different strategies for handling various critical junctures — defining a patient as in his last weeks or days, pre-announcing his probable death, "deciding" whether to prolong or hasten his dying, and engaging in and arranging for farewells and last looks. Such critical junctures may be only episodes during the last phases of the trajectory, or they may be turning points in the final evolution of a dying patient's trajectory. Moreover, a given critical juncture may appear more than once, and repetition itself alters the character of the juncture and may raise special problems.

FAMILY HANDLING

MAJOR PROBLEMS

Most patients belong to families. If kinsmen appear at the bedside of a dying relative during last days, their presence can pose severe problems for the medical and nursing personnel, and may actually interfere with the efficient care of patients. Problems tend to center around four issues: the family needs to be prepared for the forthcoming death; they may need to be persuaded to delegate responsibility for the dying person to the hospital; they may require coaching in proper modes of behavior while at the hospital; and they may need to be helped in their grieving, either for their own sake or for the sake of preventing disruption of ward activity. The nature of these central problems suggests that the personnel may be considerably engaged in working with the family during the last days.

Sometimes work with families is unnecessary or minimal. If there is no family or none close enough to visit the hospital, no family problems arise. In American geriatric hospitals, for example, family-handling problems are minimal. Many families never visit, either because they live too far away or because they have already abandoned the patient. Often kinsmen arrive at the hospital only at the very point of death; if they visit earlier, their visits tend to be short and infrequent. Since the dying relative is elderly and perhaps has been dying for a long time, visitors are likely to grieve but little, and quietly. In a ward populated largely by senile and comatose patients, these intrusions have minimal effects.

In some countries, especially in economically underdeveloped areas, close kinsmen customarily provide the comfort care to dying relatives, thus relieving nursing personnel for other duties. In these hospitals, moreover, families often provide feeding, bathing, and general routine care to recovering patients, so staff are accustomed to their presence. Grieving kinsmen tend to support one another, and when several work around one patient they may grieve collectively.

In striking contrast are those conditions that tend to maximize disruption of the staff's work and the ward's atmosphere. At a small hospital in Gubbio, Italy, we witnessed the following drama. Just as we entered the ward, a daughter ran out of her dying father's room, screaming loudly for a doctor: "My father is dying!" Other patients and their kinsmen quickly gathered and stared at the developing scene. Two nurses also quickly appeared, then scampered into the dying man's room, closing the door behind them. In the hall the distraught daughter was comforted by her husband. A few moments later, a physician scurried down the corridor, entered the room, and soon came out and told the excited couple nothing could be done for the old man, that he only had a few days to live. Then he left them, returning to his interrupted work. In cases like this, the family often spirit their relative away from the hospital, wishing him to die at home — and thus inevitably hastening his death. But if he does not die within a day or two, they may bring him back to the hospital, thinking he may be saved, not recognizing he has only had a reprieve.

As we have seen, unexpected death can cause the family to act drastically toward the physician or nurses. If a family is to be prepared for a patient's death, it must be forewarned. The physician is responsible for disclosing probable death. His timing depends on many variables. Chief among them is the nature of the expected dying trajectory. If, for example, surgery can — perhaps — give a few extra years of life, but only at great risk, then parents customarily are told that their child may not survive the operation. If a patient suffers a stroke, is brought to the hospital, and is judged to have only a few remaining days or weeks, then, too, the family is likely to be warned of the virtual certainty of death. On the other hand, extensively lingering trajectories allow the physician great

254

latitude in timing his preannouncements to the family. Indeed, he does not know exactly when the patient will die and may not be able to predict whether there will be temporary reprieves, plateaus, and even reversals. His first preannouncement of death may be long delayed, or consist initially of cues to which the family can respond with gradually growing awareness. He may make several preannouncements during the last weeks and days, indicating that death is getting closer.

Some physicians develop considerable skill at pacing out these preannouncements. Ineffective pacing — or insufficient trust by the family — may result in their shopping around for a "better" doctor, one with a cure, even though cure is really not at issue. Good strategy usually requires that the physician makes his first preannouncement to the "strongest" family member, who then has the responsibility of disclosing this (and subsequent) information to other relatives as he judges they can take it.

During the last days, family members may ply the hospital staff with queries bearing not only on time (how many days, hours, has he got to live?) but also on mode of dying (will he die peacefully, will he be entirely out of pain?). Those queries must be handled. If they are not, scenes are likely to erupt on the ward.[1]

Some families have sufficient internal resources for accepting the forthcoming death of a relative, but sometimes the staff finds it necessary to help them come to terms with the event. The staff then offers them loss rationales or supports those created by the kinsmen: "Yes, it will be a blessing if he goes soon." "Yes, he's lucky that he has no pain at all." If the last days stretch into last weeks, the staff can sustain the relatives' acceptance by displaying equanimity and by giving undiminished comfort care to the patient. (They may even act out a drama like that portrayed in the previous chapter when the husband would not "give up" on his wife.) The staff can give assurances that the patient will die peacefully. They can correct unfounded expectations concerning his mode of dying. When plateaus or reprieves occur, staff can show pleasure without encouraging false hopes, signaling quietly that death is still on the way. If need be, the nurses can put pressure on the physician to "explain again" to a close relative who will not really face the facts. On one pediatric ward, we observed a staff discussion in which nurses pressured the resident to make a mother "begin grieving," make her "really realize" that her child was not going to recover. On this ward, it is a standard tactic to get the grieving started long before the anticipated death.

[1]For fuller discussion of preannouncement of strategies and problems, see *Awareness of Dying* (Chicago: Aldine Pub. Co., 1965)

Relatives' acceptance of a forthcoming death is likely to be linked with whether they have already partly gotten over their grief or have at least gotten it under control. By the last days of an extremely slow trajectory, virtually everybody may be fairly well "grieved out," especially if the patient's social loss is relatively low. Occasionally a latecomer arrives who has only recently heard the news, and who displays his grief; this in turn may prompt other kinsmen to renew their grieving, or to put on an act in which they show more grief than they really now feel, or to explain that they are all worn out and past his stage of grieving.

If at all possible, a tactful staff allows close kinsmen plenty of time with the dying person, especially during the very last days, so that they can quietly live through their grieving. Sometimes personnel do not recognize the grieving as such — it has many individual and cultural variants. But by and large they do understand that a wife must be with a dying husband, children with a dying parent, that separation would be more painful than "participation" in the dying. Some hospitals have convenient rooms where relatives may wait when they cannot stay at bedside. At one Scottish hospital, staff members offer the relatives "spirits" and overt consolation; in American hospitals, sedatives are more likely to accompany the consolation.

When the family or the staff believes it advisable that the dying person remain ignorant of his forthcoming death, family members must take care not to display their grief before the patient. Staff members may have to warn kinsmen about this danger or take steps to prevent its occurrence. Since grieving may begin the instant that close kinsmen are told about the probability of death, the staff may immediately begin giving support. In one Greek hospital that we visited, this supportive tactic was highly institutionalized: the head of the nursing service customarily made the preannouncement in her office and then supported the stunned kinsmen.

As we have noted, nursing personnel often find their role as sympathetic listener or comforter a major one during the final days. They are especially empathetic when they regard the patient's death as a grave social loss, or when their compassion is especially aroused by an association with their own personal past, or, sometimes, when a grieving family member has behaved admirably in the face of the ordeal. Occasionally a mother has lost another child, or perhaps a sister, from the same herditary disease; the social-loss aspect adds both to the mother's grief and tc the staff's efforts to console her.

In American hospitals, social workers tend self-consciously to become "grief-workers," attempting with professional deliberateness

to "work through" the grief of relatives; this is perhaps most noticeable on pediatric wards. Priests, chaplains, and nuns also engage
in such activities; indeed, they may be called on by a desperate
nursing staff afraid of the disastrous effects of death and unable themselves to help the relative. We have observed a chaplain intervene
during the last days in a situation of growing animosity between
staff and a wife whose unacceptable behavior apparently was due to
her failure to come to terms with her husband's oncoming death.
In American hospitals, psychiatrists may also be called in to work
with family members.

The staff's third problem of family handling — getting suitable
behavior from the family members — is linked closely with whether
the family is adequately prepared for the death, and does its grieving "on schedule." As we have seen, a wife may cause upsetting
scenes if she is not at all prepared for her husband's death when it
finally draws near. A relative who grieves too early and openly
may disturb the patient; even if the latter is quite aware of his forthcoming death, he may not yet be sufficiently resigned to it.

The staff may also have to coach relatives in appropriate bedside behavior. If family members visit in too great numbers, a
rule may be laid down that only close kin can visit "from now
on" — especially as death becomes imminent. A family that is too
noisy may need to be reprimanded; the staff may forbid access to
the ward to all but the closest kin. Once we observed the nurses
intervene in a situation in which a lower income family noisily
"carried on right in the room as if the patient were not dying"; the
physician was prevailed upon to allow only the mother and father
visiting rights to the bedside.

On large, open wards, visitors must be especially careful not
to disturb nearby patients with chattering or loud sobbing, even
when they and the dying man are hidden behind a screen. When
the patient has a private room, kin still may need to be taught
not to "get in the way." Often a nurse will ask someone to leave
the bedside or the room when she suspects that a nursing or medical procedure may disturb the onlooker. Visitors may also harass
the staff by making what the latter considers unjustified, overanxious, or just plain fussy demands. Various tactics are used to
make the offending person behave properly or, if that proves impossible, to avoid contact with the person as much as possible. What
is considered unjustified or fussy depends not only on the behavior
itself, but also on how attached the personnel have become to the
patient, how well they have come to know the family member, the
nature of the patient's evolving story, and so on. The staff may
call on other family members to restrain the over-demanding person.

It may also rely on kinsmen to restrain each other's improper use of space and to control each other's noisiness, as well as to help each other to grieve on schedule, and to make judgments about who should not visit the hospital or how close the patient is to his final moments.

The staff's fourth great problem is that the kinsmen may not willingly delegate the patient's care during his last hours. Unwillingness to delegate may vary in seriousness. At its most extreme, the patient simply is withdrawn from the hospital, usually against professional advice. He may even literally be kidnapped before the staff is quite aware of what has happened (or so we have been told by nurses at foreign hospitals). Unwillingness to leave a patient in the hospital during his last hours may derive from the family's fear that he will die there rather than at home, where they feel he belongs. But their unwillingness may also be associated (as with Malayan villagers) with religious practices that they know cannot be carried out within the hospital. Sometimes an American family takes a patient home during his last days because it believes it can provide adequate care there; the family may discover its error later and return him to the hospital.

Even families who know very well that their dying kinsman should remain in professional hands may try to interfere with the staff, suggesting or demanding that certain things be done differently. The staff requires countertactics to cope with this behavior More generally, however, the division of labor in American hospitals allows close kin to carry out routine comfort care while the nursing staff gives the more difficult or professionalized care. As the last days draw to a close, sometimes the staff tactfully allows a mother or wife to take over the comfort care almost totally if the mode of dying permits such latitude. Nurses may sense that the active kinswoman needs to give this care; she would suffer more from inactivity. In many Asian and European hospitals it is standard practice to leave to family members almost complete responsibility for the comfort care of dying relatives. In a Japanese hospital, for instance, we talked with a patient dying of cancer, whose mother had accompanied him to Tokyo from a distant northern region in order to care for him during his last weeks and days. At this hospital, such an arrangement was usual.

STRUCTURAL CONDITIONS

Neither the severity of problems that a family will present the hospital staff nor the degree of success the staff will have in managing a family during the last weeks and days are entirely predictable. Yet it is possible to state in general terms the kinds of structural conditions that militate against the relative tranquility and success of the staff's efforts at management. Among those conditions are the number of visiting relatives, the distance from which they come, the experience they have with hospital customs and rules, the amount of trust they have in the professionals, and the amount or kind of ward space.

An especially important structural condition is created by the combination of type of dying trajectory and type of ward. We see the impact of this conjuncture clearly in the ICU, where a fair proportion of patients are likely to be in their last days, sometimes with rather short warning to relatives. Space limitations and the intensive character of staff work, plus the maximum visibility of patients to each other, make it necessary to keep bedside visiting very brief. Nurses develop special tactics for gentling the relatives out the door and for avoiding the pleading faces of relatives sitting restlessly in the nearby waiting room.

Prior to severe surgery or when an emergency operation is in progress — a touch-and-go situation with a strong potential of last days or last hours — family members tend to wander from the surgery waiting room to the nursing station, bombarding personnel with anxious queries and expressive chatter. Although personnel have developed standard tactics for handling families, these tactics are not always successful in these conditions. With unexpectedly quick or potentially nonrecoverable trajectories, for example, the family's queries may have to be evaded until the trajectory is more certain or until the physician can disclose it to the family. (We remember vividly how an extensive Gypsy family swarmed over a ward during an emergency operation on a kinsman. The family gave the staff a very difficult time. There were not enough staff members, and not enough time was available, to permit efficient use of the standard tactics evolved for handling more normal sized and more "disciplined" families.)

Even in such trying situations, however, a staff can sometimes count or call on some other family member to exert a controlling hand. Staff members can also draw on various resources of the ward: the telephone may call them away; they can set up spatial barriers to keep a family at arm's length; they can escape by throwing themselves with obvious gestures into their work; if need be, they can invoke rarely used hospital rules. The staff may even turn to the families of other patients, who sometimes can be counted on to help restrain or reassure an upset family.

We should not think of the structural conditions, which lessen or enlarge problems of family handling, as static. If they were, the staff's control would, paradoxically, be rendered both more difficult and much easier. The longer a lingering trajectory is, the more structural conditions are likely to change; some changes help the staff, some hinder it. Indeed, many of the most disturbing events stem from evolving conditions so unusual that the staff does not anticipate them, and may not be able to do much to prevent their recurrence. Handling the immediate situation necessitates that the staff grasp an unusual structural condition.

Here are a few examples of such conditions: first, a structural condition that is expected to change but does not. When a hospitalized child dies over a period of months, the staff ordinarily expects the parents to become more prepared for the death. But in a Roman hospital, nurses told us of parents who caused upsetting scenes during their child's last days because they could not believe he was dying, even though he had been hospitalized a year before with a diagnosis of certain death. The same hospital provides an example of an unanticipated structural condition and its consequences: The nursing personnel claim to have special difficulties with southern Italians, who are "more expressive" in their grieving and who are not familiar with proper standards of behavior in hospitals. They press for long visiting hours and for visits at inappropriate times. The standard tactics that nurses employ to control such families sometimes break down when the responsible staff physician also happens to be southern Italian; rather than becoming their ally, he may actually allow the offending family special license to visit as they wish. The nurses must then devise new tactics to handle the family.

In a Scottish hospital, by contrast, an overly expressive Italian family's visits and visiting time were cut down because of its noise, in order to minimize further disturbance of the ward. In another Scottish hospital, a nurse described how one family's queries about their kinsman's condition were enormously difficult to handle because the patient happened to be her own uncle — a structural condition that remained relatively out of her control during the entire course of his dying.

Occasionally, a responsible family member may distress the staff not by what he does but rather by what he does not do. When, for example, a wife begins to visit her dying husband less and less frequently, the staff may be sufficiently disturbed to ask the staff physician or the chaplain to intervene, either to discover "what's wrong" or urge more attention by the wife.

LEAVE-TAKING

As the last weeks move into last days, and the last days into probable last hours, a critical juncture arises that can be particularly hazardous for the work and sentiments of personnel. That juncture comes when close relatives say final (or tentatively final) fare-wells to the dying patient or — if he is not aware — when they take their last looks at him while he still lives. Told through a prean-nouncement that he has not long to live, or warned by their own senses, they take leave silently or openly.

These leave-takings are likely to be awesome ceremonies, even when the dying man is comatose, has been socially dead for some time, or is elderly. Each day's separation implies the possibility that *this* may be the last time visitors will see the patient alive. When family members travel considerable distances to visit at the hospital, as is characteristic at regional hospitals and metropolitan medical centers, they may be able to visit only on weekends or at intervals of at least several days. They must make each farewell not knowing whether they will return before their relative has died.

The anguish of visitors' farewells may be shared by some staff members. We saw this in the dying of a lovely teenaged girl who lingered long. Her mother visited each day, and stayed all day. The staff members became as attached to the mother as to the daughter. When the dying continued to stretch out over many days, each one possibly the girl's last, the collective mood of the staff grew increas-ingly tense. Each night when the mother left for home staff members felt — and some showed — great empathetic anxiety. Eventually, a solution to the daily leave-taking was found. Since the mother was a practical nurse, possessing sufficient skills to care for her daughter at home if given proper equipment and instruction, the nursing staff negotiated with the physician; and together they agreed that the mother, who increasingly wished to have her daughter spend her last days at home, should be allowed her wish. After that decision was implemented, the entire staff breathed more freely, but its ten-sion took a few days to dissipate. The most important immediate change was that the ward's normal temporal order, which had been disrupted by time spent with the mother or daughter and by time spent talking about one or another of them, was reestablished. On wards where "final" leave-takings are frequent and anguished, the disruption of temporal work and sentimental orders is sometimes devastating.

MANAGING THE PATIENT'S TRAJECTORY

During his last weeks and days, the patient is much more likely than his family to be the center of the staff's attention, unless he is comatose, scarcely sentient, or so ill as hardly to be reacting as a person. Under these latter conditions, the staff's juggling of its tasks, around him and around its relationships with him, need only be minimal. Major problems, however, are set for the personnel when the patient's expected last days stretch out interminably on wards organized for faster turnover of patients, or when a patient's mode of dying is so extraordinarily unpleasant as to disturb staff members.

If the dying person is sentient but unaware of his impending death, then the staff's major problems may be associated with keeping him unaware, or at least keeping his suspicions sufficiently damped down so that his trajectory can be shaped as seems wise.[2] If his pain is so great that the staff can stand neither his physical anguish nor his obviously increasing awareness of his waning life, the patient can be "snowed" with drugs during his final days. We shall look now at only a few of the major problems faced by staff, or family, or the patient himself during his last days.

If the patient has become aware that he is dying, through direct or indirect preannouncement, or through his reading of staff's behavioral cues and his own symptoms, his awareness necessitates his coming to terms with dying. If by virtue of a slow trajectory he has had many months to face his mortality, he has probably entered or reentered the hospital better prepared than if his period of awareness has been short or sudden. If he is not elderly and has not already come to terms with advanced age (or even with death), a quick trajectory is likely to precipitate crises of awareness for the sentient patient, as well as for his family. Such crises affect the management of his trajectory.

Even in slow dying, the breakthrough of awareness during last days can be traumatic. The staff sometimes has little control over the structural conditions that determine the impact. For instance, a patient may know he has an extremely serious illness, but not regard it as fatal. The preannouncement suddenly is made to him, or a disclosure is made inadvertently. We observed, for example, the last days of a teenager who had learned of his imminent death from a friend who had learned it from a friend, whose parents in turn had received the information from the patient's parents. The blinding news, combined with a deep sense of his parents' betrayal, resulted, as staff members put it, in the boy's almost complete "withdrawal" and "apathy." Consequently, the staff could do almost nothing to shape his trajectory as they would have wished. Even the psychiatrist whom they called in could accomplish nothing.

During the hospitalization of another patient, however, the personnel were partly responsible for creating a structural condition that genuinely prevented their shaping of her trajectory. This woman, who was lingering in great pain, was far less afraid of death than of dying with uncontrollable pain. She had good reason for

[2]For fuller discussion, see *Awareness of Dying, Ibid.*

her fear, for she did not trust the nursing staff to control her pain, much less prevent its increase. The house physician in charge was desperate both because he could not control her growing pain and because he was in the crossfire from his patient, who respected him, and the nurses, who wished him to discipline her complaining. Finally, aware that she was dying, the patient allowed him to arrange an operation that might lessen her pain, although it was not likely to have any direct bearing on the course of her illness. She permitted the operation although she was intensely afraid that it would leave her "a vegetable." This woman's complaints about tardy and ineffective medication for her pain, her fear of dying in pain, her indecision over whether to permit the final operation (she died during surgery)—all conspired to rock the house staff, to cause considerable strain between nurses and the house physician, and to prevent the staff from shaping her trajectory.*

THE MEANING OF DEATH

On the other hand, a slow trajectory often gives the patient opportunities to come to terms with his own mortality, for his awareness and understanding may develop sufficiently early so that he can confront his dying. Such coming to terms involves two separate processes. The first consists of facing the annihilation of self, of visualizing a world without one's self. The second process consists of facing up to dying as a physical and perhaps mental, disintegration. Some people are fearful of dying in great pain, or with extreme bodily disfiguration or with loss of speech, or are perhaps afraid of "just lying there like a vegetable." Some people think hardly at all about these aspects of dying, but tremble at the prospect of the disappearance of self. Moreover, some patients who have come to terms with the idea of death may only later focus on dying, especially when, as the trajectory advances, they are surprised, dismayed, or otherwise affected by bodily changes. On the other hand, someone who lives with his dying long enough may become assured that he will "pass" peacefully enough, and only then fully face the death issue.

These two issues, which generally loom large during the last sentient days, are certainly not unrelated; nor does coming to terms with them always constitute a final settlement. Unexpected turns in the trajectory are likely to unsettle previous preparations. With unexpected bodily deterioration, patients panic or begin to lose recognition of themselves as known identities. In one instance of great insight, a patient told a nurse she feared "comfort" surgery would cause her to "die twice." It might help to relieve her pain for a period, but eventually she would have to face dying again.

*Anselm Strauss and Barney Glaser, Anguish: *A Case History of A Dying Patient* (San Francisco: The Sociological Press, 1970)

Most frequently, perhaps, patients come to terms by themselves or with the participation of close kin. Nurses, however, may be drawn into the processes. The patient typically initiates the "death talk"; the nurse tends to listen, to assent, to be sympathetic, to reassure. The nurse may even cry with a patient. Occasionally, a patient repeatedly invites nurses into conversations about death or dying, but they decline his invitations. Their refusals tend to initiate a drama of mutual pretense: neither party subsequently indicates recognition of the forthcoming death, although both know about it.

Other parties, too, sometimes play significant roles in these processes. In one such situation, an elderly patient was rescued from the isolation of mutual pretense by a hospital chaplain who directly participated in his coming to terms; eventually he also persuaded the wife, and to some extent the nurses, to enter into the continuing conversation. Patients sometimes rely on members of the clergy to move their spouses to faster acceptance of the inevitable and thus ease their own acceptance.

On the whole, American nurses seem to find it difficult to carry on conversation about death or dying with patients. Only if a patient has already come to terms with death, or if they can honestly assure him he will die "easily," if he is elderly, do they find it relatively easy to talk about such topics with him.[3] Unless a patient shows considerable composure about his dying, nurses and physicians lose their composure, except when they are specially trained or specially suited by temperament, or have some unusual empathy with a patient because of a similarity of personal history. When the patient's conversation during the last days is only obliquely about death and dying — consisting, for instance, of reminiscences of the past — and is not unpleasant or unduly repetitious, he has a better chance of inducing others, including the nurses, to participate in his closing of his life.

Clergymen are also expected, in most countries, to play major roles in this phasing-out of patients. A dying Greek patient who belonged to the Coptic faith completely upset the machinery of a Greek hospital by insisting late at night that he needed a Coptic priest immediately to give him his final communion. The request was almost impossible to fulfill at that hour, but the staff felt obliged to do so. A priest was found, but only just in time. In the United States, psychiatrists also sometimes perform analogous functions during the last phasing-out of more secularized patients.[4]

[3]Jeanne C. Quint, *The Nurse and the Dying Patient* (New York: Macmillan, 1967); "Mastectomy — Symbol of Cure or Warning Sign?", *GP*, XXIX (March, 1964), pp. 119-24; "The Impact of Mastectomy." *The American Journal of Nursing*, 63 (November, 1963), pp. 88-92.

[4]Personal communications from several psychiatrists.

An important aspect of a patient's coming to terms with impending death is the closing off of various aspects of everyday business. These include material and personal matters, like the drawing-up of wills and the making-up of quarrels. Physicians seem apt to allow businessmen to close off their business dealings, though a patient may have to insist on his right to do so, and to permit distraught families to urge reluctant patients to draw up, alter, or sign wills. A lawyer is sometimes brought in by the family or physician to help persuade the patient to make or alter his will. A chaplain or priest sometimes considers that his professional duties include bridging relationships between the dying person and an alienated spouse or offspring. One chaplain elatedly described how he had been instrumental in bringing a patient, her husband, her parents, and her children to face death together. This patient had gone ahead of her kinsmen in facing her death, and could no longer really talk with them. The chaplain bridged over the awkward relationships.

Sometimes the patient accepts his forthcoming death even before the staff has quite come to terms with it. Moreover, the patient's "social willing" may shock his family or the staff precisely because he has imaginatively reached his life's end before they have. One patient, for instance, relied on the intervention of his sister (who happened to be a nurse) to will his library to a neighboring college; his wife would never discuss the matter with him. A more extreme instance of social willing, which shocked personnel, was when a patient, during his last days, insisted on signing his own autopsy papers. This action struck the staff as singularly grotesque, despite the accepted similar practice of willing one's eyes, brain, or entire body to hospitals.

TEMPORAL INCONGRUITIES

Still another great barrier may block even the best-intentioned nurses and physicians from providing adequate help to a patient when he faces his demise: the immense difference between the staff's and the patient's conceptions of time. As we have noted repeatedly, the staff operates on "work time." Their tasks are guided by schedules, which on most wards are related to many patients, both dying and recovering. More important, and more subtle, work time with a given dying patient is a matter of timing work according to his expected trajectory. He is supposed to die more or less "on time," even when that time is uncertain. Our data, as well as accounts by dying patients or by kin who have participated intimately in relatives' dying, suggest that a patient's personal sense of time, undergoes striking changes once he becomes aware of his impending death. This occurs whether he becomes aware very early or very late.

The last days become structured in highly personalized temporal terms. The future is foreshortened, cut out, or abstracted to "after I am gone." The personal past is likely to be reviewed and reconceptualized. The present takes on various kinds of personal meanings. Author Bernice Kavinovsky noted, for example: "All week, although I teach my classes, arrange for a substitute, put the dinner on, telephone my son at his apartment, shower, mark manuscripts, I perform each act almost clinically aware of the obstruction in my breast." She was "at the same time assailed on every hand by beauty's endless argument — an arc of light, or the curve of my husband's cheek . . . or the noise of the children's games on the roof next door" — the sights and sounds of the world taking on sudden and astonishing beauty.[5] Various semi-mystical experiences may be associated with the new temporal references. Things previously taken for granted are now savored as unique but unfortunately transitory. Occasional reprieves, recognized as only reprieves, evoke temporally significant reactions running from, "Oh, God! take me, I was prepared and now will not be prepared" to gratefulness for unexpected time.

The important point is not so much the variability of temporal reconstructions as the difficulty, and sometimes complete inability, of outsiders to grasp these personal reconstructions. One cannot know about them unless privy to the dying person's thoughts. He may keep them to himself, especially in a context of mutual pretense. He may not be able to express them clearly, especially when he becomes less sentient. A busy staff may have little time to listen or to invite revealing talk, particularly if patients are competing for attention. In many American hospitals nursing aides spend more time in patients' rooms than the nurses do, even during last days. When aides manage to grasp a patient's temporal reordering of his life, they may be unable to pass along this knowledge to the nurses, or not feel free to do so, or assume that the information is unimportant.

When the patient's personal time and the staff's work time are highly disparate, considerable strain may be engendered. Nor is the source of the trouble necessarily evident to either. Sometimes, of course, the staff does sense something of a patient's reconceptualizations, without necessarily realizing their deep import, and may somewhat adjust its own work time to his requirements. Thus on a medical ward housing many cancer patients, which we studied, there was a ward ideology of "letting them set the pace," with work time considerably structured around the patient's relatively slow tempo.

5 *Voyage and Return: An Experience with Cancer* (New York: W. W. Norton, 1966), p. 20.

Within limits, cancer patients could negotiate, for instance, to eat or have their temperatures taken later than when ordinarily scheduled.

ISOLATION

A staff's failure to understand a patient's attempts at achieving psychological closure in his life contributes to another process: the patient's increasing isolation, whether or not he perceives it. He may, of course, understand very well that staff members are not interested in his awesome problem, or cannot grasp its nature even if they wish to. If he has tried to communicate with the staff, he may despair of their understanding. Or he may prefer to communicate with his family or his minister, although he may actually be unable to "reach" them either.[6]

However, it is not only the communications problem that produces isolation. In all the countries where we have observed, we found strong tendencies to start isolating a dying patient during his last days in the hospital. Isolation techniques — perhaps "insulation" is a better term — have their source in various structural conditions. For instance, if everyone agrees that a patient should be kept unaware, then attempts to buffer him from knowledge immediately set in motion a train of insulating mechanisms.[7] The isolating process is also called into play if the patient is aware but accepts or invites mutual pretense about his dying. The isolating mechanisms are blunted, however, if the patient is openly aware; even then, staff may begin to avoid death talk or even the patient's room.

The patient who will not accept his dying or is dying in a socially unacceptable way also arouses avoidance — sometimes by his family as well as the staff. One of the clearest examples of this that we saw was an ICU nurse's brusque handling of a quite sentient patient who looked only a few hours away from death. The nurse described him as "ornery"; in brief, he was "asking for it." Personnel on the medical ward from which this dying man had been transferred had also regarded him as difficult and unreasonable.

During a patient's last days, the staff lightens its work and increases the probability of giving good comfort care by moving him closer to the nursing station. Of course, he may be grateful for the added security of being near the staff, but the move may frighten him despite the nurses' explanations. And in large wards, the move

6Cf. Jeanne Quint, *op. cit.,* "The Impact. . . ."
7See *Awareness of Dying, op. cit.*

267

not only tells the aware patient that he is nearing his end, but it also may isolate him from satisfying friendships he has made with other patients. Because of unpleasant odors or perhaps uncontrollable groans and sobbing, he may even be moved into a separate room, or may be shielded from the ward by a temporary screen. This is sometimes done even before the last hours, especially if he is judged disturbing to other patients. In hospitals where patients are housed in smaller rooms, the staff tends during the last days to put the dying patient either into a single room or with a comatose patient. If the roommate is not comatose, he may complain about the dying patient's behavior, and this stimulates the staff to move one or the other. Of course, when patients are moved to an intensive care unit, they are quite isolated from people other than the staff, including their families.

All these conditions contribute, without any necessary deliberation by the staff, to the isolation of dying patients. Although a patient may welcome being alone, or alone with kinsmen, he may fight against his insulation. He may plead successfully to be left with friends and acquaintances, and the staff will wait until he is no longer sentient before moving him. A patient who is already in a single room may devise tactics to get personnel into his room and to increase the time they spend with him, by making urgent demands and complaints or by managing to charm the personnel.

The limits of demand tactics are suggested by what happened to a woman who, like Coleridge's Ancient Mariner, customarily fixed her listeners by the repeated tale of her life. This tactic drove them to countertactics or nonresponse while they busily took care of her creature comforts. A patient can also gain more attention from the personnel if he can charm them. The better they like him, the more contact they are likely to give him anyway, unless his dying distresses them so much that they cannot bear to be around him. As we noted in discussing slow trajectories, a staff member may pull away from a patient not just to minimize contact with him, but to minimize her own emotions and reactions to his story. By avoiding him, she is attempting to lessen the chances of his biography having a lasting impact on her own. On the whole, then, under the kinds of structural conditions noted above it is much easier for patients to gain relative privacy from staff intrusions than to get attention. To the extent that patients fail in either aim, they lose the contest over the shaping of their own trajectories.

We have touched earlier on the staff's occasional efforts to cut down on family visits and banish certain kinsmen from the bedside, as well their attempts to pressure close kin to visit more often. The patient himself may also need to develop tactics to engage or put off his visitors, or to ally his family against the staff or the staff against his family. He complains to family members about his isolation, and gets them to intervene by requesting that they talk with the nurses or protest directly to the responsible physician. With or without prodding, families may attempt to "bribe" the personnel, sometimes successfully, so that their relatives are left less isolated. Or the patient may wish less or more attention from concerned visitors, and accomplishes his aim through negotiation with nurses or physician.

Licensed Behavior

Another phenomenon characteristic of the last weeks and days is the license granted patients to engage in otherwise forbidden activities. To the patient previously unaware of oncoming death, this license may help disclose his dying. To the patient already aware, the license may reveal how close his final hours are. However, it may not: for instance, a teenager was allowed to play with a boyfriend on her bed quite out of sympathy for her, but she did not perceive this as license given because she was so near her death. License consists of granting to a patient, sometimes without his requesting it, the opportunity to engage in activities such as eating what he wishes, leaving the hospital to go "for a drive," or going home for the weekend. A nursing student or nursing personnel new to the ward may not recognize that the staff has given up hope for the patient, and may be scandalized at what the patient is allowed to do; the newcomer does not recognize the activity as one "licensed" by certain death. Ulterior motives may be involved in the staff's granting of licensed behavior. By pleasing the patient, they lessen his complaints and make him more tractable and cooperative. Certainly, however, this is not the chief or only motive for granting special dispensations.

As we have noted, a patient sometimes accepts his demise more readily than does the staff. He may press for privileges that the staff is reluctant to grant. The nurses may even warn him that he will hasten his death, but he may not care; he may have devised his own calculus based on a different weighing of values, such as worthwhile living time versus worthless living time. A similar outlook lies behind some patients' refusal to be hospitalized until their final hours, preferring to "live it up" rather than become invalids. Sometimes they hope to die while enjoying themselves, or to die "with their boots on" while working. The patient who knows how to negotiate with the staff, or has various structural conditions working in his favor, can gain more license. Sometimes, however, he may need to obtain it by surreptitious means.

Earlier, we touched on the kinsmen's emotionally charged farewells. The patient also may make his farewells. These may not coincide with the leave-taking of his kin; they may not even be visible to his kinsmen. On the other hand, the leave-taking can be mutual and open. Sometimes it is highly ceremonious, as when a European-born American bade his family farewell with a loving, formal speech. He sent them home, said goodbye to his nurses, and died shortly thereafter.

Leave-taking can be terrible for both patient and family, also affecting the interaction between staff and patient. Farewells are especially harrowing when the patient has a while to live but he and his close kin realize how unlikely they are to meet again. Similarly, when the visitors make frequent but not necessarily final farewells, the strain can be quite as great on the patient as on them.

Staff members, too, may suffer both from a patient's poignant farewell, and from their own potential or repeated farewells, whether visible to him or not. A nurse who is much attached to a patient may go off on her weekend or annual vacation uncertain whether the patient will still be in his bed when she returns. While she may prefer *not* to be on duty when he dies, her silent farewell may effectively ruin her time away from the ward. On the other hand, if she dreads his dying when she is away, the leave-taking may be equally difficult for her. Private physicians have also indicated the impact of farewells from patients of whom they are fond.

As we have already pointed out in discussing families, repeated leave-takings can visibly affect the staff's work and collective mood. The effects occur even when a patient has evidenced excellent preparation for his death. The impact is particularly evident when his dying is seen as a considerable social loss. Sometimes when such a patient goes home to die, staff goodbyes are open and poignant.

DECISIVE JUNCTURES

Finally, there are two major critical junctures in the dying trajectory which have immense potential for disturbing either the patient or the work and sentimental orders of a ward. The first occurs when someone decides to prolong the patient's life although others believe he should be allowed to die quickly; the second juncture occurs when someone decides to hasten a patient's death although others believe this intervention should not be made. These decisions sometimes involve the patient's participation — especially the decision to prolong his life, as, for instance, in the choice of an operation that *may* prolong life at the cost of reduced mobility.

The patient's role in the decision not to prolong his dying, or perhaps even to hasten it, is not limited to negotiating with the physician. Patients directly shorten their own lives by various actions — by not eating, or by fatally exposing themselves to cold air at open windows, or, more overtly still, by suicide. Patients who are being kept alive through intravenous feeding or machinery are less likely near the end to kill themselves by pulling out the tubes or by asking that the machinery be turned off; but we have known a successful instance of each of these actions. As we have seen earlier, when patients choose suicide, staff members may be neither unsympathetic nor greatly shocked, providing they can discern an adequate rationale. Unrelenting pain or other physical suffering may seem a sufficient reason for taking one's own life. What would have been upsetting or shocking earlier in the trajectory now is more likely to be condoned. However, the more passive methods by which a patient hastens death are often especially distressing to nursing personnel, for they are cheated of a principal satisfaction in care during the final days: keeping the patient alive and in reasonable comfort and receiving his gratitude for their efforts. Instead the patient is essentially saying — sometimes loudly and clearly — "Go away, there's nothing more you can do for me, let me die."

During most patients' last days, decisions to prolong or shorten life usually are made by the close kin or by physicians, rather than by the patients themselves. Physicians know what patients and families often do not: life can be extended or shortened for at least a few hours or days, and sometimes longer, by various medical tactics. (The ordinary comfort care given by nursing personnel also can extend life, and decisions to reduce that care can reduce the length of a patient's life. By and large, however, nurses and physicians do not seem to think of comfort care alone as requiring deliberate decisions about prolonging or shortening life.)

Several factors bear upon the physician's decision. The nature of the illness is one determinant. During the last days of certain dying patients — for instance, geriatric cases — physicians customarily make no great attempts to stretch out the dying. In general hospitals, however, physicians are more likely to keep life going as long as they judge it sensible to do so; institutional pressures constantly remind them that this is their professional task. Indeed, if a patient unsuccessfully attempts to end his life, physicians are very likely to take drastic steps to prevent renewed attempts. In one instance, at a VA hospital, an elderly patient cut his own throat; a nurse and physician rushed to his rescue, and saved him before they realized that perhaps the rescue made little sense. "Why did we do it?" they asked each other afterward. Another physician remembers a lesson taught him years ago by a patient who literally almost starved him-

271

self to death before the physician saved him by forced intravenous feeding. Later the physician was brought up short by the patient's severe questions, asking whether the doctor realized how much will power was involved in deliberate starvation, and did he suppose there was no reason for it?

Like everything else pertaining to slow dying, the decision to prolong or shorten life may need to be made more than once. If kin intervene and beg the physician not to "go all out" for a patient already comatose, or if they are anguished and the physician himself considers a few more days or hours of life senseless, he may take steps not to prolong life. He may cut down on life-prolonging procedures or drugs, may stop blood transfusions, and may even order that some piece of necessary equipment be stopped. Nor is it unknown for a doctor to pass onto a nurse the decision whether or not to prolong life, by signaling that she should or may withhold (or give a bit too much) medication when it seems appropriate.

Nurses in all countries seem to be caught in a structural bind over prolonging or hastening the dying process. By and large, they tend to resist prolongation. They do not always agree with the physician that a patient's life should be prolonged. "What is the sense of it?" they ask among themselves, sometimes even asking the responsible physicians. In American hospitals, nurses frequently show their disagreement openly and may exert direct pressure on physicians. When they do not attempt to influence doctor's decisions, they may harbor disturbing doubts about the paradoxical power of modern medicine, which can not only sensibly extend life but can also extend it to no good end. We quote from one nurse on a urology ward who unconsciously summed up the dilemma:

> If a patient wants to live, then keep giving IV's. This eases it for him and the relative because you are *doing* something. But if he's incurable, why keep him alive? Just ease him out. The difficult stage is not at the very end, anyway. It's before. The period when the patient keeps wanting you to do something more than you're doing. At the end most are unconscious. When they are conscious — saying "save me!" — it's harder — you have to be a stoic not to feel some emotion. It's just as hard when you have one beg you to "let me go!"

She ended her remarks: "I've no answer really."

The probability of nurses' disagreements with physicians increases when a patient consents to becoming a research patient. The physician then is much more open to accusations that he is keeping the patient alive only because of his own research interests. Another condition encouraging disagreements (presumably a rare one, but all the more interesting by contrast) is evident in a situation we encountered in which a nurse, newly graduated from school and also new to the particular ward, found that one of her patients had begun to die. She rushed out and found the resident, but he refused to prolong the patient's life. She was indignant, not knowing the reasoning that lay behind his decision. She believed him simply callous. She did not take into account her own inexperience.

Family members sometimes have a major share in shaping this last phase of the patient's trajectory. Occasionally there may be a conflict between the physician and the family over the family's desire to shorten the ordeal. Thus, one physician brusquely denied the pleas of a mother whose child lay dying inside an oxygen tent. He vowed it was his job to keep patients alive as long as possible. If the patient is dying at home, the family may rush him to the hospital in order to give him a few more weeks or days of life. They may ask the doctor to bring in a consultant, or shop around for another doctor, though usually he cannot prolong the patient's life. In foreign hospitals where family members help with the patient's care, they may help prolong his life through their attentive providing of comfort care. In hospitals in all countries, as we remarked earlier, kin often request the doctor not to prolong the dying. But the doctor in turn may force on them a direct decision as to whether to shorten or prolong life. Rather than precipitate a direct confrontation with the moral decision, the physician may gently ask whether there is "any more we should do," and the relative, sadly or gratefully, or with some other emotion, probably signals "no." Perhaps most often, close relatives either leave the decision up to the doctor, or are unaware that he and the hospital staff explicitly exercise control over shortening or lengthening life.

Which patients, then, are likely to have their lives shortened or prolonged during the last days? We have touched upon most of the structural conditions relevant to that question. The nature of the trajectory, the mode of dying, and the patient's awareness are key variables. Other things being equal, a patient of high social value is likely to elicit staff activity designed to keep him alive longer. The adequacy of hospital and ward equipment has a bearing. Knowledge about this can enhance the patient's or family's power to prolong his life.

The essential issue in these last days is: Who shall have what kinds and degrees of influence in shaping the end of the patient's trajectory? That issue involves not merely how the patient shall die, but also how he shall live while dying. A dying person can hold almost complete control over how he lives his last days by

273

not entering a hospital, or can regain it by leaving the hospital. Lael Wertenbaker's vivid account of her husband's decision to die at home shows how he firmly rejected his doctor's offer of a comfort-giving and life-prolonging operation because of his continued determination to live while dying; as his trajectory departed from his expectations of it, it eventually required rethinking.[a] What is true of patients also is true of doctors, nurses, and families: their decisions also may need to be modified or even reversed during later phases of the trajectory, especially during last days. Insofar as the trajectory takes new directions, new tactics are needed by the agents who try to shape its next phases. However expected may be the physical aspects of a trajectory, the predictions of its psychological aspects — for staff and family as well as for the patient — tend to be less accurate.

Above all, to shape the trajectory during the last days requires juggling tasks, people, and relationships. The legerdemain also requires juggling time: time for tasks, time for people, time for talk. Most subtle of all, the staff is juggling the time still allowed by "fate," since control over aspects of the trajectory may be manageable only for a short time, but not forever. These various contingencies are immensely unstable: the patient can be kept unaware just so long; and his family can be kept under control just so long; his family can stand the strain of waiting or of continual farewells just so long; staff can stand for just so long a patient acting unacceptably in the face of death. During the last days, every major person in the dying drama operates within a total context of multiple contingencies. Maintenance of a measure of stability in the ward's temporal order depends on skillful juggling within that context.

[a]*Death of a Man* (N. Y.: Random House, 1957)

THE ROTATIONAL SYSTEM: ITS IMPACT UPON TEACHING, LEARNING, AND THE MEDICAL SERVICE*

Every educational institution must find means for introducing its students to a wide variety of subject matters and skills. Logically, and of course in fact, it is possible to vary greatly the number and kinds of teachers, the sites where learning takes place, and the ordering of subject matters. In the lower grades of our public schools, the pupils are taught by one teacher and, more or less, within one classroom.

American medical education has been committed to what may seem, at first glance, a very different and quite unique kind of procedure. Because of the multitude of medical specialties and the great differences which they demand in skill, training, and perspective, but also quite definitely because in medical education a clinical training is deemed absolutely necessary, classroom instruction is supplemented and indeed superceded in importance by actual experience on the wards. Hence in medical schools, all the students whether graduate or undergraduate rotate around the hospital, working and learning while they practice the arts of medicine.

Like those procedures of other educational institutions that are designed to widen the scope of the student's vision, and his knowledge and skill, the medical rotational system is based upon the assumption that the more varied the learning situations, the more numerous the teachers, then the better education will be achieved. Despite the difficulties inherent in running a hospital with a continually shifting junior personnel (the housestaff), probably few professors of medicine would seriously consider changing this striking feature of medical education.

*Unpublished Memo, 1958, Written for the Research Staff of
BOYS IN WHITE
(Howard S. Becker, et al.)

At KU there are three rotational cycles — respectively the internes,' the residents,' and the students.' These differ in scope, speed, sequence, and other ways. (The students' rotation is discussed in BOYS IN WHITE.) The internes have, when they first enter the hospital, a choice of services upon which they may elect to work. They must select three or four, and among these may be included the medical specialty which they plan to practice later. Allocation of the internes to these services follows no particular sequential order: if possible the men travel around in the order of their choice, but it is not always possible to arrange this. On some services the interne will find himself working with one resident, but sometimes with two or more; and when a service for some reason is understaffed, he may even be put in charge of a ward. Rarely, if ever, does he work directly with another interne. There is one service — the emergency room — which each interne must administer (although there are occasional exceptions to this rule). It can, in summary, be said that each interne during his year travels widely — if rapidly — about the hospital; so that he gets to know a good deal about the total hospital, albeit his knowledge of its workings necessarily cannot be profound.

The rotation of the resident is quite different. Because he is at the hospital to study a specialty, he circulates almost wholly within his department of specialization. That is, he is attached to a department like obstetrics, medicine, general surgery, or even to a narrower domain like urology or orthopedics. His rotation about the department usually takes him to other hospitals associated with KU — sometimes as far distant as to another state. His training is more graded than the interne's, for as he moves up in seniority he takes on more advanced or difficult tasks and tends to be excused from less advanced ones. In some departments, he takes on added administrative responsibility, but he may also be absented from administrative work for periods of time, while he does research or studies special skills. His contacts with other medical departments and their residents are minimal (reflecting the relative autonomy of the departments at KU). Of course he may know a number of residents from other departments, either because they live near him, or because he has had contact with them during the course of his administrative duties: the most frequent cause for such contact, probably, is that the men are called in as consultants by another department. On the whole, the resident's rotation about his department is somewhat slower than the interne's around the hospital, and of course it is much more confined in locale within the hospital.

These basic facts about the house staff's movements are easily ascertainable, and the field worker picked them up during his first days at the hospital. Then, as he followed the housestaff closely around the wards, he gradually became aware of the complicated, and unsuspected, workings of the rotational system. At first he recognized only that the residents and internes, like the students themselves, gravitated throughout the hospital; but the very reasonableness of this educational procedure was so convincing that he merely took its workings for granted. Besides, at first, the field worker was too preoccupied with feeling his way and with the matters that more obviously touched upon the concerns of the housestaff. But as he stumbled across certain curious events, the rotational system per se intruded itself upon his consciousness. What he saw as he moved from station to station were various combinations of personnel working together. But once these medical teams are conceived not only as impermanent but — in some sense — accidental in composition, then the grand march of junior physicians around the hospital can be seen as an immensely important characteristic of any teaching hospital.

THE LOGIC OF ROTATIONAL SITUATIONS

Rotation throws residents and internes (and students) together in ever-varied combinations. This variability will quickly be comprehended if it be imagined that each of these three rotational cycles are intersectable by the other two at numerous points of contact. For instance, a given interne will work during his year at KU with at least four residents, and under each resident his conditions of work may be dissimilar. The resident may be relaxed, he may be tense; the service may be tightly controlled by the senior staff man or it may not; the resident may delegate much responsibility to the interne, or he may not; the interne may be passionately interested in the service, or bored by it; he may on occasion too, know more about the service and its medical affairs than his resident. Such conditions contribute toward making the life of the housestaff on any particular service what it is: harassed, tense, "spastic", relaxed, enjoyable, satisfying, or what not. These conditions are not entirely idiosyncratic: some recur. If a full scale study of the rotational system were to be designed, it would be necessary to specify all such relevant conditions that throw personnel together in varied combinations, and then the consequences of this process would need to be traced. Our data fall far short of this ideal. However, much can be done with them to show the workings of rotation, and to some degree the conclusions drawn can even be woven together in systematic fashion.

To begin with, we need to visualize certain combinations of hospital conditions as logically possible outcomes — even if we should never come across them. Others, we shall recognize immediately as existing beyond any doubt. A few diagrams will serve to suggest some of these many possibilities.

(1) *One set of possibilities has to do with the skill and knowledge of the housestaff.* Assuming, for simplicity's sake, that there is only one resident and his interne on any given service, we can infer various possibilities. For instance, both can — by the faculty's standards — be "good" or competent workers (see diagram #1). (The resident of course is officially the superior, and his knowledge and skill are supposed to be greater than the interne's.)

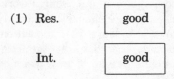

(1) Res.　good

Int.　good

Diagram #2 suggests a difficult situation for the faculty man: each of his housestaff is incompetent.*

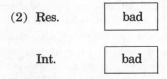

(2) Res.　bad

Int.　bad

Diagram #3 suggests a difficult situation for the resident (his interne is incompetent); or if an interne is quite uninterested in the service his resident may be led to think of him as lazy or incompetent. Diagram #4 suggests a situation that runs against the grain of authority, for the interne is better than the resident.

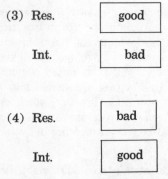

(3) Res.　good

Int.　bad

(4) Res.　bad

Int.　good

*In order to keep these diagrams simple, we are using only dichotomies, such as "good and bad".

Diagram #5 is a variant of the preceding three, assuming only that foreign residents are not very competent — although they often are by American medical standards. (If this seems a drastic assumption, yet one ought to allow the fiction: for our data will soon illustrate what happens when indeed they are incompetent; but if they are, competent, then we need only apply one of the preceding diagrams.)

(5) Res.

foreign	Amer.	foreign
foreign	foreign	Amer.

Int.

(2) *The next set of diagrams has to do with services that are understaffed or overstaffed with personnel.* The resident can be without an assisting interne (diagram #6).

(6) Res.

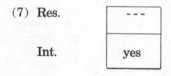

Int.

yes
- - -

The interne can be given charge of a service in the event of a shortage of residents (diagram #7).

(7) Res.

- - -
yes

Int.

Diagram #8 merely makes understaffing more complicated: the students — who often do necessary minor tasks — are absent, so that the housestaff cannot draw upon them for their labor. (We could make this yet more complicated by diagramming whether or not the students' work is important for the service.)

(8) Res.

yes	yes	- - -
yes	- - -	yes
- - -	- - -	- - -

Int.

Students

But a service can also be overstaffed. Diagrams #9 and #10 suggest what sometimes happens on certain services. (Overstaffing and understaffing are not a matter of numbers, but also of peakloads of patients and "slow periods." We shall not burden the diagrams with this complication.)

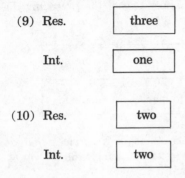

| (9) Res. | three |
| Int. | one |

| (10) Res. | two |
| Int. | two |

(3) *The next set of diagrams has to do with the degree of control exerted by the reigning faculty member.* Diagram #11 and diagram #12 chart tight and loose control as they combine with some of the variables pictured in preceding diagrams. We can begin to infer here the range of differences that this control may make in the life of the housestaff.

HIGH CONTROL

(11) Res.	yes	good	bad	good
Int.	- - -	bad	bad	good

LOW CONTROL

(12) Res.	yes	good	bad	good
Int.	- - -	bad	bad	good

(4) *The next set of diagrams pertains to which of the personnel arrives first upon the scene:* for they may be assigned together (diagram 13), or the resident may precede the interne on the service (diagram 14), or vice versa (diagram 15).

	ARRIVES FIRST	ARRIVES SECOND	ARRIVE TOGETHER
(13)	—————	—————	X
(14)	Resident	Interne	—————
(15)	Interne	Resident	—————

But a resident who precedes an interne on the service may be succeeded by another resident before this interne is reassigned; hence the interne spans the life of two residents (diagram 14a). This situation, of course, can also occur in reverse (diagram 15a).

(14a)

(15a)

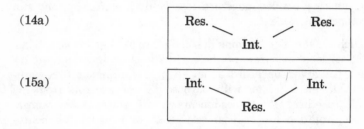

The same sets of diagrams could be paralleled if we aligned a resident and groups of students.

(5) *The final set of diagrams has to do with sequences of rotation:* the resident or interne may go from one that is generally considered difficult to one that is easy; or vice versa (his synonyms are "spastic" and "relaxed"). Diagram #16 pictures this situation:

(16) FROM   TO

	Easy	Mod. Diff.	Diff.
Easy			
Moderately difficult			
Difficult			

All the above diagrams portray only the simplest possible combinations that result from rotation (with the exception of diagrams #11 and 12 which dealt with the faculty physician's control of the service). Visualize now any diagram from one set simultaneously with any diagram from the remaining five sets. Thus (diagram #17) which involves a "good" interne:

	Easy Serv.	Mod. Diff.	Difficult
Easy Service			
Mod. Difficult Service			
Difficult Service	X		

FROM TIGHT CONTROL   TO LOOSE CONTROL
      BAD RESIDENT   GOOD RESIDENT

Here the competent interne goes from a difficult service governed closely by a faculty man who closely watches his incompetent resident; to an easy service, governed loosely by a staff man, and run by a competent resident.

So much for the diagramming of some of many possible situations. Now let us look at a few of these situations as the field worker (Strauss) observed or heard about them, recording at first without clear design but later with purpose. These excerpts from his notebook, together with his commentary, will suggest some consequences of rotation for medical service as well as for the housestaff's teaching and learning in this hospital.

ROTATIONAL SITUATIONS AND THEIR CONSEQUENCES

FOREIGN RESIDENT AND AMERICAN INTERNE

What happens when a foreign resident with slight command of English is put in charge of a ward? Ordinarily, the resident's duties require that he elicit information from patients, reassure their relatives and communicate decisions to them; also that he instruct his nurses, teach his students; also under normal circumstances share with his interne certain observations and experiences, as well as delegate to the interne the major administrative and medical decisions for the ward. A foreign physician thrust into this complex administrative role is handicapped by the language barrier, and possibly also by his "different kind of" medical training — to use an euphemism often employed around the hospital when referring to the foreign members of the housestaff.

One day the field worker fell to talking with an interne:

Gusfield said that he has been on his first service as an interne with Dr. Saki, the Japanese resident. Dr. Saki had suffered because he was inexperienced in clinical medicine. (Gusfield had said also that the foreign residents are not very good.) I pressed him, and he said that what he was saying was that the internes do the work then.

He admitted he had read orders, and talked to the relatives, but that he did not actually have to dictate the orders for Saki went along with almost anything he suggested. Gusfield said it took a certain amount of tact to handle this situation. I said this meant probably there had been a lot of talking in an indirect manner with indirect suggestions to Saki. He said, "and not so openly." I said, "that means you used the conference room and talked away from the open stations." He said, "yes, thank God for that conference room." I asked whether the staff knew about this situation and he said they did. I also asked if he had done any teaching at that time of students, but he did not. He also said pretty bluntly that although two or three sessions were scheduled with the students, he was quite sure Saki did not teach that often. I asked whether the students tended to ask him a lot of questions in the halls during the day. He said they certainly did.

In short, the resident abdicates his command to the interne, (whom the staff generally rated as fair or satisfactory). Formal teaching falls to a minimum, and the interne takes over among his duties a certain amount of informal instruction — if he feels like doing this, and if the students press him to do so. But there is a certain embarrassment attending this reversal of medical hierarchy — even though everyone expects perhaps the patients are aware of the open secret; hence the quasi-private conferences between interne and resident. The interne, as one might expect, is tolerant of the failings of the resident; after all, this own upgrading enables him to learn more than if he were doing his regular tasks. From the relatively sparse information given us in the field worker's notes, we can only speculate about other possible consequences: probably, for instance, the resident learned much from his interne, and in addition had ample opportunity to study his books. Probably, too, the senior staff kept an especially watchful surveillance upon this ward.

A Foreign Resident At The Out-Patient Clinic

The out-patient medicine clinic at KU is manned by one resident and a group of fourth year students. The latter are supposed, when working on this clinic, to be gaining independence of judgment, for they are already virtually graduates of the medical school. Hence there is a general agreement among the staff and house staff that the students be given genuine responsibility. During the morning, each sees his quota of patients — who come in great numbers and therefore cannot be given extensive examinations. After a relatively brief session with the patient, the student is supposed to confer with either the resident or with one of several "outside men" who have volunteered their services to the clinic. The student reports his findings, suggests the treatment, the physician hears him out, may question him, and when agreement is reached on therapy, signs the prescription. He may also go to see the patient with or without an explicit request from the student. The field worker spent one morning at this clinic watching, and talking with, an Egyptian resident. Two weeks previously he had followed a competent American resident around the same terrain. When excerpts from his field notes on these two men are juxtaposed, certain implications for the teaching of students become very clear.

(April 12th). I spent from 7:30 to 12 in the clinic. The resident is Pharoh, an Egyptian, who has been on about ten days. Nobody was there when I first arrived. At about 8:05 two boys came and picked up charts from the main desk nearby. One said, "I guess I'll take this one." The other took another. One began to put a check on the listings of patients they are assigned and are supposed to have seen; but the second student corrected the listing, making a line down the side of yesterday's listing, and added a new check for today. Then they both made marks opposite their names, but the one student did not erase the credit that he gave himself for supposedly taking an extra patient yesterday. I asked when the resident comes and was told, "Well, he usually is late." He said this as if: what can you expect?

When the resident came at about 8:30, I began to question him. He brought over some charts from the main desk, began to put them in the box, and checked some assignments on the list. I asked him about the students. He said they were very good. I felt he meant it. They were fourth year and soon would be out, and you could trust them. He spent the first 15 minutes going back three or four times getting the charts, and putting them in students' boxes as he assigned them, the students getting them and going off to their patients. There was no interchange between resident and students, no joking, and scarcely a question. Later, I asked one of the students where Pharoh was and he pointed out that he did not see much of him, and that they worked mostly with the outside physicians.

Later also, I went with a student and the resident to see a patient. The resident interviewed her very briefly and it was amusing because she was a colored patient with a bad sense of grammar and a marvelous southern accent, which

284

was matched by the Egyptian's accent and grammar. On the whole they got through to each other except for a couple of times when the student helped out. We went outside and held a conference, which ended with the resident asking the student what he wanted to do. After the student said various things, he agreed and made a couple of strong suggestions himself. During the next two examinations which followed the same brief pattern, I noticed that the resident hardly looked at the patient's charts.

When Pharoh and I went back to the station, we continued our conversation. Meanwhile there were about three students nearby, and I think only one or two outside doctors. We were left undisturbed by the students (although they were eager to make reports).

(March 26). I got to the clinic at 9:00 and introduced myself to Weber, the resident. Before I introduced myself I watched him with a student, he was asking him questions about a case, holding the history in his hand. The resident was busily stuffing charts into the students' boxes, but cheerfully answering.

Right behind him in a small room, students were coming and going. Weber went in to listen to a student who gave a patient's history, and then he asked him a few direct questions and they both smiled over some discussion about a prescription. I asked him why, after the student left, and he said "you get further by joshing. These students are really very intelligent. You can't push them around, if you do they will make it hard for you and you won't get anywhere with them. The main thing is that on a clinic like this they get sloppy and you have to remind them, keep them in trim. With all the turnover of patients, they get sloppy — anyone would. It's a human tendency."

When we went in with students to see patients, he also examined them, using a kindly general practitioner manner. He used verbal forms to the students like: "what she needs is —" and "I think she should have —." The students also thought, in one instance, that she needed a picture of the chest, and he said "I agree with you —." Then, to my surprise, they said to each other, the resident first, "thank you." With another patient, on the way out he noticed her fingers and showed them to the student, saying to the patient, "That's what a feller gets as he grows older. It's not a crippling kind, the best thing for it is aspirin."

285

Also he found what he thought was a venus murmur, and used it to teach the students about this. They had found it, but he discovered it was very local, and it increased as she moved from a flat back position to her left thigh. The students had to go through all these motions to hear it. Then the resident said to me that it was a good lesson for them. Outside, one student asked him a question about her and he answered. Afterward, every once in a while I noticed his getting a few more charts, once he talked to a Negro woman who had not enough money to get some lab tests done and he wrote a prescription for her himself.

If we utilize the second set of field notes to highlight what happens when the foreign resident is in charge, we can observe certain striking consequences. Because the resident arrives late, the students can more easily cheat on their work loads; but they are also thrown more on their own resources. They must use the outside physicians more, which in turn means partly that the entire service is slowed down and partly that the students grow more impatient over the slow speed of the supervision. Hence they cut corners when examining, and have less time to get information out of their interchanges with their supervisors. Between the foreign resident and the students, communication is held to a minimum: its contest is mainly supervisory. The students neither press him for information nor does he go out of his way to teach them anything. The American resident has drawn the boundaries of his job far more widely, with consequent effects for the administration of medical service and for teaching of students. To redress the balance of this judgment, it can perhaps be said that when the foreigner is in charge the students experience more independence and undoubtedly gain certain satisfaction from that unwonted responsibility. We may assume, in light of the observations by the other field workers, that when working under the foreign resident the students may more easily extend this license to signing his name on the patient's prescription.

A Mediocre Resident and a Competent Interne

Let us see now what transpires when a mediocre American resident takes charge of a medical ward with the assistance of a competent interne. Schmeil, the resident, had been preceded on this service by an interne, who described him as staying well in the background for five or six days until he learned the ropes.

The interne said the situation had ended up with about 55% to 45% sharing; that is, the resident ended up with 55% of the responsibility. I asked what would have happened if Lincoln, one of the best residents, or somebody like him had come in instead. "Oh, he would have asked questions for fifteen minutes and then it would have been 60% to 40% sharing!" The interne laughed loudly at this.

The field worker had observed Schmeil some weeks before and concluded he was not overly competent, either in medical and administrative affairs or in his teaching. This tentative judgment was sustained by the resident's superior, who characterized him as "immature."

I said Schmeil struck me either as easy going or having a pose . . . that I suspected the latter. He burst out, "and carrying, I would bet, an ulcerous condition about to break out." Schmeil had surprised him by taking more responsibility than he had thought he would, but there have been mutters about him in the last service. "I don't like to see first year residents put on this service. That's the trouble with the rotating system." But you can't tell him "you're not mature." He added that another resident, although first year, could be trusted because he was mature.

Meanwhile, a very able interne had been brought to the service by the exigencies of rotation. Almost two months later, the field worker held another conversation with the same faculty member whose service this was.

That interne, Klapp, is a brilliant boy. He has worked very well, he has taken responsibility. That was one of the troubles. Schmeil resented Klapp. (I gathered this came to a head near the end of Schmeil's stay on this service.) And so we got even more passive resistance. He resented Klapp's making what amounted to policy decisions. He thought he should have come to him and then he would make them himself.

I said this was a nice dilemma for him himself, because obviously this interne knew as much or more than the resident and that the hierarchy got in the way. "Yes that was it." I asked how he handled it when they had an interne who was better than the resident. "Get them together, as, say when I go out of town, and I would tell them about a patient and what I want done and so on. In that way I was sure the interne would see that it got done. As for Schmeil, we will have to make a decision on him right now whether he can go on, if we are going to turn him out we should do it now."

287

Here we see the staff man handicapped by the hazards of the rotational system which have brought an incompetent resident to his service, and by the formal hierarchy of authority which forbids giving the interne open authority over the resident. We may suppose that the staff man's trick of bringing both men together whilst in reality talking to the interne is supplemented by other devices. And we may be sure that the additional strain on the staff man is correspondingly great.

Two Foreign Residents On A "Resident's Service"

At least in the above instance the staff man had a talented interne to lean upon; but in the situation that we are about to discuss next, there was neither a staff man nor an adequate housestaff physician in command of one of the "resident's services." The rotational system had brought together two foreigners, neither of whom could manage English very skillfully. Unfortunately the field worker did not happen to observe this combination of personnel at work, but he heard about some of the consequences a few weeks later from an interne who had been on night call.

Quite spontaneously he said, "You should have seen that service with Ling and Ama, when they were on." He began to laugh at the recollection. After describing their accents and the difficulty of understanding them, he went on to say that the nurses would call after Ling and Ama had left for the day; then he would go in and write the orders for that service. I expressed amazement. The point was the nurses finally grew desperate and called in the housestaff on night call. This was precipitated by the case of a patient who had come in on emergency. His order had not been changed for sixteen days. The resident on call when the patient had come in through emergency remembered what he had ordered and was amazed later too. I asked this interne whether he himself did not feel funny about trespassing when writing these orders for Ling. "No. Not after sixteen days!" Did Ling know that he was writing the orders? "Yes, he did, and he did not mind" (a big smile). "His brand of medicine is very different. His idea is that you wait and see."

The interne had had no dealings with the faculty man in nominal charge of the service, only with the nurses. I asked whether he did any of this during the day, and he said, "Oh, no." At this time he was on call every other night, and he assumed that the other interne wrote orders on alternate nights. He indicated the situation had been

288

saved because of good nursing. I asked whether one of the students had not said something, after all sixteen days was sixteen days; but he said students really couldn't be expected to say anything. After all they are just students. (Though I have no proof they did not.)

This situation hardly requires much comment. Nurses and house staff on night call must take up the slack, write the orders, make the decisions, see that the service runs with at least a modicum of dispatch. The field worker who arrived on this service a day or two after it had received its next combination of resident and interne found them intensely busy. The resident was focused above all upon getting patients out of their beds and out of the hospital. He was expressing dissatisfaction with the "turnover" of patients; and talking (to the field worker) about "tightening up the service" — meaning among other things getting more discipline into the students. One very obvious consequence for the second pair of housestaff was that they hardly had any time to spend on their own studies until they had gotten the service squared away.

Apropos also of this second pair, it should not be supposed that a combination of competent housestaff men is rare. With this kind of combination — other things being equal, although they often are not! — the resident has much more opportunity to read his books and to spend time with his students, and of course the interne has an opportunity to extend his range of authority and initiative.

A COMPETENT RESIDENT ON AN UNDERSTAFFED SERVICE

In the OB service, the students are an essential segment of the labor force: they sit with the expectant mother, take her measurements down to the last moments before she is transferred to the delivery room, and they check the placenta after birth for possible tears in it. At the associated OB and GYN clinics, the students do the dog-work of examining the patients, calling upon residents for their signatures on prescriptions and for checkups upon their own examinations. When the students leave the hospital for their summer vacations, and before the new housestaff appears during July, the entire OB service is exceedingly understaffed: This year particularly so, for more than the usual number of residents had been rotated to hospitals elsewhere.

A day or two after the students had gone for the summer, the field worker seized the opportunity to see how an excellent resident might handle a birth during their absence (the resident had been anticipating this situation for several days). Observe how the field worker himself becomes part of the work team; and how the resident treats him as a target for instructional comments.

The whole matter of how the students fit in came out very nicely. The OB clinic was being manned by the interne and by the resident, Dewey. The interne, Dr. Cressey, sent for Dewey within a few minutes. Dewey came in and gave the gas. I believe also another resident (ordinarily on GYN duty) had doubled up for him at the OB clinic, but not for the whole time. At one point Cressey asked whether this other resident was in surgery, but Dewey said he was in the clinic. "Good, that's a square deal." After a time, Dewey showed me the child's whisk of hair showing up in the birth canal. He tried to relax the mother's muscles by three injections, and from time to time would pinch her around the opening with clamps to see if she had feeling — mostly she had. He pointed this out to me and to the nurse, once telling me that her right side muscle had relaxed but the left side had not and that was why she sagged a bit on that side. There were other such things that he would normally show the students, I guess.

After the baby was born, Dewey asked me to do what he was doing which was massaging her uterus, while he went back to the clinic. I did this, while Cressey sewed. The nurse and he laughed about this, and he told me one or two things about sewing up.

There was also the business of the placenta, looking at it and weighing it. Again he explained to me, the student, about the various possibilities of tearing; also that he expected a large blood loss with a baby this large. These occasional explanations continued while he filled out the charts out in the hall. As he wrote, new things would occur to him and he would, thinking about them, say them to me. For instance, that the blood loss was higher than it should have been because the placenta did not come out sooner.

Aside from the resident's and interne's instructional momentum, observe how this service must shift its housestaff around, and how the clinic which is already very shorthanded is made more so by the necessity of proper staffing for each birth. This kind of make-shift will continue for another three weeks until the new residents arrive — but the situation will grow increasingly worse; for at the end of the next week the interne on OB finishes his year at the hospital, and Dr. Dewey will grow increasingly tense as he anticipates having to break in a large number of new students. He has already begun to fantasy about how he is going to handle this trying period.*

AN ACUTELY UNDERSTAFFED SERVICE

We turn now to a surgical ward, one run solely by senior residents where there was acute understaffing despite the presence of students. This situation was brought about through a conjunction of circumstances. For one thing, the press of patients was very great; for another, the assignment of a foreign resident who was virtually incapable of any contribution cut down the available manpower. Yet the resident in charge is a very superior and, as we shall see, conscientious physician. He is assisted by two other residents, and an interne (besides the foreign resident). First, we hear the field-worker reporting his interview with the junior resident.

> He said that they worked as much as nineteen hours a day constantly now. However they did not have rounds with the students as there was simply no time for the students. It was work but he enjoyed it. He was learning a lot. There was no resentment in his voice as he talked about the amount of work.

On the following day, the resident who is second in command is overheard addressing himself angrily to his senior resident.

> He said that Holmes (the senior resident) should jump on Hawakaya (the foreign resident) to get him to pull his weight. Holmes said mildly that probably he was better than Aka last month; that whereas Aka was better than nothing, probably Hawakaya would be able to carry out some duties. The other man said he had worked with him in the Wichita hospital and the same thing had happened, so he had had it out with Hawakaya that either he did some work or none at all. Holmes said he would speak with him. The senior resident turned to me and said last month when Aka was on the service they had simply disregarded him because he could not keep up at all.

Later in the afternoon, the sociologist interviewed Dr. Holmes about himself and the service. The conversation turned eventually to the students.

> It disturbs him greatly that he has not done a better job of teaching. Ordinarily he spends a lot of time and is con-

---

*We might briefly contrast all this haphazard and hazardous shuffling of housestaff with the situation on the orthopedic services. Here the role of the student (and even the interne) is negligible, for this field requires such specialization that the newcomer to the service for the most part can only stand by and observe.

cerned with the students, but they have been so short-handed and have had so many operations that he was afraid the students had not had much attention paid to them, and of course they have understandably, no doubt, reacted to this. However this bunch of boys is a good group. (Around the coffee table earlier Holmes expressed great concern because they had not done a very good job of teaching this bunch, because they are still short-handed, and that this bothered him a good deal. His assisting resident broke abruptly into the conversation, full of emotion, expressing himself and simultaneously explaining to me that this of course was one of their problems, and that he was close enough to his student days to recapture it. Holmes said now that, beginning tomorrow, they had one more resident, they should schedule things so someone would be with the students on rounds.)

The interview with Dr. Holmes then touched upon the divided chores of his junior resident and interne. Ordinarily the senior resident rotates to this ward with his entire team; but his assisting resident entered a month late because he was held up at the Wichita hospital.

His junior resident, whom Holmes characterized as very intelligent, had worked out very well. This first year resident and the interne, Broome, had worked things out remarkably well between them. They had, in short, divided the interne's job, which they had to do because they were so shorthanded, and because they had so many beds, and because the beds were scattered all over the hospital.

In other words, the interne has been upgraded virtually to the rank of resident, or at least is doing many of the tasks of a resident. But:

then Holmes said a most interesting thing. The new second year resident, Chase, who has just come, after some years in general practice, has disappointed him because he is so slow at picking up the junior resident's jobs. In other words, Holmes expected that Chase and the interne would get worked out between them the writing of orders and the handling of patients; but Chase is apparently not going to be this good. I remarked to Holmes that I noticed he himself was making decisions on the orders.

Since we already know that the students are not being taken on rounds or having much attention paid to them (and can therefore assume that they are resentful or at least disinterested in the service), it's especially pertinent to see what work role ordinarily is assigned to the students by this resident:

Conventionally some of the work done on the floor is done by the nurses, some by residents, some by the internes, and some by students. If the nurses are not cooperative then somebody else has to do these jobs. If the students are good, then some of the work can be done by them. If the students are uninterested or not good, then their work must be done by somebody else. And so on up and down, so that all the lines of hierarchy are blurred. Of course, in actual cases, sometimes (this is the fieldworker commenting now) some of this work does not get done, and this is where a lot of the cutting of corners, cheating, mistakes, and just inferior medical service probably occurs. But when you get a conscientious person like this resident, tension and anxiety rises up.

On the following day:

The new resident is spending a fair amount of time dictating chart summaries, because as Holmes has told me, "He can do that very well without more experience on the wards." Holmes has him really acting (and he said this in so many words), like an interne for a while. So it is the interne's job to see that this resident gets to know his way around. I remarked that this means the interne will, in a sense, be teaching the resident rather than informally spending time teaching the students. Holmes answered that he teaches the students too, but that was true he would be teaching the resident. The idea is that in two weeks when the interne rotates to another service, this resident will have to take over "until another interne is broken in". What a worried look appeared in Holmes' eye as he tried to tell himself that things were going to be all right!

A short time afterwards the sociologist interviewed the interne, who was all unaware of the senior resident's doubt about the new man. This interne expressed no dissatisfaction over the heavy load of work, but rather gratitude for what he was learning. He regarded his senior resident as easy-going although hard pressed.

He thinks that the next two weeks is going to be much easier however. This of course, is quite a different notion than Holmes'. The reason he conceives of it as being relatively easy is that there is another resident with him now. Then he told how, when things last month were quite tight because of lack of residents, a staff man had suggested they use one student as an interne. They had picked Becker. This was when the students had only two or three weeks remaining on this service, after being there almost two and a half months; and after he himself had been there only a couple of weeks. The interne took the student aside and told him that he "was practically an interne." He could even almost write the orders. The student said ok, but the interne hastened to tell me that "no doubt sometimes he had to supervise the students and they resented it, they really rebelled, it was really a hell of a mess." All this was expressed by the interne explosively. This student left with the rest of his group at the end of the month. The surgical team had wanted Becker to continue and he had agreed to, but the night before the students left he called up and said he couldn't. The interne said to me, "He had to live with those fellows for another year and a half. It's pretty competitive, med. school." I asked whether he had not himself anticipated that they would be upset. "Well, he and we thought they would a bit, but we didn't expect it to last."

We can read volumes into these last comments! Remember, too, that this is a service manned by men who have genuine interest, perhaps more than is usual, in the students. The two ranking residents are disturbed by the situation (the fieldworker is certain of this), the junior resident is especially oriented toward teaching students, and the interne struck the sociologist as also having an eye out for students. Perhaps, though, some of his concern is sharpened by some sense of guilt brought to a head by the student rebellion.

In short: a great load of patients; and a shorthanded, excellent, but harassed senior resident — hence a doubling up of duties, an upgrading of the interne, and in the height of emergency the recruitment of an extra interne from the ranks of the students. with consequent turmoil. And, since there are patients to be operated upon and to be cared for, teaching vanishes except in its informal forms.

An Excellent Resident On A Tightly Controlled, Understaffed Service

To complicate further the picture of what happens when a service is understaffed, observe now the same general kind of situation when the resident is closely governed by a senior staff man. The field worker stumbled upon precisely this confluence of events long before he was aware of the consequences of rotation.

He observed during the day that he followed an extremely busy resident around, that although this man was very tense he seemed quite efficient. He darted here and there on administrative and medical tasks with the sociologist close upon his trail. He was running the ward without the assistance of an interne.

During the teaching rounds Dr. Wohl, the resident, did not stay most of the time. He explained later that he does run back and forth, joining them. (On another day, I noticed that he did.) During the interview with him at lunch he responded well enough but was very tense, constantly picking on his finger and finger nails, as indeed he did all through grand rounds the next hour, and later in the day during another interview with him.

Dr. Wohl, who is highly regarded by the senior staff, expressed great admiration for his superior, Dr. Goffman:

> This physician, he said, is the really outstanding man in the hospital. He is a great physician but gets very tense and cracks down on people. Right now he is working up to a peak. "He gets more irritable and begins to press people; he works up gradually and stays that way for a couple of days and then it blows over." The resident seemed to take this as a fact of nature. I asked why they had not been able to do something about getting an extra man on the service. He said his superior had done all that he could.

Later in the day, the field worker observed that this resident taught the students conscientiously, presenting to them some very abstract medical information. The following day, the resident was seen now and again by the sociologist, who was following someone else in a nearby service. He appeared then equally busy but much more relaxed.

Two weeks later while conversing with two other residents, Dr. Wohl's name came up:

> I said something about Wohl being short of an interne and rushing around. They both snorted with glee asking whether he had told me he was short? "It's always like being a freshman on that service. Discipline — iron discipline." One of them said, "It may make you so sleepy that you can't tell the difference between a man and a woman, but—!" One of these residents had nothing but the greatest admiration, though for this faculty physician.

A month later, the field worker sought out Dr. Wohl — who now had obtained his so greatly desired interne. The resident was not particularly busy, for it was a Saturday and he was about to leave for the library.

> The contrast between today and the first day with him was startling. He spoke freely, and conversationally. He did a bit of nail biting and scissor cutting but without the ferocity of last time.

The conversation touched upon a number of points, including one raised by the interviewer about the conflict between time and study and time spent upon administering a service:

> He blurted out with pride how a couple of weeks ago when he was so shorthanded he'd griped and grumbled for quite a while about this, and finally threatened to leave the hospital entirely. With a smile, "It was a bluff —. I'm not sure I would have done it." I'm not sure that he would have either. Since I expressed naivete and curiosity about how this had been worked, he explained it had been pretty complicated. They had gotten an interne from surgery, and he guessed that one of the staff men there had to be handled. I sensed that this was quite a victory for him, as well as sheer relief from work. I said he had led me a merry chase a couple of weeks ago, because he had been so tense and rather uncommunicative on this. I said something about not being able to learn much under those conditions and he denied it flatly, saying, "Oh, I can learn."

We can take this last bit of information, surely, with some disbelief. Control over this service by the faculty man is so tight, the work done there is so meticulously supervised and scanned, that at least during the peaks of tension the resident must mind his p's and q's. As one of the students said, "Dr. Wohl is intense but he's very good and smart. He gets it from Dr. Goffman worse than we do. We've got only three or four patients apiece, but he's got all of them." Another student, who was queried casually about the resident five minutes later: "Wohl? He's smart. He's good. He gets it worse than we do. He has the whole floor to do."

Why the resident needed —and finally demanded — an interne may appear self-evident. Is the resident not simply shorthanded? But sometimes a service is run by a single resident, and sometimes even by a single interne, without this kind of tension. (We find Dr. Wohl saying to the fieldworker that soon he is to get a very fine interne on the associated service — which he himself is partly responsible for: and the fieldworker notes that "he says he is going to turn the service over to the interne and simply supervise it. This, he smiled in anticipation, would leave him more time to study." We must recognize that Dr. Wohl is working with a senior staff physician who simultaneously delegates less responsibility to him (although rating him highly) and holds him more responsible for details of ward administration. On such a service the resident is more apt to receive rebuke for error. Not that he is more on his toes, necessarily, than he would be elsewhere; but if he errs, he must expect to be confronted more bluntly than if he were on a more

"relaxed" service — and if the truth be told, elsewhere it is sometimes easier to cut corners with impunity.

What the resident needs the interne for on this service is to take
many minor procedural details off his hands. This service is known
among the internes as a place where the interne does a great amount
of scut work, where he gets demoted virtually to doing students'
work. We need not accept their view of the service — which is not
shared, anyhow, by all the internes — to see that even an eager and
competent interne can expect somewhat less play for his initiative
on this service than he might be allowed elsewhere.

The students also may be assigned, as on other services, a supplementary place in the labor force. But, as always, the students are
less relied upon if they are judged mediocre or "not much good,"
and on this closely supervised service, perhaps the standards of
"goodness" get affected by the pressure exerted upon the resident
from the top.

> I asked whether having bad students in a way did not give
> him more time to spend administering the service. He said
> yes, in a way, that it did but repeated that if he had good
> students it relieved him of certain kinds of detail for which
> he was responsible to his superior. I asked whether the differ-
> ent expectations of senior staff and himself did not some-
> times come into conflict. He did not seem to get this so I
> used the example of "detail" and "wanting to study," and
> he shook his head vigorously in assent. He said this is
> one of the things about this particular service, that there
> was such a lot of such detail. He pointed to the difference
> between this service and another specific one.

A few minutes before, the resident had been telling of some specific
rules laid down by his superior. The sociologist observed to himself
that "He talked about teaching the students the ground rules, about
being very firm the first week or so." The point here is that the students can easily get the resident into trouble because he is held to
such strict accountability for their behavior. But, anyhow, if he
can depend upon them to do certain specific procedures which his
superior insists be done, then the students save the resident the
trouble of doing it himself, and he can depend upon them even to
know and supply certain bits of information when his superior, on
rounds, requests it.

Now it happened during this period that the students were judged
by resident and faculty men to be an inferior bunch. Consequently
there was even more pressure upon the resident than there need be.
He was, in short, not only doing his absent interne's work, but some

of the detail ordinarily delegated to students. Whether the students were really inferior, or whether this evaluation of them stemmed also from events that occurred because the resident was already tense and harassed and the senior physician was more than usually concerned about the smooth operation of his service, this we do not know. But it is certainly possible, and more than a little probable.

Loosely And Tightly Governed Services: Permanent Nurse And Rotating Residents

As the housestaff physicians rotate around the services, they are brought into contact with nurses who are permanent members of each service. This sets problems of diplomacy and control for the young physicians; but the nurses, especially the head nurses, have comparable problems with the housestaff. The head nurse can rather naturally be expected to believe that her longer stay on the service has given her greater knowledge of how it works and ought to work. In this hospital, as elsewhere, the doughty head nurse is a problem to the resident who officially is her superior.

When the service is unquestionably a "resident's service," then his official authority is maximized. At the other extreme, we might visualize a service that is almost completely given over by the senior staff to the head nurse, whatever the formal ranking of authority. Listen first to the head nurse on the former kind of service, and note what the rotation of housestaff means to her.

> I asked whether the interne was important to her. He is, because the students are supposed to draw the bloods, and sometimes they do not do it on time or so readily; and the interne is important to her because he is responsible for getting on them. She said you have to keep on the interne to do these kinds of jobs. She said the interne that she had before the present one was not so good in this respect. He did not keep up to snuff. She had to keep on him. This fouls up things for the nurse; because if she does not get the IVs done, this means she has to delay on breakfasts, and then she gets behind generally. She said the interne is likely to change every month; meaning that it is about half over before he knows the ropes entirely. When I pressed her on this she said it only takes two or three days for him to kind of know his place, but I think the first statement more accurately represents her viewpoint.

> As for the residents: she spoke of idiosyncracies. Recently one resident when he first came on wanted short needles for IV's (she said with kind of a snort). So she got him

short needles. In this way she gets on his right side. It is, as she said, a matter of sizing up what they want and pretty much giving in to it. But in return, of course, she gets certain concessions. "You order them short needles, and they write you the orders when you want them." For if she does not have the orders when she wants them, it upsets her whole scheduling. The idea is to get orders written ahead of time in case they have to be used when the residents are not around. This nurse, however, has an arrangement with other services, who bed some of their patients with her: then she finds things need to be done with their patients, rather than calling them up and having them come down to write orders, she is allowed to go ahead and do what she wishes, and then later when the resident appears he will write the orders. On these particular services the residents are much more stationary; on the resident's service they rotate, of course.

The major difference between a service run by a resident and one run by a staff man seems to be that on the former service the nurse depends more upon whatever relationship she can build with each new resident. Her control over him probably is less firm, more unstable.

Be that as it may be, observe now a nurse who has a very great deal of control over her residents. Hers is an unusual position and an unusual service. She is in charge of the premature baby service. She has no assisting internes, and only one resident (and one student) at a time. The care of premature babies apparently calls for considerable skill, for the margin between death and life is very slight. Whether or not the faculty men have given this nurse de facto authority over residents on this service, it is clear that she believes they have.

The sociologist first came across her domain when a pediatrics resident told him about Miss Geer:

He said she had been there for fifteen years and she knows a very great deal about new born babies, that she is quite good just out of sheer experience. As a consequence she practically writes the orders. She will say to the residents, "Here are the orders." If you cross her and give her other orders, she simply will end up not doing most of them. You can complain about her and she'll be alright for perhaps a month and then you are back again in the same position. Also she will withhold information so that it will embarrass you. For instance, there was a jaundiced child, and you come into the room with the staff man and discover it, and she says she had told you the day before — but she had not. So I said to this resident that in other words she pretty much runs the nursery and he said that was right; but it was not proper she should do this. On the other hand the residents, it would seem, have very little defense against this. He was cheerful about this, but displayed a strong air of resentment.

The sociologist, when he went to visit Miss Geer, was much less interested in the amount of her control over the nursery than he was in her attitude toward that control. By now he was well aware of rotational consequences, and wished to know how her perspective influenced the life of the resident while he was assigned to the nursery.

I let her know from the very first what I thought her problems with residents were: saying I realized she has been here for some time, whereas the residents were constantly rotating. How in the world did she ever handle the situation? Within five or six minutes she was talking freely, talked for thirty minutes without much of a break, and ended up at my request enthusiastically showing me the nursery. Her whole demeanor and style of speaking indicates that she thinks this is her own terrain, at least as far as anything but research on these babies is concerned; and research is done by the staff itself. Right now she has a "good resident." "We work together." Some residents do not work with her. But on the whole "we cooperate and get along." She stressed experience as important in handling premature babies, for it takes a good deal of experience to handle them and to know just what is going on. There are frequent emergencies, when one has to act very quickly to save the baby's life. Now the point here is that, as she noted, you supposedly have to get hold of a resident, and he is not very often around, but you have to act quickly. It was quite clear from the way she said this, that she does act on her own accord. I asked, what if she gets a resident who will not cooperate and will not write orders quickly and so on? She said that she can — if she has to — call on the faculty man. I got the impression that he is a great source of authoritative strength in such show-downs. "It makes a big difference that he is behind me."

She went on to describe the difficulties that residents sometimes made for her, as when they are not tactful to parents of the babies. She made a point of remarking that some residents regard the babies as cases rather than as patients. She spoke of a resident who had ordered three times too much drug for a baby. She said something to him about it and he asked whether they should give more. She disgustedly imitated his question, and said "you have to know your babies."

It is evident that if the resident can get on good working terms with Miss Geer — mainly her terms, of course — then he can learn a good deal both from her and from the greater freedom of movement within the nursery that he will enjoy. But what of the students? Presumably they too can learn something from this specialist — providing that they will forget she is a nurse and regard her as a clinical teacher; and providing they play the game according to her rules.

> I asked if she had much contact with students. She spoke, her voice one big exclamation: "One every week!" Some do not even know enough to wash their hands to put on their gowns. She added, "I sometimes wonder why they are here." They do the physicals and then the residents are supposed to check them. I asked whether she got any benefit out of these physicals, suspecting not from her tone of voice. She said "no," and with a kind of weary patience added that physicals got done three times: once by the student, once by the resident, and once by the private pediatrician. Then I asked whether students ever asked questions of her about the babies. She said "no, they don't ever ask anything of us, except occasionally they may say that this is a nice baby."

Her remarks do not tell us about the amount of learning — and teaching — that may go on but they do suggest something of the consequences of rotation when an established nurse is given considerable authority. Even an outsider like the field worker, can sense quickly that this is a ward where medical service is paramount, and teaching and learning is quite secondary. Since the babies are important subjects for research also, we may guess that research also takes precedence over teaching functions.

SEQUENCES AND ROTATION

Rotation sends the housestaff to services which the young doctor may judge are unequally demanding or deserving of his time and effort. We shall say only a word or two about the effect of interest upon his work, and then turn to the effect of his judgments about how demanding a service is.

Obviously when a man is interested in a given service and the medicine which it practices, he will — other things being equal —

work more energetically and assiduously than when he is disinterested or acutely dislikes the service or its type of medical practice. But the man's interest is, as we have seen, only one variable among many: we must hasten also to add that the breadth of interest displayed by these young men is sometimes surprisingly wide. For instance, an interne will not necessarily be less interested in surgery merely because he is going to specialize in internal medicine; for the ideology of medical training is such that it becomes easy for him to tell himself, and be told, that one can never tell when this information and training will become useful. (Perhaps too it is important that one feels he is learning, not wasting time, so that learning for its own sake gets a kind of priority.) The field worker found remarkably little griping about work being disinteresting because it was not actually, or potentially, useful. It would be wise to consider "interest" the product, as much as the cause, of the total gestalt of a service during the houseman's term on the service. Whether he will find the work interesting must also, although we have no very good evidence concerning this, be related to the order in which services are encountered.

But without any question this order or sequence does enter into how much effort he will expend upon service, regardless of how interesting the work may be. For one thing, interne after interne arranges matters so that he encounters one "easy service" just before, or just after, another which is reputed to be demanding. These easy services are regarded as periods of relative rest before or after periods of hard work. Occasionally, the interne is surprised to find the service more exacting than anticipated, but generally his plans are not disappointed. If he finds the work more interesting than anticipated, of course he will expend more effort — within reason. From time to time the field worker would come across a member of the housestaff relaxing on such services — or unexpectedly relaxing somewhat on services which followed more "spastic" ones, but the latter is, so to speak, an unearned increment. However, this regularized relaxation is negatively consequential for the hospital whenever more effort is expected of the interne (or resident) than he anticipates. This is not at all the case when he takes off a month to learn a bit of orthopedics, say, for here he is expected to remain peripheral to the operation of the service.

The interne or resident also often expects to learn different things on different services. Sometimes his expectations are fairly specifically formulated, sometimes less. His expectations may affect the sequence of services that he asks for (although the interne has generally greater choice in this matter, because the residents' sequences fall more under departmental jurisdiction). To the housestaff itself it is perfectly clear that certain services, falling as they do after others, are not only more valuable — but more restful, more exciting, even more freeing. The surgical services are particularly striking because the four year residency program is rather strictly controlled by the department. The surgical residents proceed by fairly regular sequences from one service to another, graded roughly by difficulty, until the final year when the senior resident is given his own ward to administer. Long before then he has had an opportunity to run a ward by himself, or virtually by himself, in one of the associated hospitals. We quote from a couple of surgical residents to suggest some of the consequences of sequential rotation, particularly those having to do with the resident's opportunities to learn.

> Dr. Hughes found his time at Wichita, during the first year, disappointing. He said this was mostly because the staff was not too good, and it was a slow period, and they did not have too many interesting cases. During this period they do bread and butter surgery, and learn to do many of the procedures. Ordinarily one would learn quite a bit, he believes, and be enthusiastic because everything is after all, so new. The two surgical specialties that he worked on that year he found easy going. He worked in the dog lab too. There they keep "good hours;" and it gives them a chance to do a lot of reading. The private patient services he characterized as "this is your big chance to see how they do it. This is it." He means, this is the time when the residents actually see the staff at work. He also indicated this as a tense, anxious time, because the staff can be very critical of your performances and your work on the floor. He said that the third year (consisting of three months in surgical pathology, six months at two VA hospitals, and three months as "underdog on ward surgery") is known as "the famine year."

Another resident concurred with his judgment of the third year, pointing out that it was the third year residents who were among the most impatient, which makes it hard on fourth year residents like himself. He added, that this is why the laboratory and pathological lab "help to cool them off." What he is referring to is the diplomacy, and restraining hand, that are called for in administering a resident's ward when the third year resident, who is assisting him, wants to do surgical procedures which the senior resident is reluctant to let him try.

The time when the fourth year resident runs his own ward at KU is for him the peak, or close to the peak, of his residency. Its satisfactions are almost self evident: he is in charge; he does such operating as he wishes, and hands over to his underlings what he does not wish to do. Yet this is a period, at least for some men, of great anxiety and tension. For one thing, it is like operating in a fishbowl, as over against running a ward in far away Wichita or at the Kansas City VA hospital; for another thing, the resident is occasionally caught between the crossfire of two staffmen. (The field worker watched one such situation where a senior resident ran head on into such a conflict: The resident was dressed down by one staff man for almost losing a patient because of a seemingly foolish and unorthodox surgical procedure; but before the operation the resident had sought advice of another faculty member and had followed that advice.) One last hazard encountered by fourth year residents is most graphically portrayed by some further comments of a senior resident.

> We walked out of the room and he said to me, "That's another of those anxious cases of the resident. It wasn't one of mine luckily! He's been around a couple of months already, and he's pretty bad. Probably it wasn't Harper's fault. He's done good work. But he, the patient, passes on to someone else and everybody knows about it for a long time — like mine upstairs. I know that will dog me!" Of course he said this with a wince and a grimace. He said that probably this patient of Harper's will get cleared up but meanwhile there he is and everybody knows about it. The whole point, of course, is that here one's failure is written as big as life for everyone to see.

The senior ward is not only a fishbowl: it is the resident's only for a short period of time, and then he must hand it — and his visible errors — over to the next resident. Worst yet, there can be competition, with somewhat measurable comparisons, with this kind of rotation. As the same young surgeon admitted when he was asked about competition:

> He said there was competition because you know how each other has done on the various wards, because you could tell by the mortality rates. He assured me that if the mortality rate went up you could tell quite quickly, so that you were always trying to do as well as the next fellow.

The moral is clear!

A CHANGE OF HOUSESTAFF, BUT THE SAME STUDENTS

Some pages ago, we described how a resident's ward could function under the administration of a foreign resident and a foreign interne, and the change in mood on this service when this foreign combination was succeeded by an American resident and his American interne.

We hinted, also, how interesting it would be to pursue what this succession meant for the medical students. This case study is also useful for helping to understand some of the problems of the American resident, whom you will recollect was at first greatly concerned with speeding up the turnover on his ward and with tightening "discipline," particularly over the students.

The field worker came upon the scene about one week after the change of housestaff. During the first day's observation, he was struck by the tremendous busyness of both the resident and his interne, who together and alone were constantly on the move: examining, speaking with patients, writing and giving and discussing orders, conferring over the telephone, making rounds with students. The resident even held a teaching conference. Something of the atmosphere of the ward is suggested by the field worker's comment (to himself) at the end of the day:

> This was an odd day. I found myself somewhat depressed after a while, following these people around with neither resident nor interne talking to me, so that I could feel like breaking in and asking questions about what they were doing. And when I tried sociable phrases, I got little or no response. But also, part of the atmosphere was that there was virtually no conversation or gestural interaction, other than business, between the two men: only consultation and orders. Most important though, because they were pressed, they spent much time just sitting and thinking about their medical problems. So instead of being informed at many steps of the way by their side comments to me, as I usually try to do, or getting information from them by asking or by more indirect means; I was limited to watching. It was also my impression that the resident used the teaching period as relaxation before he again swung into action — if he did, he was wise considering the whirl of activity that met him after he left the class. On the other hand, this resident is skilled at setting for the service a feeling of informality, and interviews his patients with a relatively gentle, pleasant, general practitioner manner. And he displayed no impatience with students, either in class or on the rounds.

But how do the students see him? Two students, separately interviewed, concurred that "Things are now much more tense." This judgment which means one thing for the efficiency of ward administration and medical supervision — and the students recognize the American resident's superiority on these grounds — can mean something quite different if one looks at his teaching as might a student. A student is mainly concerned with how good the resident is at providing maximum opportunities for the learning of medicine. Hence when students get to comparing the foreign resident and his successor on this ward, they can say things like this:

This resident pays more attention to detail and so you have to be prepared to know all kinds of things about the patient. With Dr. Lin, things were much more easy going. But with this resident you hear him telling the patients what is wrong with them, and this is much more informative; and he talks more with you about these things. Lin rarely told the students anything, and he never spoke to the patients, so the students didn't hear anything. The current resident, the student said, is a very good diagnostician, so they can learn a good deal from him. But you can never ask him anything and get an answer because he then asks a question in turn and keeps you at it, and then asks you to go look it up. For instance, you can't ask him why he put something down in an order because he will ask you what you think, and you end up having to go look it up. Lin would answer you directly. The student also said that with this resident you have to know everything about the patient, including the minutae; and he said this with mixed feelings, I thought. Whereas, with Lin, since you were not responsible this way, the students could spend their time studying their books; and he thought this was good, because in many ways you could better spend your time that way than knowing all the details of your patient. And, again, now you can never get a direct answer to a question on the rounds.

The second student made almost identical remarks, and added a detail or two. For instance:

This student likes the more relaxed or looser atmosphere; likes to have time to read for himself in the text, likes to be much more on his own; likes to be able to do more with his patients. With Dr. Lin, because he did not tell you so much about the patient, or teach you, you had then to go to the text and figure it out for yourself. So you were really less like a student; which was good. Of course, now however, there is much more turnover of patients, so actually you see more patients. But then again, this resident insists you know everything about them, including some pretty irrelevant things. Instead of spending all that time on one case — he cited a rare disease that was interesting but irrelevant to practice — it would be much better to be reading about things more important and more prevalent. And at the same time he said he's tired of looking things up — not that that isn't useful or good — but he would rather be "spoonfed." He would much rather they laid it out for you. You could look it up, but it would take four or five hours to track it down, whereas they could tell you in five minutes.

In short, this American resident is providing not only more patients to be looked at but certain other conditions which appear favorable to learning medicine; but at the same time the "relaxed" atmosphere provided by the foreign resident allowed the students to obtain more direct answers to their questions, and greater freedom to allocate their own time and energy. Inevitably the two residents are compared with each other — naturally along the axes of student interests.

The Interne Who Was Not An Interne

There is no end to depicting these complex combinations of circumstances that are brought about by the rotational system. We shall satisfy ourselves with one more instance: an interne who was really not an interne. He had been a failure as a medical student but had not been denied his diploma; for his graduation had been made unofficially contingent upon his returning for one more year at the hospital, nominally as an interne. Hence whenever this interne, whom we shall call Dr. Zero, was assigned to a service, then that service was at best short-handed and was at worst burdened with a liability. The fieldworker was interested in how these situations were handled — regarding Dr. Zero as a kind of "tracer" who could be easily trailed through service after service. He was; he left his mark.

There was no particular secret about who this man was, or why he was an interne (although until the fieldworker indicated that he knew who Dr. Zero was, by name, people were loathe to mention his name). The most common reaction was to relegate him, immediately or within a short time, to something like the status of a student. As one man said: "I had him on service, and I tried to teach him, but it was hopeless. I ended up telling him that he could do the bloods, and the physicals, and that was all." He added that Zero was more likely than not to be found in his room than on the service: that is, there was tacit agreement to withhold the usual demands (and punishments). Another resident described how a service was protected against the potential danger inherent in his mere presence:

> Dr. Lindesmith said, "Would you like to know how I handled Zero? I stayed ahead of him all the time." What this resident did was to do a procedure, and then he would tell Zero to go ahead and do it; meanwhile he was doing the next thing and so staying partly ahead of him — and

in a sense never giving Zero any trust or discretion at all. Also when Zero was on night call, Dr. Lindesmith arranged with the emergency room to have himself telephoned if anything serious came up, making clear they should call Zero only in the event of something quite minor.

We see that the resident possesses great powers in this situation for demoting the interne in order to protect himself, the patients, and the service. But, as with any incompetent interne, the resident must take up the slack and do extra work. As with other internes, also, Dr. Zero's reputation preceded him, so that when he came to the service he was not entirely an unknown figure.

Before he came to the service, it seems that the residents in this department talked him over among themselves and agreed to share this burden. They decided also to put him where he could do the least harm. They did this. And the resident says they shifted him around at least once, to distribute the problem.

There is one service where no resident can quite so directly protect the hospital and that is the emergency room, for there only an interne is in charge. Eventually Dr. Zero was rotated to this administrative post. The field worker spoke with the nurse who was assisting him in the emergency room; in the cautious conversation which ensued, both spoke about Dr. Zero with only slightly veiled allusion.

She made a distinction between the more intelligent internes and the less. She thinks that the intelligent learn pretty rapidly which residents to call and when not to call residents and — as we shall see in a moment — they learn to lean upon the nurse's experience. I asked her about the lazy internes. She pointed out that they could of course use the students, having them do much of the work. I asked whether lazy internes tend to make more use of students and she said they did. The lazy interne also may not bother to spend so much time in examining the patient. It is apparent that he can cut corners with some impunity. He does not have to have the resident come down either but can assume responsibility for sending the patient home after not much of an exam. Also he can call a number of residents down and they, of course, cannot know whether the case is an acute one until they get down. I gather that there can be considerable friction between the interne and the resident who is unnecessarily or too often called.

I asked about the internes and whether they used her longer

experience on emergency. She said the intelligent ones tended to use her, that they would even sometimes get her advice on diagnosis and therapy. She would tell them that various residents had done it this way or that way. The less intelligent ones — about whom she seemed less inclined to talk — she admitted when pressed, did not ask for this kind of advice or stayed in the background and just let things happen. I have the impression that then tension rises and cases just pile up. For she said one of the important things on emergency is that there are periods of nothing happening, and then cases pile up. A good interne will keep the turnover going but if he does not, then an acute case may come in suddenly and then there is a mess. It was graphic enough what happens when an inexperienced interne does not ask her advice. This nurse, who is young, did not say any of this with relish or a sense of resentment.

A week later, an already over-wrought resident up on the third floor blurted out angrily that: "Zero is calling all the residents down to do the work, and the student does the sewing up of lacerations."

Thus the student gets to do more actual medical procedure — but can learn less medicine from observing and querying the interne — while all over the hospital the residents must bear the brunt of the faculty's decision to protect the wider civic community against a poorly trained graduate. The alternatives, to flunk the student or to deny him his diploma, are paths apparently not easily chosen by this state school.

SOME CONCLUDING REMARKS ABOUT ROTATION

We are far from having discussed all the consequences of rotation for the hospital and for education, but this much is unquestionable: the commitment of medical schools to the rotational system is immensely important. On the negative side of the ledger: the hospital suffers because its various services must operate with unstable work-teams — the teaching hospital must forever have built into it this ingredient of organizational inefficiency and strain, as long as students and housestaff circulate from service to service. On the positive side: the teaching hospital is, after all, an educational institution and — quite as the prevailing medical ideology has it — rotation does widen the scope and breadth of students' knowledge. Between these two very obvious poles of vice and virtue, one can place those other observations necessary to any more subtle evaluation of the rotational system of education.

Our diagrams and the accompanying analysis of case materials help to clarify how, and why, the teaching of undergraduates by the housestaff must often suffer — especially that kind of teaching which consists of informal interplay of question and answer, remark and counter-remark, during periods of work on the wards. The studying, and frequently the learning, of the housestaff itself must often decline in quality and in efficiency under the pressure of taking up the slack of understaffing and incompetency — combined with some additional contingencies outlined in the preceding pages. That the quantity and quality of ward administration is also affected is a point that needed no underscoring, although our case materials bear pointedly upon what situations reduce (and increase) the effectiveness of the work. They also demonstrate quite clearly how administrating takes precedence over the house staff's studying, and how studying in turn takes precedence over teaching the undergraduate.

There are several further quite relevant points, not perhaps sufficiently brought out by our comments upon the field worker's notes. One point has to do with the limitation of authority brought about by rotation. The resident is vested with certain powers by virtue of his hierarchized position: however, because he is always newer to the service than some of his assisting personnel (especially the nurses), he is periodically (and sometime permanently on certain services) handicapped. (He is handicapped also in his role as a teacher because he can never get the kind of discipline over students, or loyalty from them, that he needs for maximum effectiveness; for they, in turn, are constantly on the move. He may teach a given group once, or twice, but rarely more; and then for only relatively short periods of time.) To return to the problem of getting and maintaining authority over the more stable personnel, the resident does not always possess actual power over his head nurse, but may share power with her — hence some of the polite verbal forms which she may use to offer her "suggestions" — or he may virtually yield authority to her. On occasion, he may share authority or yield to his interne. The rotational system, in other words, effectively helps prevent the crystallization of sharp hierarchial distinctions between resident and interne, and to some extent between housestaff and head nurse.

Another weighty consequence of continual circulation about the hospital is that strong loyalties to specific faculty members occur with less frequency than if such circulation were curtailed. It is useful to recollect that although medical education is sometimes described as a kind of "apprenticeship," that "genuine" apprenticeships frequently result in intense attachment: of student to teacher, and often vice versa. But the rotation of students and housestaff throughout the hospital makes it more difficult, though not impossible, for such attachments to develop. When they do, (especially we have in mind those of the housestaff) then they sometimes make life just that more difficult for the man and his associates. Ideally, each resident or interne should approach each new service with an open mind: he should seek to learn quickly what each new faculty physician believes is good medicine and good administration, and he should work hard and well for this man. The more committed the resident is to some other faculty man's brand of medicine, the more difficult it will be to throw heart and energy behind the ways of the new man. Occasionally it happens that some resident is too committed, and so friction does develop around this discrepancy between medical standards. Of course when departments are small, or dominated by the chief, then the residents can afford to develop strong loyalties with relative impunity.

Rotation also ought to be viewed in relation to personnel "failure" as a perennial institutional problem. Every institution must handle the contingency that some personnel fail to measure up to expectations formulated at the time they were hired, or when placed into positions for which they were judged fit. The problem of failure is met, for instance in armies or industrial concerns, by such mechanisms as kicking a man upstairs, creating a special post where he will do no harm, giving him a title but little or no working function, sending him to another department; or he can be frankly demoted — or fired. The KU teaching hospital rarely fires outright, although members of the housestaff have been let go occasionally. But rotation allows each faculty physician the luxury of being able to draw a deep breath every few months, as he passes along one of the hospital's bad choices to the next service. (This is the obverse of his not being able to keep an excellent man permanently and of running the risk of getting, although temporarily, a worse resident than he currently possesses.) On occasion, a faculty man may simply refuse to accept on his service a proven or certain failure: one such case came to the attention of the field worker (the "failure' was a foreign member of the housestaff). In sum: a kind of "buck passing" mechanism is permanently built into the rotational system.

Conversely, rotation allows the housestaff to gain considerable autonomy which might otherwise not be granted. This is revealed most clearly by the "choice" of services: for instance, the internes may choose which services they wish to work upon. Choice thus operates to minimize friction and to maximize interest. (This institutional mechanism is highlighted by what happens when an interne unacquainted with the medical school chooses as his first service one which proves to be disappointing. At the spring meeting of the internes, which was called by the committee on internes, one of the chief complaints against the hospital was directed by some non-Kansans against the head of a service. In effect, the choice of these particular internes was limited by their lack of acquaintance with the service — although their complaint was couched in quite other terms.) What an interne cannot avoid so easily is having to work with a specific resident. Whereas it is possible beforehand to get a line on the staff and on the service itself, he must patiently wait to see who will be his resident. The residents possess less freedom perhaps, at least during their first year or two; but there is considerable latitude of choice thereafter, especially must we recognize that the resident may decide to work harder, or less hard, on particular services; and that he can better implement those decisions because his superior is, to some degree, limited by the resident's rotation.

Here is yet another consequence of rotation: every service has the problem of "breaking in" new personnel. The physician in charge has this problem with his residents. So do the nurses, and especially the head nurse. But so does every specialized functionary — the social worker, the dietician, even the women in the admitting department (which handles also the consignment of beds). These functionaries usually are women, and of course they are not physicians; this means that they must handle each new resident and interne in especially delicate, and frequently oblique, ways. The social worker speaks of "building relationships" and patiently teaching them to see how she can be useful to them, and getting them to think a bit like a social worker. The dietician also has problems of getting cooperation from the housestaff.

The problems of these special functionaries are not unlike those of the nurse who diplomatically coaches the novitiate resident in the ways of the chief of service — except the nurse at least has more apparent claim to being at the heart of the medical process. The dietician and the social worker are latecomers to the hospital, and more marginal to its workings so far as the resident seems often to be concerned. Their marginality is probably magnified, if anything, by some aspects of this rotational system.

We shall end by noting briefly that, like the housestaff itself, the hospital gains certain unexpected dividends from the rotational system. Because the internes circulate more widely than do the residents, they sometimes function as unofficial "consults" for the service on which they are working. In other words, when a point is too minor to call in a resident from another service for his specialized knowledge, the resident (say on obstetrics) will harken to the words of a competent interne — especially perhaps if he has just come off the relevant medical service. If the interne continues at KU, his previous rotation around the hospital comes in handy in another way. As a resident, it will pay him to know a good deal about certain features of the hospital, and it is additionally helpful to know some of the personnel in other departments. The resident must deal with these places and must call in residents and staff from other departments as occasional consultants. Although this part of the resident's education is not a calculated part of the medical curriculum it is useful to him, to his superiors, and certainly adds to the hospital's efficiency.